MW00628673

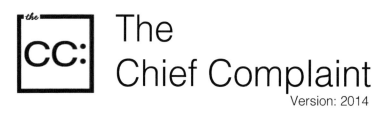

The
Chief Complaint

Version: 2014

Author

Chris Feier M.D., Pharm.D.
Clinical Assistant Professor of Emergency Medicine
Dept of Emergency Medicine
Keck School of Medicine at LAC+USC Medical Center

5150 Publishing
Hermosa Beach, CA

"Everything should be made as simple as possible, but not simpler."
Albert Einstein

TABLE OF CONTENTS

TABLE OF CONTENTS

Personally, I don't like to refer to patients as complainers (I would say a 55 yo male "presents with", NOT "complains of"), but the terminology is so ingrained in medicine and so widely used at the bedside that the phrase has become iconic. Having noted that, Chris Feier's book of that title is really something totally new in the medical education world. This pocket sized book does something many have tried to do but few have achieved, which is to create an orienteering guide to the med-ed landscape while launching your thought processes AT THE BEDSIDE when confronted with a new undifferentiated and undiagnosed patient. And it is truly pocket sized, not like some of the brick shaped (and brick weighted) books you see dragging a residents white coat into a lopsided drape from some Edvard Munch painting. This book can actually be put in your pocket with reasonable ergonomics and retained balance. This is really important for a book like this to be a functional companion to your stethoscope. When I was medical student and intern it was The Washington Manual that served this purpose, but now this book is too Internal Medicine oriented, and it no longer fits in the pocket of a white coat.

The size also means that the book is not encyclopedic. Rosen's it isn't, and that is good because you need BOTH a wheelbarrow and a diagnosis to use that thing (or burning curiosity, a burning fire, and a long cold winter night trapped inside a cabin with a good light source) and Rosen's is not chief complaint oriented. While this book will never replace the comprehensive tomes of EM, it WILL follow students and residents into the clinical landscape. This pocket manual also links young doctors to dozens of updated algorithms, podcasts, CME Download, EM-Rap, HIPPO-EM, the NNT, ACEP guidelines, AHA guidelines and the Abstracts of EM and serves to orient them when faced with a patient. In this manner it is more of a map and compass which are crucially important orienteering tools when you are lost in a forest of differential diagnostic considerations. The connectivity of this book is quite unusual because it rapidly bridges to a place all new medical practitioners want to go which is the on-line world. It lets the computer resources come to bear on the understanding process, which lets this manual be both small AND powerful. This map and compass leads directly into convenient computer resources. It also fits better into the "real world" of on-line learning, visual comprehension, and on-line images that the modern student and resident are so much more comfortable with.

The original cover of The Chief Complaint was a picture of the old (1933) Los Angeles County hospital which is the site of the first academic department of Emergency Medicine (1971), and the second oldest training program in the country. Arguably it is the birthplace of academic EM in the United States. Many of the links represent work by LAC+USC physicians over the years including WR Bukata, Jerome Hoffman, Mel Herbert, Stuart Swadron, Diku Mandavia, and me. Mel Herbert has been busily making textbooks irrelevant and is "inverting" the classrooms of EM medical education around the world with on-line teaching. "County Hospital" as it is known has trained more EM residents than any other training program in the US, and Chris Feier

FOREWORD: MALLON

(class of 2008) drew heavily on this heritage when creating his manual.

   The audience for this book is clinicians at the beginning of their careers. Medical students rotating on an EM clerkship, EM interns, Non-EM interns with an EM service month, and junior EM residents will all find The Chief Complaint to be a useful resource. This little book will open their world to great educators, on-line resources, and help them answer the pesky "What's your plan?" question that will be asked of them repetitively when they see a new patient with a common chief complaint in the ED. This book will also lead them to data that challenges the traditional dogma like the NNT (the Number Needed to Treat for benefit and harm) by David Newman, and on-line debates by experts in Emergency Medicine. In this manner The Chief Complaint moves quickly from the black and white binary world of algorithms into the clinical reality of grey tones, study design, evidence based medicine, expert opinion, and controversy while retaining utility at the bedside.

   I hope you will enjoy The Chief Complaint which will continue as a living document in its on-line version where updates and rewrites can keep it current. Print versions will follow annually. As a self-published book on-line updates can be added seamlessly. I congratulate Dr. Feier on what I see as a new type of clinical tool that fits the learning style of new clinicians in the field I love, Emergency Medicine.

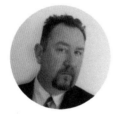

William K. Mallon MD DTMH FACEP FAAEM
Professor of Clinical Emergency Medicine
Keck School of Medicine at the University of Southern California
LAC+USC Medical Center, Los Angeles, California

ACKNOWLEDGMENTS

PEER REVIEW

William K Mallon MD DTMH FACEP FAAEM
Professor of Clinical Emergency Medicine
Keck School of Medicine at the University of Southern California
LAC+USC Medical Center, Los Angeles, California

Stuart Swadron MD FAAEM
Professor of Clinical Emergency Medicine
Keck School of Medicine at the University of Southern California
LAC+USC Medical Center, Los Angeles, California

Mel Herbert MD MBBS FAAEM
Professor of Clinical Emergency Medicine
Keck School of Medicine at the University of Southern California
LAC+USC Medical Center, Los Angeles, California

Edward J Newton MD
Professor of Clinical Emergency Medicine
Chairman, Dept of Emergency Medicine
Keck School of Medicine at the University of Southern California
LAC+USC Medical Center, Los Angeles, California

Ilene Claudius MD
Associate Professor of Clinical Emergency Medicine
Keck School of Medicine at the University of Southern California
LAC+USC Medical Center, Los Angeles, California

Paul Jhun MD FAAEM
Associate Professor of Clinical Emergency Medicine
Keck School of Medicine at the University of Southern California
LAC+USC Medical Center, Los Angeles, California

Edward Kwon MD
Assistant Professor of Clinical Surgery (Trauma)
LAC+USC Medical Center, Los Angeles, California

ACKNOWLEDGMENTS

SPECIAL THANKS

Creative consult: Ariel Bowman MD [PGY2 USC]

Editing: Craig Torres-Ness MD [PGY1 USC] & Erik Akopian MD [PGY1 USC]

Content: Ariel Bowman MD, Ryan Raam MD [PGY4 USC], Brian Doane MD [USC class of 2014]

Illustrations: Sonia Johnson MD [USC Class of 2010]

Dr Mel Herbert for access to EM:RAP and Essentials of Emergency Medicine

Dr Diku Mandavia for allowing access CMEDownload.com and Resuscitation Conference

Dr David Newman for use of his website: thennt.com

Figure1 for providing cover pictures (figure1.com)

Red Blanket Society for initial funding/donation of books

To my wife and daughter for all your love and support. Thank you for putting up with me locking myself away in the office for hours on end.   Also, thanks to my wife for helping me edit the OB/Gyn section.

cmedownload

PREFACE

WHY THIS BOOK?

(Adapted from: West J Emerg Med. Jan 2008; 9(1): 47–51)

"The Chief Complaint" book was born out of my frustration with the educational process in medicine. In medical school, professors teach us by a disease-based system. We read textbooks and learn about Takayasu's Arteritis and Diphyllobrohtium latum. We then enter our clinical rotations with confidence that we know the minutiae about the most uncommon disease processes. This is when it hits us--patients don't walk into the hospital saying they are having acute mesenteric ischemia in the distribution of their superior mesenteric artery. They say their stomach hurts.

This is when we learned of the "differential diagnosis," a list of diseases that may present with a certain symptom. This is not what I needed; the differential for a patient with low back pain including zebras like Scheurmann's disease on the same list next to common entities like Spondylolisthesis, which is next to emergent entities like Abdominal Aortic Aneurysm. I am no better off in my understanding of how to approach these complaints. What I needed was an algorithm. While searching through different textbooks for algorithms, I became even more confused.

Traditional medical algorithms seem so complicated with arrows in every direction. This is where the concept of "The Chief Complaint" book was born. The goal was to structure algorithms in a way an emergency physician would approach a patient's complaint. They are very simple in their structure and comply with the EM mantra of "worst first." In constructing them, I have found that each complaint is approached in its own unique way and that "one size does not fit all." They are not meant to be all-inclusive, but rather to provide a framework upon which to build future knowledge. They are ideal for those new to medicine or just beginning emergency medicine training. They can even help experienced practitioners to be more thorough and efficient.

I initially started writing this book just for myself as a 2nd year resident so that I could become a better physician. Eight years later, I realize that I am still learning new things every day and am continuing to expand on the book.

HOW TO USE THIS BOOK

There is no set structure for each algorithm, much like an emergency physician will approach each chief complaint (Chest pain, Syncope etc...) differently. However, there are some general guidelines. Each complaint is broken down into 3-7 steps that describe how to approach the complaint. The first step is usually the ABCs which includes resuscitation if they are critically ill. After that, you want to start ruling out the major life threatening diseases. This is usually done by looking for red flags for each disease that you are worried about. For example, in the Low Back Pain algorithm, you would start by ruling out the life threatening diseases (AAA, epidural compression, epidural abscess, vertebral fracture etc...). Then, using the history and physical, evaluate what the likelihood of each disease process would be. If your suspicion is high enough, you would proceed with the work-up (PVR, MRI etc...).

The text based portion of the book follows the same outline as the algorithm but allows a deeper dive into each of the steps with further explanation and evidence based decision points. Where there is controversy in medical decision making, (which is quite often in emergency medicine), a review of the evidence is given in the form of a "Journal Club" box. Each point in the algorithm is heavily evidence based and documented throughout the text. References are also made to some of the best learning resources (EM:RAP, CMEDownload etc...) in emergency medicine for more details on a topic.

PREFACE

The Chief Complaint is my personal book that I use every day in the ER. I originally started making this guide for myself as a 2nd year resident to help me through my shifts. The algorithms then became so popular with the other residents that I continued to make them and even started a mini lecture series. I have continued to edit the book over the years as more studies became available. Parts of this book have been internally published for the USC residents as "The ER Survival Guide" since I was a resident. One of the algorithms was also published in WestJEM (West J Emerg Med 2008;9(1): 47-51). Due to ongoing demand from the residents, I decided to make it available to the public. I interviewed multiple faculty members about their own approaches, and integrated this with the literature and my practice. I also sought after the residents about their greatest difficulties with the workup and treatment of different complaints and set out to help resolve those issues.

Everyone's medical practice and approach to patient care is different. This book represents only one of many approaches. It represents MY approach and should not be taken as gospel. I implore the reader to check all facts/figures/doses/recommendations/sources etc. If you are not willing to do that, then please do NOT buy this book. Immediately stop reading and return this book for a full refund.

This book is and always will be a work in progress. Medicine is an ever changing field and every effort has been made to ensure the information in this book is accurate, easy to use, and up to date. Errors, however, are expected. Even a misplaced comma can have life threatening consequences as evidenced by the following statement:

Let's eat, Grandma
Let's eat Grandma

So, I urge readers of this book to give feedback, not only on grammatical and typographical errors, but also on medical decision making. If a critical study was left out or there is a better approach to a complaint, I implore you to send feedback.

Please direct all comments and suggestions to:

Email: info@thechiefcomplaint.com
Facebook: https://www.facebook.com/thechiefcomplaint
Website: thechiefcomplaint.com

All post publication errors/omissions/corrections will be placed on thechiefcomplaint.com

Thank you,

Chris Feier MD

PEA

Initial Evaluation

- ☐ History-(events of code, meds given, history)
- ☐ Confirm PEA (pulse, respirations, monitor)
- ☐ Large bore IVs/Central line
- ☐ Cardiac US: true PEA vs cardiac standstill vs pseudoPEA?

Continuous

1 Rapidly Reversible Causes?
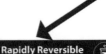

- ☐ H1: **Oxygen** → prepare to rapidly intubate
- ☐ H2: **IV Fluids** → NS resuscitation
- ☐ H3: Hypothermia → **Warm** patient

CPR/Epi

- ☐ **CPR** – ETCO$_2$ goal of >10-20mmHg
- ☐ **Epinephrine** 1mg IV/IO q 3-5 min

2 Chemical Resuscitation

- ☐ H4, H5, T1: **HCO$_3$** (1 amp)
- ☐ H5: **CaCO$_3$** (1 amp)
- ☐ H6: **D50** (1 amp) or Accucheck

3 Needles vs US

- ☐ T2, T5: Lung US → Bilateral Needle **Thoracostomies/Chest tubes?**
- ☐ T3, T5: Cardiac US → **Pericardiocentesis?**

4 Thrombolytics?

- ☐ T4: PE/MI → Consider tPA
- ☐ US to √ for DVT

Reversible Causes of PEA

- **H1**-Hypoxia
- **H2**-Hypovolemia
- **H3**-Hypothermia
- **H4**-Hydrogen ion (acidosis)
- **H5**-Hypo/Hyperkalemia
- **H6**-Hypoglycemia
- **T1**-Toxins(TCA, Dig, CCB, β-blocker)
- **T2**-Tension pneumothorax
- **T3**-Tamponade, cardiac
- **T4**-Thrombosis (PE/MI)
- **T5**-Trauma

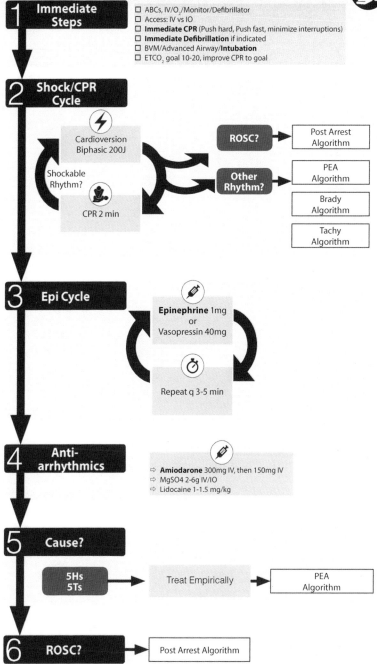

1 Immediate Steps

☐ ABCs, IV/O₂/Monitor/Defibrillator
☐ Access: IV vs IO
☐ **Immediate CPR** (Push hard, Push fast, minimize interruptions)
☐ **Immediate Defibrillation** if indicated
☐ BVM/Advanced Airway/**Intubation**
☐ ETCO₂ goal 10-20, improve CPR to goal

2 Shock/CPR Cycle

Cardioversion Biphasic 200J

Shockable Rhythm?

CPR 2 min

ROSC? → Post Arrest Algorithm

Other Rhythm? → PEA Algorithm
Brady Algorithm
Tachy Algorithm

3 Epi Cycle

Epinephrine 1mg
or
Vasopressin 40mg

Repeat q 3-5 min

4 Anti-arrhythmics

⇨ **Amiodarone** 300mg IV, then 150mg IV
⇨ MgSO4 2-6g IV/IO
⇨ Lidocaine 1-1.5 mg/kg

5 Cause?

5Hs 5Ts → Treat Empirically → PEA Algorithm

6 ROSC? → Post Arrest Algorithm

1 True Shock?

- ☐ Ill appearing/AMS
- ☐ Tachycardia /Hypotension > 20min?
- ☐ Met acidosis (lactate>4 or Base def <-5)
- ☐ Tachypnea (RR>22 or PCO2<32)
- ☐ Oliguria: UOP<0.5ml/kg/h

2 Resuscitation

- ☐ ABCs, IV, O2, monitor, vital signs
- ☐ Correct emergent causes (PTX/HTX, tamponade, PE)
- ☐ Stop hemorrhage
- ☐ Fluid resuscitation/PRBCs?

3 Cause?

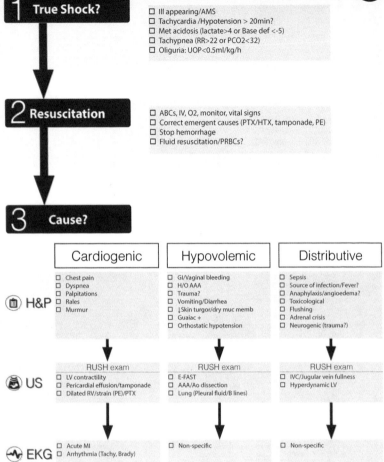

	Cardiogenic	Hypovolemic	Distributive
H&P	☐ Chest pain ☐ Dyspnea ☐ Palpitations ☐ Rales ☐ Murmur	☐ GI/Vaginal bleeding ☐ H/O AAA ☐ Trauma? ☐ Vomiting/Diarrhea ☐ ↓Skin turgor/dry muc memb ☐ Guaiac + ☐ Orthostatic hypotension	☐ Sepsis ☐ Source of infection/Fever? ☐ Anaphylaxis/angioedema? ☐ Toxicological ☐ Flushing ☐ Adrenal crisis ☐ Neurogenic (trauma?)
US	RUSH exam ☐ LV contractility ☐ Pericardial effusion/tamponade ☐ Dilated RV/strain (PE)/PTX	RUSH exam ☐ E-FAST ☐ AAA/Ao dissection ☐ Lung (Pleural fluid/B lines)	RUSH exam ☐ IVC/Jugular vein fullness ☐ Hyperdynamic LV
EKG	☐ Acute MI ☐ Arrhythmia (Tachy, Brady)	☐ Non-specific	☐ Non-specific
CXR	☐ Pulmonary edema ☐ PTX	☐ Wide mediastinum ☐ Hemothorax	☐ Pneumonia
Labs	☐ ↑Troponin/BNP ☐ ↑Lactate	☐ ↑ BUN/Cr ☐ ↓H/H → Type and Cross ☐ ↑Lactate	☐ ↑Lactate ☐ Cortisol, TSH
Tx	⇨ ACLS algorithms ⇨ Thrombolytics ⇨ Cath vs CABG ⇨ Pressors/afterload reducers/IABP	⇨ IV Fluids ⇨ Warmed blood products (PRBC, FFP, Platelets) ⇨ Stop the bleeding (OR, IR) ⇨ Consider Massive Transfusion protocol	⇨ Antibiotics ⇨ IVF/Blood products ⇨ Vasopressors ⇨ Steroids? T4? Antidote?

SHOCK

1. TRUE SHOCK?
(CMEDownload "Modern Concepts in Shock" USC Trauma 2009)(Essentials 2013 "US in Shock")

General
- The goal for the patient in shock is rapidly identifying that the patient is in shock, finding the cause of shock and treating the cause while simultaneously resuscitating the patient

Clinical Presentation
- Ill appearing/AMS
- Tachycardia /Hypotension>20min?
- Met acidosis (lactate>4 mg/dl or Base def <-5)
- Tachypnea (RR>22 or PCO_2<32)
- Oliguria: UOP<0.5 ml/kg/h
- Base deficit, lactate and sublingual capnometry ($SLCO_2$) can help identify patients in early shock and are a predictor of mortality (J Trauma 2007;62:120)

2. RESUSCITATION
- ABCs
- IV/O_2/Cardiac monitor
- Foley
- Crystalloids
  - ⇨ 20ml/kg boluses
  - ⇨ Caution in CLOCK (CNS, Liver, Older, Children, Kidney disease)
- Antibiotics empirically
- Blood (before Pressors)
- Vasopressors (from $\alpha{\rightarrow}\beta$: PNEDDI) (**EM:RAP** 5/10 "Pressors")

PNEDDI ($\alpha{\rightarrow}\beta$)
• Phenylephrine
• Norepinephrine
• Epinephrine
• Dopamine
• Dobutamine
• Isoproterenol

3. CAUSE OF SHOCK

Assessment
- Correct emergent and reversible causes
  - ⇨ Tension PTX → needle thoracostomy
  - ⇨ Cardiac tamponade → pericardiocentesis/thoracotomy
  - ⇨ Arrhythmia → shock?
- Vital signs
  - ⇨ Shock index: HR/SBP > 0.9 abnormal
  - ⇨ SIRS: HR>90; RR>20; T<36 or >38; WBC<4 or >12 (>10% bands); $PaCO_2$ <32
- Pediatrics assessment
  - ⇨ Pediatric assessment triangle
    - ✓ Work of breathing
    - ✓ General appearance
    - ✓ Circulation to skin
- RUSH protocol for sonography (Emerg Med Clin N Am 2010 Feb;28(1):29-56)
  - ⇨ The Pump: Pericardial effusion, LV contractility, RV strain
  - ⇨ The Tank: IVC/Jugular vein fullness, FAST, Lung (PTX, Pleural fluid, B lines)
  - ⇨ The Pipes: AAA, Ao Dissection, DVT

Classification of shock
- **Hypovolemic**
  - ⇨ Low CVP, Low CI (Cardiac index), High SVR
  - ⇨ Volume depletion type
    - ✓ Vomiting/Diarrhea, Heat stroke, Burns, decreased intake
    - ✓ 3rd Spacing Pancreatitis, Burns
  - ⇨ Hemorrhagic type
    - ✓ GI bleed/Vaginal bleed, AAA rupture/Dissection, Trauma
- **Cardiogenic**
  - ⇨ High CVP, Low CI-cardiac index, High SVR
  - ⇨ Cardiomyopathy
    - ✓ MI/Ischemia
  - ⇨ Arrhythmias
    - ✓ Tachy (AF/VT), Slow (Brady, blocks)
  - ⇨ Mechanical
    - ✓ Valve defect, atrial myxoma, ruptured ventricular aneurysm
  - ⇨ Obstructive
    - ✓ Massive PE, tension PTX, constrictive pericarditis, cardiac tamponade, pulmonary HTN

- **Distributive**
  - ⇨ Low CVP, High CI, Low SVR
  - ⇨ Sepsis/SIRS (See Sepsis Algorithm)
  - ⇨ Anaphylaxis, Toxic shock
  - ⇨ Drugs
  - ⇨ Addisonian crisis
  - ⇨ Myxedema coma
  - ⇨ Neurogenic shock

BRADYCARDIA

1 Unstable?

Unstable Criteria
- ☐ Hypotension
- ☐ Hypoperfusion
- ☐ Pulmonary edema
- ☐ Altered mental status

2 Level of Block?

SA Node

Sinus rhythm
- ☐ Are P waves present
- ☐ Can be normal variant
- ☐ SSS?

Above AV-node

1^0 or 2^0 (Wenckebach) AV block
- ☐ Usually stable
- ☐ Narrow QRS
- ☐ Responsive to atropine

Below AV-node

$2°$ (Mobitz II) or $3°$ AV block
- ☐ Usually unstable
- ☐ Wide QRS
- ☐ No response to atropine

3 Treatment

Treat Bradycardia
- ⇨ **Atropine** 0.25-0.5mg IV increments (3mg max)
- ⇨ **Epinephrine** (2-10mcg/min)
- ⇨ Dopamine (2-10 mcg/kg/min)
- ⇨ TCP (Transcutaneous pacer)
- ⇨ Transvenous pacer (ED vs cath lab)

Treat Causes

Drugs/OD
- ⇨ β-blocker OD → glucagon 3mg IV
- ⇨ CCB OD → CaCl 1-2 gm IV
- ⇨ Digoxin OD → Digibind

(K+) Electrolytes

Hyperkalemia Tx
- ⇨ CaCl 1 amp IV
- ⇨ D50 1 amp/Regular Insulin 10 units IV
- ⇨ Albuterol 15mg NEB
- ⇨ HCO3 1 amp IV
- ⇨ Lasix 40mg IV
- ⇨ Kayexalate 30gm PO
- ⇨ Emergent Dialysis

Ischemia
- ⇨ Treat as MI → Cath Lab

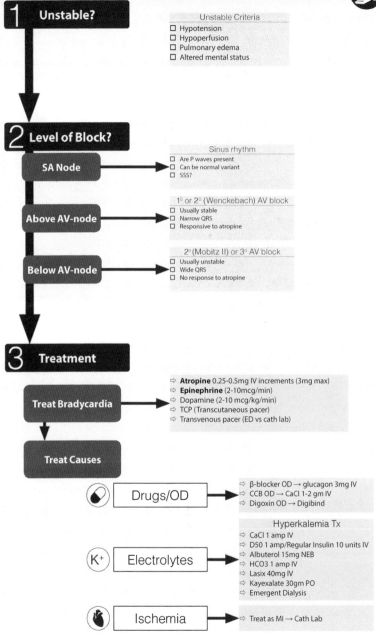

6

BRADYCARDIA

1. STABLE VS UNSTABLE
(CMEDownload Resus 2006-Mattu)(EMRAP.TV Episode 55-Herbert)

Treat only unstable bradycardia
- Hypotension/Shock
- Acute CHF/pulmonary edema
- Altered mental status
- Ischemic chest pain (angina equivalent)

Asymptomatic: observation

2. LEVEL OF BLOCK

SA Node
- Bradycardia may be normal in athletes, young
- Increased vagal tone- can cause vasovagal episode
- SSS Sick sinus syndrome (primary disease of SA node)
- Acute MI (inferior wall)
- Drugs (β-blockers, CCB, Digoxin, Amiodarone)

1° AV block
- Normal in 5% of population

2° AV block- Wenckebach
- At level of AV node, narrow complex → progressive prolongation of PR interval until a QRS is dropped
- Stable and transient

2° AV block- Mobitz II
- Sudden unexpected loss of P wave conduction → Likely to go into asystole, 3°AV block
- Below AV node

3° AV block
- Narrow complex → block at AV node
- Wide complex → bad

	Narrow	Wide
Level of Block:	AV Node → Bundle of His	Below AV Node (usually slower)
Response to Atropine:	Frequently responsive	Usually not
Stability:	Usually stable	Unstable, usually progress → asystole

3. TREATMENT

Atropine
- Dose: 0.5mg IV while awaiting pacemaker
  - ⇨ May repeat to max 3mg; can dose higher in cholinergic OD
- Caution
  - ⇨ Cardiac transplant → atropine ineffective, can make worse
  - ⇨ Caution in Mobitz II and 3° AV block → may make worse
  - ⇨ Not useful in hypothermia → must rewarm patient

Bradycardia Causes
- ☐ Drugs
- ☐ Electrolytes
- ☐ Ischemia

Pressors
- Epinephrine (2-10mcg/min)
- Dopamine (2-10mcg/kg/min)
- Use while awaiting pacer or pacer ineffective

Trans-cutaneous pacing
- Indications
  - ⇨ High failure rate → be ready to move onto next modality
  - ⇨ Unstable bradycardia not responsive to atropine
  - ⇨ Mobitz II or 3° AV block
  - ⇨ Do not use in hypothermia → irritates myocardium → arrhythmia
- Use
  - ⇨ Apply electrodes to chest, set rate at 70-80 bpm, set amps high then drop down until capture is lost.
    - ✓ Check for **electrical capture** (monitor) and **mechanical capture** (pulse)
    - ✓ Use immediately for high degree block (type II 2° or type 3° AV block)
    - ✓ Place pads at least 10cm away from implanted pacemaker

BRADYCARDIA

Trans-venous pacer
- Insertion sites R IJ > R supraclavicular > L subclavian (EMRAP.TV Episode 73)
- Contraindicated in prosthetic tricuspid valve (↑likelihood in pt with hx IVDA)

Specific treatment
- Glucagon
  - ⇨ Use: β-blocker or CCB OD
  - ⇨ Dose: 3mg IV x 1 then 3mg/h
- CaCl
  - ⇨ Use: CCB OD and hyperkalemia
  - ⇨ Dose: 1-2 gm IV over 10min q20 min x 5 doses (CCB overdose)
  - ⇨ Special case: Patient taking Digoxin? Ca^{++} causing stone heart in Digoxin overdose may be questionable (J of Emerg Med 2011;40:41-46)
- HCO_3
  - ⇨ Use: Acidosis, hyperkalemia, toxic ingestion (TCA etc.)
  - ⇨ Dose: 1-2 amps IV (if patient acidotic→ other treatments not work well)
- Digibind- dosing based on amount of digoxin ingested

Other Causes of bradycardia
- Hypoxia, hypothyroid, increased ICP, hypothermia, SSS

TACHYCARDIA

1 Unstable?

- ☐ ABCs
- ☐ IV/O₂/Monitor
- ☐ Immediate Cardioversion
- ☐ Resuscitation

2 P waves?

+ P waves → **Sinus Tachycardia** (look for underlying etiology)

No P waves

3 Narrow vs Wide?

4 Regular vs Irregular?

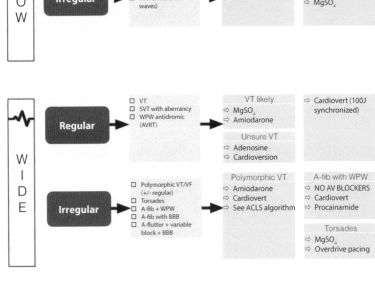

	Ddx	Stable Tx	Unstable Tx
NARROW — Regular	☐ PSVT (AVNRT) ☐ A-flutter ☐ Orthodromic WPW (AVRT)	⇨ Vagal maneuvers ⇨ Adenosine ⇨ CCB ⇨ β-blocker	⇨ Cardiovert (50-100J sync) ⇨ Adenosine
NARROW — Irregular	☐ A-fibrillation ☐ A-flutter/ variable block ☐ MAT (multifocal P waves)	⇨ CCB ⇨ β-blocker	⇨ Cardiovert ⇨ Diltiazem ⇨ Amiodarone ⇨ MgSO₄

	Ddx	Stable Tx	Unstable Tx
WIDE — Regular	☐ VT ☐ SVT with aberrancy ☐ WPW antidromic (AVRT)	**VT likely** ⇨ MgSO₄ ⇨ Amiodarone **Unsure VT** ⇨ Adenosine ⇨ Cardioversion	⇨ Cardiovert (100J synchronized)
WIDE — Irregular	☐ Polymorphic VT/VF (+/- regular) ☐ Torsades ☐ A-fib + WPW ☐ A-fib with BBB ☐ A-flutter + variable block + BBB	**Polymorphic VT** ⇨ Amiodarone ⇨ Cardiovert ⇨ See ACLS algorithm	**A-fib with WPW** ⇨ NO AV BLOCKERS ⇨ Cardiovert ⇨ Procainamide **Torsades** ⇨ MgSO₄ ⇨ Overdrive pacing

TACHYCARDIA

THE APPROACH TO TACHYCARDIA
(EM:RAP 9/08 "Tachycardia"-Herbert)(EMRAP.TV Episode 62-Herbert)

- **Step 1**: IV, O₂, Monitor, advanced airway to bedside
- **Step 2:** Stable vs. Unstable
  - ⇨ Not a dichotomous decision→it is a spectrum
  - ⇨ Based on: Chest pain, Hypotension, AMS, Pulmonary edema,
- **Step 3:** P waves
  - ⇨ P waves=sinus=no defibrillation=1 to 1 with QRS=normal axis
- **Step 4:** Rhythm: Regular or Irregular?
  - ⇨ Irregular = mostly supraventricular, block the AV node, usually not VT
- **Step 5**: Complexes: Wide vs Narrow
  - ⇨ Narrow= supraventricular, block the AV node, not VT, <0.12 sec (3 small squares, <0.08 sec in children)

GROUP 1: NARROW, REGULAR, NO P's

Differential:
- PSVT (AVNRT; exquisitely regular)
- Atrial flutter with consistent block (not variable-usually 150bpm)
- Orthodromic WPW (95% of WPW, no Δ wave)
- Narrow complex VT (very rarely)

PSVT (AVNRT)

Define
- AVNRT (Atrioventricular nodal reentrant tachycardia)-Reentrant rhythm that uses the AV node
- AVNRT is one type of paroxysmal SVT (supraventricular tachycardia)

Cause:
- Electrical circus movement within the AV node

Treatment
- Treat narrow and regular tachycardia as PSVT
- AV nodal blocker (Adenosine) can also be used to slow rate and diagnose other arrhythmias (atrial-flutter)

SVT types
☐ AVNRT
☐ AVRT(e.g. WPW)
☐ Atrial Tachycardia (AT)

Stable Treatment: Block the circus movement
- Adenosine (EM:RAP 3/11 "Adenosine in the 2010 ACLS Guidelines" – Herbert)
  - ⇨ 6mg IV push → 12mg IV push → 12mg IV push
  - ⇨ Push fast with a flush, raise arm
  - ⇨ Potentiated by: central line (3mg IVP), heart transplant (1mg IVP), Carbamazepine, Dipyridamole
  - ⇨ Inhibited by: Theophylline, Caffeine
  - ⇨ Beware: Asthma/Active pulmonary disease
- Diltiazem
  - ⇨ ACLS: 15-20mg over 2 minutes
  - ⇨ Alternative: 2.5mg/min to total of 50mg
- Other treatments: Verapamil, β-blocker, MgSO₄ (J Assoc Physicians India 1995;43(8):529-31), Amiodarone, Procain-amide

Unstable treatment:
- Consider Adenosine (Ann Emerg Med 1993;22(4):709-13)
- Cardioversion: Can start at 50J and double every time
  - ⇨ Sedation??? Etomidate/Fentanyl vs Versed vs Propofol/Brevital

GROUP 2: NARROW, IRREGULAR, NO Ps

Differential
- Atrial fibrillation
- Atrial flutter with variable block
- MAT (give fluids/treat hypoxia, do not shock/no CCB!) (Essentials 2011 "Fib vs Flutter" – Orman)

Cause
- Increased automaticity

Stable treatment
- Rate control → Long acting AV-nodal blocker
- Diltiazem
  - ⇨ 10mg and repeat q 5-10min (max 60mg)
  - ⇨ Can start a drip at 5-10mg/h
- β-blockers
  - ⇨ Metoprolol 5mg IV q 5min

- Digoxin
  - ⇨ Slow onset, not great for rate control acutely
  - ⇨ Consider use for patients in CHF or unable to take CCB or β-blocker
- ED cardioversion?
  - ⇨ Pharmacologic: Similar conversion rates in all classes (50-70%)
  - ⇨ Electrical

Unstable treatment

- Cardioversion: 200J synchronized
  - ⇨ Sedation
    - ✓ No Propofol, may drop BP
    - ✓ Consider Ketamine (0.1-0.15mg/kg) + Etomidate (5-10mg)
  - ⇨ Anticoagulation-Consider Heparin IV if unknown/prolonged time in AF
- Diltiazem – slowly
- Magnesium 2-10gm (Heart 2007;93:1433-40)
- Amiodarone? Digoxin?
- Hypotension?
  - ⇨ Push dose pressors? Phenylephrine (50-200mcg IV q 1 minute until DBP > 60)

ATRIAL FIBRILLATION/FLUTTER

(CMEDownload "UCSF 2012"-Snoey)

Rate Control

- Diltiazem
  - ⇨ 10mg and repeat q 5-10min (max 60mg)
  - ⇨ Can start a drip at 5-10mg/h
- β-blockers
  - ⇨ Metoprolol 5mg IV q 5min
- Digoxin
  - ⇨ Slow onset, not good for rate control acutely
  - ⇨ Use for patients in CHF or unable to take CCB or BB
- Rate control preferred over rhythm control (N Engl J Med 2002;347:1825)(N Engl J Med 2008;358:2667--2677)
  - ⇨ Trend towards better outcomes with rate control
  - ⇨ Patients still need anticoagulation
  - ⇨ Avoid anti-arrhythmic side effects
- Who may benefit from rhythm control
  - ⇨ Failure of rate control
  - ⇨ Younger patients requiring optimal cardiac performance (Lone AF)
  - ⇨ One shot at NSR? (30% of patients converted to NSR will never revert back to AF)

Rhythm Control

- **Low embolic risk pt** (<48 hours of sx)
  - ⇨ Rate control as above
  - ⇨ Early Cardioversion
    - ✓ Embolic risk 0.7% in patients treated without peri- or post-cardioversion anticoagulation (J Am Coll Cardiol. 2013;62(13):1187)
  - ⇨ Ottawa aggressive protocol (EM:RAP 11/11 "A fib: Ottawa Aggressive Protocol – Stiell), (CJEM 2010;12(3):181-91)
    - ✓ Procainamide 1gm IV over 60 min (60% conversion rate) then→
    - ✓ Electrical cardioversion (92%) conversion rate→
    - ✓ D/C Home, no anticoagulation
    - ✓ 96.8% were discharged home and of those → 93% were in NSR
- **High embolic risk pt** (>48 hours of sx)
  - ⇨ Define: >48-72 hours of sx or unknown, no LV dysfunction, no mitral valve disease, no previous embolism
  - ⇨ Immediate cardioversion option
    - ✓ Immediate TEE (r/o thrombus) + Heparin → Cardioversion 100-150J → Coumadin x 4 weeks
  - ⇨ Delayed cardioversion option
    - ✓ Coumadin x 3 weeks → Elective Cardioversion → Coumadin x 4 weeks post

CHADS2 Score	
Clinical Parameter	Points
CHF (history)	1
Hypertension (history)	1
Age > 75	1
Diabetes	1
Secondary prevention	2

CHADS2 score	Risk CVA/yr
0	1.9%
1	2.8%
2	4%
3	5.9%
4	8.5%
5	12.5%
6	18.2%

Unstable treatment options (EM:RAP 7/10 "Atrial fibrillation: a critical review"-Weingart)

- **Cardioversion**:
  - ⇨ 200J synchronized
  - ⇨ Sedation
    - ✓ No Propofol, may drop BP
    - ✓ Use Ketamine (0.1-0.15mg/kg) + Etomidate (5-10mg)
  - ⇨ Anticoagulation
    - i. Pre-cardioversion Heparin bolus +/- TEE depending on stability of patient
- Diltiazem – slowly as a gtt (start at 2.5mg/h)

ATRIAL FIBRILLATION ALGORITHM

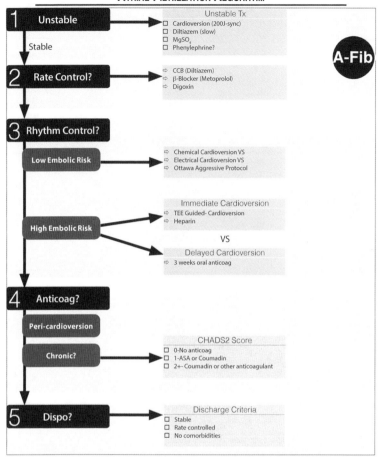

- Magnesium 2-10gm (Heart 2007;93:1433-40)
- Amiodarone? Digoxin?
- Hypotension?
  - ⇨ Push dose pressors? Phenylephrine (50-200mcg IV q 1 minute until DBP > 60)

Anticoagulation

- Thromboembolism risk varies between 1.5 to 17% per year depending on pt risk factors
  - ⇨ Same risk in chronic vs paroxysmal AF → risk defined by CHADS score (AFFIRM and RACE trials)
- Coumadin
  - ⇨ Risk of Coumadin complication ≈ 1-2%/yr
  - ⇨ Reduces stroke risk by 2/3
- ASA
  - ⇨ 50% of benefit of Coumadin → CHADS 1 only
- Peri-cardioversion (consider)
  - ⇨ High risk of embolism after cardioversion regardless of method (6% in first week)
  - ⇨ Risk drops to 0.6% if A-fib <48h (ACUTE and RE-LY studies) (except in CHF, mitral valve dz, or h/o thromboembolism)

- Chronic
  - ⇨ CHADS2 vs CHA2DS2-VASc score (JAMA 2001; 285:2864)
    - ✓ Low risk : CHADS = 0; no benefit with ASA (stroke rate 0.5-1.7%/yr)
    - ✓ Intermediate risk: CHADS = 1; Recommend Anticoagulation > ASA (stroke rate 2%/yr)
    - ✓ High risk: CHADS ≥ 2; Oral anticoagulation recommended (stroke rate ≥4%/yr)

Disposition

- Admit criteria
  - ⇨ Expedite work-up (ECHO etc...)
  - ⇨ Not stabilized (hypotensive, difficult rate control...)
  - ⇨ Monitor, cardioversion, eval effects of anti-arrhythmics
  - ⇨ R/O ACS? (AF is rarely a manifestation of ACS)
- Discharge
  - ⇨ No comorbidities (underlying heart disease, structural heart disease)
  - ⇨ Stable and rate controlled

GROUP 3: WIDE, REGULAR, NO P WAVES

Differential:

- Ventricular tachycardia (until proven otherwise)
- SVT with aberrancy (bundle branch block)
- Antidromic WPW (5% of WPW, Δ wave)

Cause: Circus re-entry in ventricles

Treatment:

- Cardioversion, synchronized
- Unsure (EM:RAP 6/11 "WCT and Adenosine Revisited" – Herbert) (Ann Emerg Med 1997;29(1):172-4)
  - ⇨ Can use adenosine 6mg, repeat at 12mg
- VT most likely (EM:RAP 2/11 "Amio vs Procain for Wide Complex Arrhythmias" – Mattu)
  - ⇨ Magnesium 2-4 grams over 2-4 minutes or
  - ⇨ Procainamide 17mg/kg slow IV or
  - ⇨ Amiodarone 150mg IV over 10 min

WIDE COMPLEX TACHYCARDIA (WCT)

What predicts VT? (Ann Emerg Med. 1987;16(1):40.)

- History
  - ⇨ Age greater than 35 years had a sensitivity of 92% and a positive predictive value of 85% for VT
  - ⇨ Known CAD/heart disease, ICD, h/o VT
  - ⇨ Medications (QT prolonging drugs, anti-arrhythmics, Digoxin)
- EKG criteria
  - ⇨ Brugada criteria
  - ⇨ Bayesian approach
  - ⇨ Sensitivity 79 to 92 % and specificity from 43 to 70 % (Acad Emerg Med. 2000;7(7):769)

WCT ALGORITHM

TACHYCARDIA

VT (VENTRICULAR TACHYCARDIA)

VT Arrest (See ACLS Section: VT)

Definitions
- Non-sustained VT (3 beats of PVCs, >120bpm, <30s)
- Sustained VT (>30s)

Treatment, Unstable
- Emergent Cardioversion, synchronized (50-100J)
- Anti-arrhythmics, see below
- Treat underlying cause (electrolytes, ischemia, drug OD, decompensated CHF)

Treatment, Stable (EM:RAP 2/11 "Amio vs Procain for Wide Complex Arrhythmias" – Mattu)
- Urgent/Elective Cardioversion (sync 50-100J)
- Procainamide 17mg/kg slow IV (25-30min) then 1-4 mg/minute by continuous infusion or
- Amiodarone 150mg IV over 10 min then1 mg/minute for 6 hours, then 0.5 mg/minute
- Lidocaine 1 to 1.5 mg/kg over 2 to 3 minutes
- Magnesium 2-4 grams over 2-4 minutes

GROUP 4: WIDE, IRREGULAR, NO P

Differential:
- A-fib with BBB (most common cause)
- A-flutter with variable block and BBB
- A-fib and WPW
- Polymorphic VT or Torsades

WPW

Wolff-Parkinson-White (WPW)

Treatment (An approach) (0.1-0.5% of general population)
- Regular tachycardic rhythm + WPW history
  - ⇨ (AVRT) Orthodromic
    - ✓ AV nodal blockers, can treat similar to AVNRT
  - ⇨ (AVRT) Antidromic
    - ✓ Avoid AV blockers (β-blockers, CCB, Adenosine, Dig) unless arrhythmia is **definitely known** to be antidromic AVRT
    - ✓ Difficult to distinguish between VT → Treat as VT if unknown
    - ✓ Procainamide 20-50mg/min for total 17mg/kg
- **Irregular rhythm: WPW + A-fib**
  - ⇨ **Unstable: DC Cardioversion**
  - ⇨ **NO AV NODE BLOCKERS!!!**
    - ✓ Atrial fibrillation is conducted to the ventricles through both accessory pathway and AV node
    - ✓ If use AV-nodal blocker→ all conduction will go down accessory pathway with a decreased refractory period → can lead to **Ventricular Fibrillation** (CJEM 2005;7(4):262-265)
  - ⇨ Cardioversion
    - ✓ DC Cardioversion
    - ✓ Procainamide
    - ✓ Amiodarone
    - ✓ Ibutilide
- Consider WPW in patients with:
  - ⇨ History of WPW
  - ⇨ Wide complexes
  - ⇨ Bizarre complexes
  - ⇨ Rapid ventricular response: R-R intervals >250 (also seen in hypersympathetic states)

POST-CARDIAC ARREST

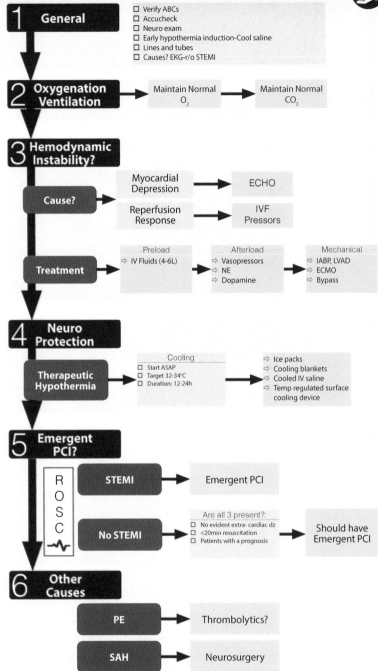

15

POST-CARDIAC ARREST

1. GENERAL STEPS

(EM:RAP 4/12-Mattu/Herbert) (Essentials 2010 "Post-arrest care"-Weingart)(Circulation 2011;123:1428)

- Verify ABCs, Accucheck, Neuro exam
- Early hypothermia induction-cooled saline
- Procedures: Lines and tubes (Central line, A-line)
- Look for Causes: EKG-r/o STEMI
- Check for Complications

2. OXYGENATION/VENTILATION

Oxygenation (JAMA 2010; 303:2165)
- Avoid hyperoxia and hypoxia
- Hyperoxia (PaO$_2$ >300 mm Hg) was independently associated with increased in-hospital mortality compared with patients with normoxia or hypoxia

Ventilation
- Hypocarbia causes cerebral vasoconstriction and hyperventilation decreases cardiac output
- Optimal respiratory parameters
    ⇨ Goal pH 7.35, pCO$_2$ 45, pO$_2$ 100, O$_2$ sat 95%

3. CIRCULATORY SUPPORT

Causes of Hemodynamic instability
- Ischemia- Reperfusion Response (Circulation 2002;106:562-568)
    ⇨ Sepsis-like syndrome with SIRS
    ⇨ Leaky and vasodilated capillaries
    ⇨ Treatment: IV Fluids and Vasopressors
- Post Arrest myocardial depression
    ⇨ Cardiac stunning is reversible if survive 24-48h (be aggressive on these pts)
    ⇨ Treatment: Dobutamine, Balloon Pump, Extra-corporeal Life Support (ECMO, Bypass)

What works in CA?
1. Early defibrillation
2. Quality compression, without interruption
3. Therapeutic Hypothermia (ROSC w/o recovery of neuro function)
4. Coronary angio + PCI (for almost everyone)

Treatment-Resuscitation
- Target MAP: 65-100 (likely in higher range of 80-100)
- Improve **Preload**: (Resus 2009;80:1223)
    ⇨ Fluid resuscitation 4-6L
- Improve **Afterload**:
    ⇨ Vasopressor support start immediately after return of pulses
    ⇨ Norepinephrine
    ⇨ Dopamine
- **Mechanical support**?
    ⇨ Intra-aortic balloon pump (IABP, LVAD, ECMO, Bypass)?
- Improve O$_2$ carrying capacity-transfuse to Hb 7-10?
- Adequate resuscitation?
    ⇨ Lactate: Serial lactate to ensure improvement
    ⇨ ScvO$_2$ >75%
- Electrolytes (Mg, Ca), do not replace K right away

4. NEUROPROTECTION: THERAPEUTIC HYPOTHERMIA (TH)

(EM:RAP 8/13-Mattu)(Essentials 2010-Eckstein, 2013-Rittenberger)
(Circulation. 2013;127:244-250)

Indication
- *Therapeutic hypothermia is the only therapy proven to improve neurologic outcome and decrease mortality in comatose patients after cardiac arrest*
- **Indication**: Comatose (lack of meaningful response to verbal commands) adult patients with ROSC after out-of-hospital cardiac arrest
- Goal: Rapid initiation and maintenance of temperature of 32°C to 34°C for 12 to 24 hours

TH for Cardiac Arrest
NNT = 6 for mortality

- Guidelines
    ⇨ **AHA Class I**: Cardiac arrest from VT/VF (Circulation. 2010;122(suppl 3):S768–S786)
    ⇨ **AHA Class IIb**: Cardiac arrest from non-shockable rhythms
    ⇨ The **European Resuscitation Council**: recommends TH for all comatose survivors of CA regardless of initial rhythm (Resuscitation. 2010;81:1305–1352)

Special Populations
    ⇨ Consider TH in pregnancy, pediatrics and patients on vasopressors
    ⇨ Trauma pts: Not indicated

POST-CARDIAC ARREST

Journal Club: TH for Shockable Rhythm

Study 1: Hypothermia after Cardiac Arrest Study Group (N Engl J Med 2002;346:549-56.)
- Favorable neurologic outcome: 55% (hypothermia) vs 39% (normothermia) groups
- ↓**Mortality** at 6 months with hypothermia: 41% (hypothermia) vs 55% (normothermia) groups

Study 2: Bernard et. al. (N Engl J Med 2002;346:557-63)
- Treatment Of Comatose Survivors Of Out-Of-Hospital Cardiac Arrest With Induced Hypothermia
- **Favorable neurologic outcome:** 49% (hypothermia) vs 26% (normothermia) groups (OR 5.25, **NNT=4**)

Meta-analysis: (Crit Care Med 2005;33:414)
- (3 RCTs) number needed-to-treat to allow 1 additional patient to leave the hospital with improvements in neurological outcome was 6 (95% confidence interval: 4 to 13)

TTM Trial (N Engl J Med 2013;369:2197-206)(EM:RAP 4/14)
- ⇨ **No Difference in Mortality**: 50% (33°C group) vs 48% (36°C group)(CI= 0.89 to 1.28; P=0.51)
- ⇨ Hypothermia at a targeted temperature of 33°C had **no benefit** vs a targeted temperature of 36°C

Journal Club: TH for Non-Shockable Rhythm

Review (Circulation 2011;123:1428)
- Largely observational, no difference in outcomes

Kim et al (Resuscitation 2012;83:188-196)
- Meta-analysis: 2 RCTs and 12 non-randomized
- Randomized trials: RR (6-month mortality) = 0.85 (95% CI 0.65–1.11; no statistical difference)
- Conclusion: TH is associated with reduced in-hospital mortality for adult patients resuscitated from non-shockable cardiac arrest

---

HYPOTHERMIA PROTOCOL

1. Initiation
   - ⇨ ASAP with target temp of 32-34°C
   - ⇨ Ice packs, cooling blankets, cooled IV saline, temp regulated surface cooling device (e.g. Arctic Sun)
   - ⇨ Method of cooling does not matter
   - ⇨ Treat shivering: (occurs between 35-37°C)
     - ✓ Wrap hands/feet/head with blanket,
   - ⇨ Sedative/analgesic options
     - ✓ Propofol infusion (20-50 mcg/kg/min)
     - ✓ Fentanyl infusion (25-100 mcg/hr)
     - ✓ Diazepam (10-20mg IV)
     - ✓ $MgSO_4$ (4 gm IV over 15 min)
     - ✓ Vecuronium (0.1mg/kg IV)
2. Maintenance
   - ⇨ Follow BP, O_2 sat, volume repletion, glucose, potassium, seizures
3. Rewarming
   - ⇨ Begin 24h after induction at rate of 0.5°C/hr
   - ⇨ Monitor BP, K^+, glucose
4. Normothermia

Complications
- Bradycardia (13%): normal with hypothermia, treat only if hypotensive
- Seizures (24%)
- Hypokalemia- reversed at rewarming, replete to K^+ >3.5
- Pneumonia (41%)

Contraindications
- Intracranial hemorrhage, severe hemorrhage/exsanguination, hypotension refractory to multiple vasopressors, severe sepsis, and pregnancy

Sedation/analgesia
- ⇨ Fentanyl/Propofol ideal, Midazolam if cannot use Propofol

Glucose control (NEJM 2009;360:1283-1297)(Resuscitation 2009;80:624-630)
- Measure hourly?
- Goal 120-180 (Tighter control not associated with improved outcomes)

POST-CARDIAC ARREST

5. EMERGENT PCI?

STEMI (Essentials 2013 "Post ROSC: Cath lab for everyone?"-Pineda)
- May not have typical STEMI EKG after cardiac arrest
- Guidelines (2013 STEMI Guidelines (Level B) Circulation 2013;127:529-555)
  - ⇨ Immediate angiography and PCI if initial ECG shows STEMI
- Consider **Thrombolysis** if PCI not available

No ST Elevation
- PCI for **ALL Cardiac Arrest**? (J Am Coll Cardiol Intv 2012;5:597)
  - ⇨ *"...anyone successfully resuscitated from out-of-hospital arrest thought to be cardiac in etiology should undergo emergent coronary angiography, regardless of their post-resuscitation ECG findings"*
- EKG no STEMI (Should they still go to PCI?)
  - ⇨ Post ROSC EKG PPV = 95%
  - ⇨ NPV = 44% (Therefore it rules in but **does not rule out STEMI**)
  - ⇨ Patients s/p cardiac arrest without a STEMI on EKG → NNT = 4 to find a lesion on PCI

Summary
- Consider all survivors of OHCA of suspected cardiac origin for primary PCI
- When emergent coronary intervention is unavailable, treatment with thrombolytic drugs may be considered

Cath Lab Indications
☐ ROSC + STEMI
☐ ROSC + Initial rhythm VF/VT

PCI for no STEMI
NNT = 4 to find lesion

Cath Lab Likely
ROSC + no STEMI + :
1. No evident extra- cardiac dz +
2. < 20min resuscitation +
3. Patients with a prognosis

Journal Club: Emergent PCI

STEMI
- Case Series (J Am Coll Cardiol Intv 2012;5:597–605)
  - ⇨ STEMI + PCI (19 studies, 1100 pts)
  - ⇨ Overall survival to discharge: 60% (vs 25-30% historical controls)
  - ⇨ Good neurologic outcome: 86% of all survivors
- French study (Circulation 2007;115:1354)
  - ⇨ 186 patients with OHCA and STEMI, primary PCI was performed routinely
  - ⇨ Survival at 6 months was 54%, with 46% of patients free of neurological impairment

No STEMI
- Study 1: (Resuscitation 2013;84:1250)
  - ⇨ No ST elevation on EKG → 33% had an acute coronary lesion
- Study 2: (Am J Cardiol 2011;108:634–638)
  - ⇨ No ST elevation on EKG → acute coronary lesion in 25% of patients

6. OTHER CAUSES

MI, Non-ST Elevation (AHA Guidelines: Circulation. 2010;122:S787–S817)
- The role of urgent PCI in patients with OHCA and non-STEMI is uncertain
- See above for ROSC + No ST elevation on EKG
- Should likely go to PCI

PE
- Consider thrombolysis in ER
- See SOB algorithm

Subarachnoid hemorrhage (SAH)
- Cardiac arrest from catecholamine surge
- Consider CT Head on all cardiac arrest patients
- Consider DDAVP to reverse antiplatelet effects?

CHEST PAIN

1 Emergent Causes?

	📋 Hx	🩺 PEX	💉 Action
STEMI	☐ Pressure like CP ☐ Radiation to arm/jaw ☐ CAD risk factors	☐ Non-reproducible ☐ Non-pleuritic ☐ N/V/diaphoresis	⇨ Immediate EKG! ⇨ Cath lab vs t-PA ⇨ (see below)
Ao Dissection	☐ Sudden onset, severe, tearing CP ☐ Risks: h/o Marfan, HTN, cocaine	☐ New murmur ☐ Pulse deficit ☐ Focal neuro deficit ☐ Limb ischemia	⇨ CXR, US ⇨ CT Chest ⇨ CT Surgery consult
PE	☐ Sudden onset **pleuritic CP** ☐ Dyspnea ☐ PE risk factors	☐ Dyspnea ☐ Leg pain/swelling ☐ Wells score ☐ See SOB algorithm	⇨ CXR/EKG ⇨ D-dimer ⇨ CTPA ⇨ V/Q scan ⇨ LE Duplex
Pericarditis	☐ **Pleuritic pain** ☐ Preceded by URI, underlying dz (SLE), uremia	☐ **Positional:** worse supine, improves on sitting up ☐ Pericardial friction rub ☐ Fever, ↑WBC	⇨ EKG ⇨ US/ECHO ⇨ Troponin
Boerhaave's	☐ Severe **vomiting** → retrosternal CP ☐ H/O recent instrumentation, EtOH, blunt trauma, caustic ingestion, HIV	☐ PEX: crepitus?	⇨ CXR ⇨ CT ⇨ Surgery consult ⇨ GI consult
Pneumothorax	☐ Acute pleuritic pain ☐ Asthenic body, h/o trauma	☐ Decreased/absent breath sounds ☐ Dyspnea ☐ H/O COPD, asthma, CF, PCP	⇨ CXR ⇨ Chest tube vs Heimlich

2 Consider ACS?

Risk Stratify: low vs high
- ☐ CAD risks
- ☐ CP History
- ☐ EKG
- ☐ Troponin
- ☐ ACP-TIPI
- ☐ TIMI risk score
- ☐ Braunwald
- ☐ Gestalt

⬇ Low Risk

Low risk therapies

Empiric Tx	☐ ASA ☐ Nitrates ☐ O₂ ☐ Morphine
R/O MI	☐ Serial EKG ☐ Cardiac Markers/Trop
R/O UA	☐ Non-invasive testing ☐ Inpatient/Obs unit ☐ 72h output

⬆ High Risk

NSTEMI/ UA	☐ Low risk therapies ☐ Heparin/LMWH ☐ Clopidogrel? ☐ GPI? ☐ PCI: Selective vs Early (high risk)
STEMI	☐ Low risk therapies ☐ Heparin/LMWH ☐ Clopidogrel? ☐ GPI? ☐ PCI vs Lytics stat

3 Very low risk/ No ACS? ⬇ ⬇

Stable Angina
VS
Non-Cardiac causes

CHEST PAIN

GENERAL APPROACH

- Always think about emergent/immediately life-threatening conditions first
- After those are ruled out by H&P, EKG, CXR or more advanced testing, then begin work-up to r/o ACS
- Patients are stratified into low or high risk ACS using certain criteria, then given empiric treatment based on their risk level
- If not concerned for ACS (young, no risk factors, atypical story), then think of other causes of chest pain and give appropriate treatment

1. EMERGENT CAUSES

AORTIC DISSECTION

(Essentials 2010 Dissection: 5 Tips) (CMEDownload UCSF High Risk- Snoey, Slovis)

General (EM Clinics North Amer 2012;30:307)
- **Mortality**
  - ⇨ 40% for immediate death → increases 1-2% thereafter per hour if unrecognized
  - ⇨ Type A (62%)
    - ✓ Ascending dissection +/- descending (10% mortality at 24 hours)
  - ⇨ Type B (38%)
    - ✓ Descending dissection (10% mortality at 30 days)
- Risk factors: (Circulation 2010;121:e266)
  - ⇨ HTN, Marfan's, vasculitis, pregnancy, coarctation, bicuspid aortic valve, trauma, cocaine/meth

Classification of Ao Dissection	
Proximal	Distal
Stanford A	Stanford B
DeBakey II	DeBakey I	DeBakey III
10-15%	60%	25-30%

Clinical Presentation (classic)
- Chest pain
  - ⇨ Sudden onset
  - ⇨ Severe tearing/ripping/sharp
  - ⇨ Pain may ease or migrate
- New murmur
  - ⇨ Aortic regurgitation → CHF → cardiac tamponade → cardiogenic shock
- Pulse deficit
- Focal neuro deficit
- Limb ischemia

↑Likelihood of Dissect	(+) LR	↓Likelihood of Dissect	(-) LR
HTN Hx	1.6	Absence of sudden CP	0.3
Marfan syndrome	4.1	Absence of HTN hx	0.5
Pulse deficit	5.7		
Migrating pain	1.1-7.6		
Focal neuro deficit	6.6-33		

History and Physical (JAMA 2002;287:2262-72) (Arch Intern Med 2000;160:2977)
- **Ascending (Type A)**
  - ⇨ Pulse deficit
  - ⇨ Pericardial effusion
  - ⇨ Aortic diastolic murmur
  - ⇨ Dramatic EKG changes (inferior MI)
- **Abdominal pain + Chest pain**
  - ⇨ Be highly suspicious if pain above and below diaphragm
- **Isolated neurological symptoms**:
  - ⇨ Altered mental status, seizure, unable to move legs
  - ⇨ Paralysis
    - ✓ No pain and presents like spinal cord injury T10-T12 (Compromise of spinal artery)
- **Stroke presentation**
  - ⇨ 95% of patients with a stroke and dissection have some type of chest pain or back pain.
  - ⇨ Caution with giving thrombolytics to a stroke patient → consider aortic dissection
  - ⇨ Consider screening CXR
- **Compression effects, local**
  - ⇨ SVC syndrome, trachea (dyspnea, stridor), esophagus (dysphagia), recurrent laryngeal nerve (hoarseness), and sympathetic chain (ipsilateral Horner syndrome)
- **Chest pain and leg pain**
  - ⇨ Type B dissection down to iliac vessels
- **Syncope** IRAD Study (JAMA 2000;283:897-903)
  - ⇨ 13% of patients with aortic dissection had syncope as their only symptom
  - ⇨ No CP/back pain/abdominal pain
  - ⇨ Consider bedside U/S to screen for pericardial effusion
- **Myocardial Infarction**
  - ⇨ Dissection flap that comes down into R coronary ostia → inferior MI on EKG
  - ⇨ CP that radiates to back with ↑ST II, III, aVF
- **Abdominal pain**
  - ⇨ Type B dissections causing mesenteric ischemia

CHEST PAIN

- **Painless dissection** (Mayo Clin Proc. 2002;77(3):296)
  - ⇨ 15% of patients had a painless presentation
  - ⇨ Failed to make a diagnosis in almost one-third
- **Cardiac arrest** (Resuscitation 2004;60:143–150)
  - ⇨ Study evaluated patients with aortic dissection or AAA that presented as PEA arrest
    - ✓ Thoracic dissection → only 48% patients had chest pain
    - ✓ AAA rupture → abdominal pain in only 52%
  - ⇨ Bedside U/S diagnostic of their process (effusion, free fluid)
- **Malperfusion syndromes**
  - ⇨ Surgery contraindicated in patients who have end organ ischemia? (Mortality 100%)
  - ⇨ Must improve perfusion to end organ (kidney, spinal cord, intestines…) prior to surgery
  - ⇨ May need to involve IR, vascular surgery, or transfer patient

Work-up
- EKG
  - ⇨ Non-specific, use to exclude other diagnosis
  - ⇨ Consider dissection in patients with inferior ischemia (II, III, aVF)
- D-dimer (**EM:RAP** 1/09 "D-dimer and Aortic Dissection")
  - ⇨ Sens 100%, Specificity 68% in one study (Eur Heart J. 2007;28:3067-75)
  - ⇨ Other studies show sens as low as 85% → not all dissection involves clotting cascade, may dissect through false lumen (Ann Emerg. Med. 2008;52:339-43)(J Emerg Med 2008; 34:367)
  - ⇨ Currently **NOT recommended as screening test** for dissection
- Chest X-ray
  - ⇨ 90% patients with aortic dissection have an abnormal CXR
  - ⇨ Sensitivity of 64% and Specificity of 86% for diagnosis of Ao dissection (Am J Med 2004;116:73-77)
  - ⇨ Use:
    - ✓ Evaluate for other causes of pain (alternate diagnosis) → no further imaging
    - ✓ Screening test (dilated aorta, bleeding) → patient will need further imaging

AAA X-ray features	(+) LR	(-) LR
Wide aortic contour	3.2	0.4
Wide mediastinum	2.2	0.6
Tracheal displacement	ns	ns
Displaced calcification	5.6	0.9
Aortic kinking	10.2	0.6
Opacified pulm window	2.3	0.8
Blurred aortic contour	ns	ns

- CTA (Arch Intern Med 2006;166:1350)
  - ⇨ Optimal imaging modality for ruling out aortic dissection in patients with a low clinical pretest probability for aortic dissection
  - ⇨ Sens 98%; Spec. 100% for dissection
- TEE (Transesophageal ECHO)
  - ⇨ Use: patients that are too unstable to go to CT, can show aortic regurgitation and pericardial effusion
  - ⇨ High sensitivity up to 98%
- MRI
  - ⇨ Equivalent to CT and TEE for diagnosis of dissection
- **Work-up summary** (Circulation. 2010;121:1544)
  - ⇨ D-dimer is not sensitive enough to r/o aortic dissection
  - ⇨ CXR- useful for establishing alternate diagnosis, decreases LR if completely negative
  - ⇨ CT, MRI, and TEE are equally effective to rule out/confirm aortic dissection
  - ⇨ If high suspicion for aortic dissection and initial test (CT, TEE, MRI) negative → second imaging study should be obtained

Treatment
- Goal is to stop extension of dissection
- Hypertensive: BP control
  - ⇨ β-blockers
    - ✓ Most important medication to give → can give empirically if high suspicion
    - ✓ Labetalol IV, Esmolol IV
    - ✓ Give to goal HR<60
  - ⇨ Vasodilators (typically after the beta blockers to reduce shear forces)
    - ✓ Use: if HR <60 with β-blockers and BP is still > 120/80 → start vasodilators
    - ✓ Caution: **do not use without β-blockers,** can cause reflex tachycardia → ↑dissection
    - ✓ Nitroprusside (agent of choice), Nitroglycerin
    - ✓ Fenoldopam: Selective dopamine-1 agonist, titratable
  - ⇨ Goal: HR< 60 and BP<120/80 (as low as possible) and pain under control
- Hypotensive
  - ⇨ Aggressive resuscitation
  - ⇨ IV fluids, PRBC transfusion
  - ⇨ Immediate surgery consult → OR
  - ⇨ Pericardial tamponade → Cardiac US → Pericardiocentesis?
- Other management scenarios
  - ⇨ Aortic insufficiency: gentle rate control, early surgery
  - ⇨ MI: gentle rate control (no ASA, anticoagulants, thrombolytics!)

CHEST PAIN

- Consultation
  - ⇨ Cardiothoracic surgery
  - ⇨ Type B:
    - ✓ Usually medically managed vs IR (grafts, stents, fenestrations)
    - ✓ Surgery indications: ongoing pain, refractory hypertension, occlusion of major arterial trunk origins, leaking or rupture, or development of local aneurysms
  - ⇨ Type A: Proximal Dissection
    - ✓ Consider Cardiothoracic surgery consult prior to CT
    - ✓ Immediate OR for surgical repair
    - ✓ Surgery decreases mortality from 56% (medical management) to 27%

PERICARDITIS

Causes (Am J Cardiol 1995;75:378-382)
- Idiopathic up to 80%, viral 1-10%, Bacterial, TB, Inflammatory, Metabolic, Neoplastic

Presentation
- Chest pain (95%)
  - ⇨ Pleuritic: sharp pleuritic pain, worsens with cough or moving
  - ⇨ Positional: worse supine, improves on sitting up
- Preceded by URI, underlying dz (SLE, uremia)
- Fever, ↑WBC, ↑ESR
- Pericardial friction rub – a superficial scratchy sound over the left sternal border

Pericarditis algorithm
1. R/O Tamponade/effusion
2. R/O myocarditis
3. High risk patient?
4. Treat as viral

EKG changes
- Stage 1: (Acute pain) diffuse ST elevation (except depressed in aVR and V1), PR depression
- Stage 2: (days later) ST returns to baseline with flattening of T waves
- Stage 3: T waves inverted
- Stage 4: (weeks-months) EKG returns to patient's baseline, +/- TWI persisting (chronic pericarditis)

Work-up
1. R/O cardiac tamponade/effusion
   - ⇨ Bedside US/ECHO
     - ✓ Effusion seen in only 60% of pericarditis patients-usually small without hemodynamic changes
     - ✓ Effusion helps confirm diagnosis, does not exclude pericarditis
     - ✓ **Tamponade seen in 5% patients with pericarditis**
   - ⇨ EKG: electrical alternans (beat to beat alternation in QRS), low voltage seen in effusion
2. R/O Myocarditis
   - ⇨ ↑Troponin
   - ⇨ New LV dysfunction
3. High risk patient?
   - ⇨ R/O medical/surgical condition associated with pericarditis
     - ✓ Neoplasia, TB, autoimmune disorders, purulent pericarditis, uremia, recent MI, cardiac surgery, HIV
     - ✓ CBC, CMP, ANA, Tb testing, HIV, troponin, blood cx etc...
4. Viral/Idiopathic
   - ⇨ Most cases are viral or idiopathic → extensive w/u not needed
   - ⇨ Brief and benign course, treat with anti-inflammatory meds

Pericarditis Dx (need 2 of 4)
☐ Chest pain-typical
☐ Pericardial friction rub
☐ ECG changes
☐ Pericardial effusion

Myocarditis Dx (need 1 of 2)
Pericarditis +
☐ ↑Troponin
☐ New LV dysfunction

Treatment
- Based on underlying cause and evidence of effusion/tamponade
- Pericardiocentesis?
  - ⇨ Symptomatic: large effusion, cardiac tamponade, hemodynamic compromise
- Viral/Idiopathic: (NSAIDS + Colchicine)
  - ⇨ NSAIDs
    - ✓ Indomethacin 50mg po q 8h, Ibuprofen, High dose ASA
    - ✓ 2 weeks or as long as symptomatic, add PPI for gastric protection
  - ⇨ Colchicine: (N Engl J Med 2013;369(16):1522) (EM:RAP 3/14)
    - ✓ Dose: 0.5mg po bid x 3 months (0.5mg po QD if <70kg) added to NSAIDs
    - ✓ Faster resolution of symptoms and fewer recurrences vs NSAIDs alone
  - ⇨ Glucocorticoids:
    - ✓ Use: only if refractory to NSAIDs + Colchicine treatment or NSAIDs contraindicated

Disposition
- Admit → High risk features?
  - ⇨ Fever, leukocytosis, subacute onset, immunosuppression, trauma, anticoagulants
  - ⇨ Myopericarditis (↑troponin)
  - ⇨ Severe effusion(>20mm), cardiac tamponade
  - ⇨ Failure of outpatient treatment
- Discharge?
  - ⇨ Asymptomatic, low risk, well appearing with likely viral etiology
  - ⇨ Can consider d/c home with appropriate follow up

CHEST PAIN

BOERHAAVE'S

Definition
- Effort rupture of esophagus → spontaneous esophageal perforation from vomiting or straining

Clinical Presentation
- Severe retching/vomiting → retrosternal chest pain/upper abdominal pain
- Patients then develop odynophagia, tachypnea, dyspnea, fever, and shock
- PMH: Alcohol abuse or gastric/duodenal ulcer, recent endoscopy

Work-up
- CXR: mediastinal/peritoneal air; air in soft tissue prevertebral space in neck, pneumothorax, pleural effusion
- CT: may show non-specific signs → esophageal wall edema/thickening, extraesophageal air, periesophageal fluid, mediastinal widening, pneumothorax/pleural effusion

Treatment
- Contained perforation: conservative tx → NPO, IV antibiotics, TPN
- Free perforation: Surgery vs endoscopic treatment

PE
(see Dyspnea algorithm)

STEMI
(see below)

PNEUMOTHORAX
(see Dyspnea algorithm)

2. ACS RISK STRATIFICATION (LOW VS HIGH)

ACS (ACUTE CORONARY SYNDROME)

Goal
- Stratify patients into one of three risk classes:
  - ⇨ **High Risk:**
    - ✓ Definitely worried about ACS and patient will be admitted
    - ✓ Includes STEMI, NSTEMI, UA
  - ⇨ **Low Risk:**
    - ✓ Somewhat worried and unsure if patient can go home
    - ✓ Will need serial troponin/EKG to r/o AMI/UA
  - ⇨ **Very low/No Risk:**
    - ✓ Not worried about patient and can go home without further workup
- Risk stratify based on 4 variables:
  - ⇨ CAD risk factors
  - ⇨ Chest pain history
  - ⇨ EKG
  - ⇨ Troponin level
- ACS continuum (Emerg Med Clin N Am 2011;29:689)
  - ⇨ Physiology: ruptured acute coronary artery wall → thrombus forms → clot obstructs the artery's lumen → diminish blood flow to tissues beyond the lesion → **myocardial injury**

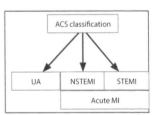

ACS RISK STRATIFICATION

1. CAD Risk factors (JAMA 2005;294:2623-2629)(EM:RAP 9/12-Mattu)
- Traditional risk factors:
  ⇨ Family history (first-degree relative with a history of early-life MI), male, advanced age, hypertension, smoking history, diabetes, hyperlipidemia
  ⇨ Limited clinical value in diagnosing CAD in the ED setting, especially >40yo
  ⇨ Useful in assessing whether or not the patient has chronic CAD (population risk) not ACS
  ⇨ Age
    ✓ Pt <40yo: CAD screening can help (Ann EM 2007;49:145-152)
- Risk factors
  ⇨ No risk factors → negative LR 0.17 (95% CI 0.04-0.66)
  ⇨ 4 or more risk factors → positive LR 7.39 (95% CI 3.09-17.67)

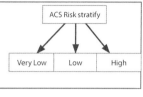

2. Clinical symptoms (JAMA 1998;280(14):1256) (Resuscitation 2010;81(3):281)
- Quality of chest pain associated with likelihood of ACS
- **Classic (typical symptoms)**
  ⇨ Crushing pressure
  ⇨ Radiating to the right shoulder and arm or left shoulder and arm
  ⇨ Jaw or neck pain
- **Atypical chest pain**:
  ⇨ Pricking or stabbing chest pain, shortness of breath, fatigue, dizziness, nausea, upper abdominal pain
  ⇨ More common in women, elderly, DM (with no CP)
  ⇨ **20-30% patients with ACS have atypical symptoms** (N Engl J Med 2000;342(16):1207)

3. Troponin
- Test for myocardial injury → positive troponin indicates myocardial damage
- Mortality increases as peak troponin rises
- Non-ACS causes of ↑troponin
  ⇨ CHF, sepsis, renal failure, PE, aortic dissection, chronic severe HTN

ACS Predictors
1. Risk factors
2. History
3. EKG
4. Troponin

4. EKG
- Insensitive but specific
  ⇨ Use Hx/PEX to eval for other causes, EKG to rule in ACS
  ⇨ **Up to 55% ACS patients have normal/non-diagnostic EKGs** → when negative, not very helpful (Ann Emerg Med 1989;18:741-746)
  ⇨ 7% AMI have completely normal EKG
  ⇨ Specificity≈80% (when positive, they're helpful)
- Repeat EKG
  ⇨ ACS is dynamic, evolving process
  ⇨ Normal EKG can evolve into NSTEMI or STEMI
- Prognosis
  ⇨ ACS (suspected) + non-diagnostic EKG=1.1%mortality
  ⇨ ST depression = 4-6x death/MI/ischemia rate

↑Likelihood of AMI	(+) LR	↓Likelihood of AMI	(-) LR
Radiation	4.5	Pleuritic	0.2
Worse with exertion	2.4	Positional	0.3
N/V/diaphoresis	2	Sharp	0.3
Similar to previous MI	1.8	Reproducible	0.3
Pressure	1.3		

Risk Scores (combine all of the above)
- **TIMI Risk Score** (JAMA Aug 2000; 284:835-842)
  ⇨ Use: 14 day event rate
  ⇨ **Historical**:
    1. Age ≥65
    2. ≥3 CAD risk factors
    3. Prior stenosis ≥ 50%
    4. ≥2 anginal episodes in prior 24h
    5. ASA in prior 7 days
  ⇨ **Presentation**:
    6. ST deviation on EKG
    7. Elevated troponins
  ⇨ Prospective validation yielded similar results, but still unable to rule-out ACS
    ✓ TIMI score 0/7 had 1.7% risk of adverse outcomes (Ann Emerg Med 2006;48:252-259)
  ⇨ http://www.mdcalc.com/ for plug-in TIMI score
- **Braunwald Risk stratification** (Heart Disease: Braunwald 2004, p 1248)
  ⇨ Low risk=
    ✓ TIMI score <3 + nondiagnostic EKG + normal Troponin
    ✓ 30 day death rate is 1.7%
  ⇨ High risk = TIMI score >3 OR ST depression OR Troponin positive
- **Gestalt:** overall clinical gestalt: one of the best predictors for ACS

CHEST PAIN

⬇ Low Risk Work Up

Rule out AMI (non-ST-segment elevation AMI)

- Cardiac serum markers
    - ⇨ **ACEP Clinical Policy** (Level B ACEP recommendation Ann Emerg Med. 2006;48:270-301)
        - ✓ Single negative CK-MB or Troponin 8-12 hours after sx onset
        - ✓ Negative myoglobin + negative CK or Troponin at baseline and 90 min if <8 hours of sx onset
        - ✓ Negative 2hour delta CK-MB and 2 hour delta Troponin if <8 hours of sx onset
    - ⇨ **ACC/AHA Guidelines 2011** (Circulation. 2011;123:2022-2060)
        - ✓ Single negative marker 12h after sx onset
        - ✓ Negative marker on arrival and 6 hr later
    - ⇨ **Clinical Chemistry Society Guidelines** (Circulation 2007;115:356-375)
        - ✓ Low risk pt → negative marker >6h after onset
        - ✓ Mod/High risk pt. → negative markers 12h after onset
- **Serial EKGs** (Level B ACEP recommendation)
    - ⇨ Initial EKG in patients with AMI can be normal/non-diagnostic up to 55% of the time.

Rule-out UA (Stress Test) (Essentials 2012 "Why Provocative tests for ACS are Stupid"-Weingart)

- ⇨ [Controversial: many different approaches to r/o MI/UA in a chest pain patient]
- Indication: (Emerg Med Clin N Am 2011;29:721)
    - ⇨ Use: Rule out Unstable Angina
    - ⇨ Who?: Low risk patient after AMI has been ruled out (serial troponin/EKG)
    - ⇨ Is stress test low yield?: http://emcrit.org/chestpain
        - ✓ Once pt ruled out for AMI, likelihood of ACS is so low that further risk stratification is difficult (Emerg Med Clin N Am 2011;29:721)
        - ✓ Non-diagnostic EKG + Trop (-) x 2 + well appearing → **<1% risk of death or MI!**
        - ✓ Further testing will likely only yield false (+)
    - ⇨ AHA/ACC Guidelines (J Am Coll Cardiol 2007;50;1-157)
        - ✓ **Recommend 72 hour stress test** (ED, Obs unit or outpatient)
        - ✓ Must be low risk: 6 to 12 hours observation, normal troponins, no recurrent symptoms of ischemia, and normal EKGs
    - ⇨ Outpatient Stress test (Ann Emerg Med 2006;47:427-435)
        - ✓ Kaiser study: Safe strategy in low risk patients after AMI ruled out, within 72h
        - ✓ ACC/AHA recommendation → **Non-invasive testing within 72 hours** (J Am Coll Cardiol 2007;50;1-157)
        - ✓ Sens 86%; Spec 81%
- Exercise Treadmill Test (ETT)
    - ⇨ Does prior stress test help? (Am J Emerg Med 2007;25:39-44)
        - ✓ Previous positive → increases admission and adverse events
        - ✓ Previous negative → **does not change** admission rate or adverse events (not reassuring)
    - ⇨ ED Treadmill Study (TST) (J Am Coll Cardiol 2002;40:251-6)
        - ✓ Negative TST: **0.2%** cardiac event rate at 30 days → can d/c these patients home
        - ✓ Non-diagnostic TST: **3.6%** event rate → further work-up and risk stratification
        - ✓ Positive TST: **14%** event rate → Admission
        - ✓ ~20% of patients are not candidates, another 20% non-diagnostic
    - ⇨ **Overall: Sens 70%; Spec 75%** (Not very good)
- Stress Echo
    - ✓ Better sensitivity vs standard ETT
    - ✓ ECHO- test for inducible wall motion abnormalities → + CAD
- Radionuclide myocardial perfusion imaging
    - ✓ Injectable radioisotope used to image myocardium at rest and with exercise
    - ✓ Sensitivity approaches 90%
- CT Coronary Arteries (Acad Radiol 2011;18:1522-8)
    - ✓ Emerging technology, very mixed evidence
    - ✓ Shows great anatomy, patient-centered outcomes lacking
    - ✓ Stats: Sens 93%; Spec 90%; PPV 48%; NPV 99.3 %
    - ✓ Possible alternative to stress test??

> **Journal Club**: 2 hour ADP (Accelerated Diagnostic Protocol)
>
> **ASPECT trial** (Lancet. 2011; 377:1077) (EM:RAP 12/12-Mattu)
> - Criteria: trop neg x 2 (at 0 and 2 hours of arrival), EKG without ischemia, TIMI = 0
> - **Sensitivity 99%**
>
> **Aldous et. al.** (Acad Emerg Med 2012;19(5):510)
> - Criteria: trop neg x 2, EKG without ischemia, **TIMI = 1**
> - Sensitivity 97%
>
> **ADAPT trial** (J Am Coll Cardiol 2012;59:2091)
> - Criteria: trop neg x 2, EKG without ischemia, TIMI = 0
> - **Sensitivity 99.7%**

⊕ LOW RISK THERAPIES

ASA
⇨ Dose: 162 or 325mg, chewed if they can
   ✓ ASA allergy: Clopidogrel 300-600mg loading dose
⇨ Indications: **ALL patients with chest pain** (GI bleed? give H_2 blocker)
⇨ Journal Club (Lancet 1998;8607:359)
   ✓ **NNT to prevent 1 death = 42**
   ✓ Harm: 0.6% had minor bleeding
⇨ Bottom Line: Chest Pain=ASA, ASA=Chest Pain

NTG
⇨ Short-term benefit unknown?
⇨ Long term → no decrease in mortality (ISIS-4)
⇨ Dose:
   ✓ PO → 400mcg SL (equivalent to 50-100mcg/min!)
   ✓ IV → start 10mcg/min and go up to max 200, 250 mcg/min (so must titrate IV dose up quickly for same effect as po)
⇨ Contraindications: hypotension, PDE5 inhibitors (sildenafil), right sided MI, critical aortic stenosis

Morphine
• Dose: Initially 2-4mg, then 2-8 mg increments
• Indication: Relieving CP in patients whom nitrate fail to relieve pain or are contraindicated

O_2
• Titrate to O_2 sat > 92%

Beta-blockers
• Benefits: lower HR, lower O_2 requirement, decrease arrhythmic events, lower potential for myocardial rupture (day 2-3, esp if given lytics)
• Harm: due to cardiogenic shock
• Contraindications: Bradycardia, heart blocks, COPD/Asthma (decrease dose), CHF
• **Summary**
   ⇨ **No urgency to give Beta-blockers in ED**
   ⇨ Give orally within first 24h (no longer a CMS quality measure)
   ⇨ Long term (secondary prevention): effective
   ⇨ Low risk in ED: may give but may interfere with treadmill

Journal Club: β-blockers in ACS
STEMI:
• Very bad, esp in CHF with systolic dysfunction (COMMIT trial-see below)
NSTEMI:
• UA/NSTEMI Guidelines (Circulation 2008;117:296)
⇨ Beta-blockers should be given in **first 24 hours** orally for ACS →↓VF and sudden death
⇨ Do not recommend routine use in ED
• COMMIT trial (Lancet 2005; 366: 1622–32)
⇨ β-blocker group → no difference in mortality
⇨ Slight reduction in re-infarction and V-fib but increased risk of cardiogenic shock
• Cochrane Review 2009 (Cochrane Database Syst Rev 2009(4))
⇨ No mortality benefit over placebo
• GUSTO-I
⇨ Early IV β-blockers associated with increased death, CHF, shock, recurrent ischemia, need for pacemakers

CHEST PAIN

⬆ HIGH RISK THERAPIES

Heparin (EM:RAP 6/12 "Heparin for ACS")
- Journal Club (Cochrane Review 2008)
  - ⇨ **No difference in overall mortality** with heparin vs placebo
  - ⇨ Short term benefit: At 7-10 days → 3% lower rate of MIs in the heparin group (NNT = 33)
  - ⇨ Long term benefit: No difference in mortality after 30 days (early mortality benefit lost)
- Bad: Severe bleeding complications 4%
- Dose: [See PDR for most up to date dosing]
  - ⇨ 60 Units/kg bolus (max 4000 U) + 12 Units/kg/h (max 1000 U)
  - ⇨ aPTT in 6 hours (goal 1.5-2.5x control)
- All benefit limited to high risk patients only
- **LMWH vs UFH** (JAMA 2004;292:55-64)
  - ⇨ Meta-analysis combining 6 trials
  - ⇨ 17% relative risk reduction in death/MI at 30 days
  - ⇨ Bleeding rates similar
  - ⇨ 6 month follow-up showed increased bleeding with LMWH, particularly in patients with 2 antiplatelet agents.
  - ⇨ Can use either: LMWH easier dosing, UFH easier to turn off if invasive strategy chosen
  - ⇨ Bottom Line: Possible intervention→ UFH; Easier → LMWH
- **Lovenox IV?** (JACC 2003;42:424)
  - ⇨ Brings ANTI-Xa levels up almost immediately

Thienopyridenes
- General
  - ⇨ Clopidogrel (Plavix), prasugrel, and ticagrelor
  - ⇨ Use: Added to ASA as another antiplatelet agent for dual antiplatelet action
  - ⇨ **No mortality benefit**
  - ⇨ Helps prevent non-fatal MI
- STEMI (Clarity TIMI 28 trial NEJM 2005;352:1179)
  - ⇨ Good: **Composite endpoint** risk reduction 21.7 → 15 (**NNT=16**)
  - ⇨ Dose: maybe increasing loading dose (JACC 2005;46:906)
    - ✓ 75mg peak effect → 5 days
    - ✓ 600mg peak effect → **2 hours!!**
    - ✓ 900mg → **even faster!!!** (Albion trial)
    - ✓ No increased bleeding with increased loading doses
- **Summary** (JAMA 2012;308:2507-16)
  - ⇨ Evidence is mixed: Should be given before PCI, but can be given by cardiology; not need to be given in ED
  - ⇨ No decrease in mortality
  - ⇨ Decreases rate of cardiac events (1 in 27 patients)
  - ⇨ Increased major bleeding rates (0.9%)

Journal Club: Clopidogrel in ACS

Cochrane Review (Cochrane Database Syst Rev 2011(1))
- Review: Clopidogrel + ASA vs ASA alone (two major trials: CHARISMA and CURE)
- **No mortality benefit**
- Decreased cardiovascular event rate (OR = 0.87)
- Increased major bleeding (OR = 1.34)

CURE trial (NEJM 2001;345:494)
- **Good:**
  - ⇨ 2% (11.4 → 9.3) absolute risk reduction in **composite endpoint** of death, MI, stroke
  - ⇨ Mortality: no significant reduction in death alone!
  - ⇨ 25% of effect seen in first 24h (maybe 4 hrs!!)
- **Bad:** increased bleeding (major bleed 2.7 → 3.7%)

Statins
- MIRACL study (JAMA 2001;285:1711)
  - ⇨ Atorvastatin 80mg given w/in 24-96h of admission
  - ⇨ Significant improvement in **composite endpoint**: recurrent ischemia and stroke at 16 weeks.
- ACS: Statin (Lancet 2001;357:1063)
  - ⇨ Decreased death/MI at 6 months
- Use: for secondary prophylaxis and doesn't matter if given in ED, as long as given at discharge.

Glycoprotein inhibitors (GP IIb/IIIa)
- General
  - ⇨ Eptifibatide, tirofiban, abciximab
  - ⇨ Use: only for high risk patients, can delay to cath lab
- NSTEMI
  - ⇨ Should we give in ED? ACUITY-Timing Trial (JAMA 2007;297:591-602)
    - ✓ No advantage in giving upstream vs selective use in the cath lab
    - ✓ No benefit if negative troponins
    - ✓ Increased bleeding if already giving heparin (NEJM 2011;365:1980-1989)
- STEMI (Cochrane Database Syst Rev 2001(4))
  - ⇨ No benefit (mortality, MI prevention)
  - ⇨ Increased major bleeding event (1 in 116)
- **Summary**
  - ⇨ Use: only for high risk patients, can delay to cath lab

PCI (PERCUTANEOUS CORONARY INTERVENTION)

NSTEMI (Routine vs Selective PCI)
- General
  - ⇨ Fibrinolytics are not used in NSTEMI/UA
  - ⇨ Early PCI shows no mortality benefit
  - ⇨ Early PCI shows an increased rate of major bleeding
- **Summary**: Early PCI (6-48h) vs selective strategy
  - ⇨ **33% RR** reduction of angina/rehospitalization at 6-12mos
  - ⇨ **2x** increase peri-procedural MI
  - ⇨ **No mortality benefit** until 2-5 yrs
  - ⇨ Benefit limited to **high risk** patients

> ### Journal Club: Early invasive strategy for NSTEMI/UA
>
> **Cochrane Review** (Cochrane Database Syst Rev 2010 Mar 17;(3))(www.thennt.com)
> - Benefits
>   - ⇨ None were helped (preventing death)
>   - ⇨ 1 in 9 were helped (feeling less chest pain)
>   - ⇨ 1 in 50 were helped (avoiding a heart attack in the next year)
> - Harm
>   - ⇨ 1 in 33 were harmed (suffering a heart attack)
>   - ⇨ 1 in 33 were harmed (suffered major bleeding)
>   - ⇨ Patients who did not have a positive troponin had increased mortality with stents
>
> **OASIS-5 trial** (European Heart Journal 2012;33:51)
> - ⇨ Early invasive strategy had increased 1yr mortality (8.8% vs 1.1%)
> - ⇨ Early invasive strategy had increased 30d major bleeding rate (8.8% vs 1.1%)
>
> **Meta-analysis** (JAMA 2008;300:71)
> - No difference in mortality (4% vs 4%) and MI (7% vs 8%) in invasive vs conservative groups

STEMI
- General
  - ⇨ Primary PCI preferable over lytics (better at establishing reperfusion and decrease hemorrhage)
- Primary PCI
  - ⇨ PCI vs fibrinolytics (Lancet 2003;361:13)
    - ✓ PCI had improved composite outcome and less bleeding (T<4.6h) over in-hospital fibrinolysis
  - ⇨ Transfer to PCI center?
    - ✓ 2013 AHA Guidelines (Circulation 2013;124:362-425)
    - ✓ Transfer for PCI if can get a door to balloon time of **120 minutes** (previously 90)
  - ⇨ PCI as standard?
    - ✓ Does delay matter? (JAMA June 2000;283:2941-7)
      - i. 90 minute delay → 42% increase relative mortality
      - ii. 2 hour delay → 62% increase mortality
- Facilitated PCI? (Drip and Ship)
  - ⇨ Definition: Give fibrinolytics prior to transfer of patient for PCI
  - ⇨ Early 90s studies mostly negative
  - ⇨ ASSENT 4 PCI trial (Lancet 2006;367:569)
    - ✓ Equivalent TIMI-3 flow post PCI in both groups of primary PCI and Fibrinolysis + PCI (facilitated PCI)
    - ✓ **Facilitated PCI group did worse in all other outcomes** (death, shock, strokes, bleeds) vs primary PCI.
    - ✓ Study stopped early because of ↑mortality with facilitated PCI (6% vs 3%)
    - ✓ **Facilitated PCI with full dose fibrinolytics NOT RECOMMENDED**
  - ⇨ Partial dose Fibrinolytics may be considered

CHEST PAIN

UA/NSTEMI

Definition
- Pathophysiology: Heart muscle necrosis caused by interruption of blood supply to a part of the heart without typical EKG changes of STEMI, but demonstrated by cardiac marker elevation

Diagnosis
- NSTEMI
  - ⇨ Clinically significant EKG changes (ST depression, T wave inversion)
  - ⇨ Positive biomarkers (CK-MB or Troponin)
- UA: CAD (known or unknown) → coronary flow limitation
  - ⇨ Symptoms that are accelerating or induced with less activity.
  - ⇨ These patients are at risk for AMI and can evolve to have a NSTEMI or STEMI.
  - ⇨ Diagnosis of UA: normal or unchanged EKGs and a negative biomarker evaluation

High risk features NSTEMI
☐ Recurrent angina/rest ischemia
☐ Elevated troponin
☐ New ST-segment depression
☐ CHF or mitral regurgitation
☐ High-risk findings from noninvasive testing
☐ Hemodynamic instability
☐ Sustained VT
☐ PCI within 6 months
☐ Prior CABG
☐ High risk score (TIMI, GRACE)
☐ LVEF less than 40%

Medical Treatment
- ASA 162-325mg po chewed
- Oxygen
- Nitroglycerin
- Morphine
- Anticoagulation
  - ⇨ Heparin vs LMWH
- Thienopyridene options (AHA 2012 Circulation 2012;126:875)
  - ⇨ Initial invasive strategy:
    - ✓ Add to ASA for dual antiplatelet treatment prior to PCI
    - ✓ Administration may be deferred to cardiologist in cath lab
  - ⇨ Initial conservative strategy:
    - ✓ Add to ASA as soon as possible after admission
- GP IIb/IIIa inhibitor
  - ⇨ Can be used instead of thienopyridene prior to PCI (per cardiologist)
  - ⇨ Eptifibatide and tirofiban
- PCI (AHA 2012 Circulation 2012;126:875)
  - ⇨ Initial invasive strategy
    - ✓ Refractory angina or hemodynamic or electrical instability
    - ✓ Elevated risk for clinical events (high risk features in table)
  - ⇨ Initial conservative strategy
    - ✓ Low risk score (TIMI, GRACE)
    - ✓ Patient or physician preference without high risk features

STEMI

Pathophysiology
- Complete occlusion of a coronary artery → full-thickness myocardial infarction
- Pathophysiology made simple
  - ⇨ 0-3 hours goal (time dependent)
    - ✓ Myocardial salvage
    - ✓ Decreased Mortality
  - ⇨ 3-12 hours goal (Time independent) → PCI
    - ✓ Plaque stabilization (PCI)
    - ✓ Perfuse hibernating myocardium
    - ✓ Prevent infarct expansion

Diagnosis (Circulation 2012;126(16):2020)
- **New ST segment elevation** at the J point in **two contiguous leads** >0.1 mV
  - ⇨ In all leads other than leads V2-V3
  - ⇨ V2-V3:
    - ✓ ≥0.2 mV in men ≥40 years
    - ✓ ≥0.25 mV in men <40 years
    - ✓ ≥0.15 mV in women
- AMI Patterns (Essentials 2012-Swadron)
  - ⇨ Anterior/apical MI
    - ✓ ST elevation V1-V6 and limb leads-I and aVL
  - ⇨ Inferior MI (ST elevation II, III, aVF)
    - ✓ Right sided MI? (Right sided leads V3R and V4R)
    - ✓ Posterior MI? (Posterior leads)
  - ⇨ Isolated Posterior MI
    - ✓ ST depression V1-V2 and ST elevation V7-V9
  - ⇨ Acute left main occlusion
    - ✓ ST elevation aVR; ST depression in limb/chest leads (diffuse)

- ⇨ de Winter ST/T wave complex
  - ✓ Upsloping ST elevations V1-V6 and persistent tall symmetrical T-waves
- ⇨ LBBB with Sgarbossa criteria (Essentials 2013-Tabas)
  - ✓ New LBBB no longer used in diagnosis of acute MI in isolation
  - ✓ **AMI Diagnosis**: Inappropriate or excessive discordance in one or more leads
    - i. Concordant ST deviation: (same direction as QRS): >1mm in any lead
    - ii. Excessive discordance (opposite QRS but too large): > 1/4 of S wave
- ⇨ Resuscitated cardiac arrest
  - ✓ Treat as STEMI regardless of EKG pattern? (See Cardiac arrest algorithm)

Medical Treatment
- ASA 162-325mg po chewed
- Oxygen
- Nitroglycerin
- Morphine
- Anticoagulation
  - ⇨ Heparin vs LMWH
  - ⇨ All patients with STEMI, regardless of reperfusion strategy
  - ⇨ Dose: [See PDR for most up to date dosing]
    - ✓ 60 Units/kg bolus (max 4000 U) + 12 Units/kg/h (max 1000 U)
- Thienopyridene
  - ⇨ Add to ASA for dual antiplatelet treatment, regardless of reperfusion strategy
  - ⇨ Loading dose ASAP: [See PDR for most up to date dosing]
  - ⇨ Defer to cardiologist
- GP IIb/IIIa inhibitor
  - ⇨ May be started at time of PCI per cardiologist

Fibrinolytics
- Indications:
  - ⇨ Unable to obtain PCI within **120 minutes** of patient arrival
  - ⇨ Can be used up to 24h after STEMI onset if ongoing ischemia or hemodynamic instability
- Problem with lytics
  - ⇨ Major bleeding 1% (usually intracranial, mortality rate of 50%)
  - ⇨ Only 50% of STEMIs recover with full patency (TIMI-3 flow)
  - ⇨ 15% of those that recover patency → will re-occlude

PCI
- **PCI is preferred treatment of STEMI, should be done ASAP**
- Indications:
  - ⇨ STEMI + Ischemic symptoms <12h or ongoing ischemia up to 24h
  - ⇨ STEMI + cardiogenic shock or acute severe HF
    - ✓ Irrespective of time delay from myocardial infarction (MI) onset
- Transfer to PCI center
  - ✓ Transfer for PCI if can get a door to balloon time of **120 minutes**

SYNCOPE

1 True Syncope?

Pseudosyncope
- [ ] Hypoglycemia
- [ ] Vertigo
- [ ] Stroke/TIA
- [ ] Seizure
- [ ] Drop attacks

2 R/O Emergent Causes

History
- [ ] **HPI:** Prodrome brief/absent
- [ ] **HPI:** Exertional/post exertional
- [ ] **HPI:** Occurs while sitting/standing
- [ ] **HPI:** Palpitations at time of syncope
- [ ] **Meds:** Meds that ↑QT
- [ ] **PMH:** (CAD/CHF/Vent arrhythmia)
- [ ] **FamHx:** Sudden Cardiac Death (SCD)

Physical Exam
- [ ] Vitals: tachy, persistent hypotension?
- [ ] CHF S/Sx (rales, S3/4, edema, CM)
- [ ] Murmur

EKG
- [ ] Ischemia/infarct
- [ ] Arrhythmia
- [ ] Prolonged QT
- [ ] Brugada
- [ ] WPW
- [ ] LVH (HCM/AS)
- [ ] e/o PE

Labs
- [ ] Troponin
- [ ] Pregnancy test (ectopic)
- [ ] Hb/HCT (anemia)
- [ ] Stool guaiac (GI bleed)
- [ ] Glucose
- [ ] CT? LP?? (SAH)

Dispo

San Francisco Rules
- [ ] C: No CHF Sx
- [ ] H: Hct > 30
- [ ] E: nl EKG
- [ ] S: no SOB
- [ ] S: SBP > 90

ACEP Guidelines 2007
- [ ] **High risk:** S/Sx of Heart Failure
- [ ] **High risk:** consider older age, structural heart disease, or history of CAD
- [ ] **Low risk:** younger patients with non-exertional syncope, no CAD, no FamHx SCD

3 Benign Cause?
- [ ] Vasovagal
- [ ] Orthostatic
- [ ] Carotid sinus hypersensitivity
- [ ] Psych

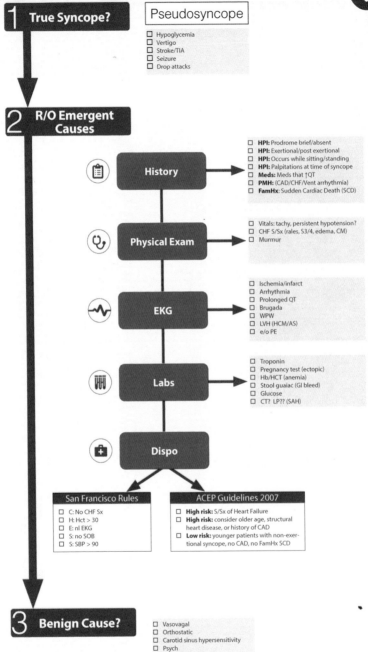

SYNCOPE

GENERAL

(CMEdownload: Syncope 2013-Mattu) (EM:RAP 12/2008)(EM:RAP 04/2013)

Approach:
- Chief objective in syncope work-up is distinguishing life-threatening cardiac causes from benign causes using the history, physical, and EKG
- Patients are risk stratified and high risk patients are then admitted for monitoring and further work-up
- Usually unable to establish exact diagnosis/cause of syncope in the ED (Unable to dx approx 50%)

Differential (Eur Heart J. 2009;30(21):2631.)
- **Non cardiac:** (1 year mortality 2-4%) Vasovagal (21%), Orthostatic (9.4%), Unknown (~20%)
- **Cardiac:** (1 year mortality 18-33%) Arrhythmia, Myocardial ischemia, Outflow obstruction

1. R/O PSEUDOSYNCOPE:

Syncope definition:
- Sudden transient loss of consciousness with a loss of postural tone, followed by a return to preexisting neurological function

Syncope mimics can usually be ruled out by history.
- **Hypoglycemia**-usually not transient event, sx resolve after glucose
- **Vertigo**-pt elicits spinning sensation, no LOC
- **Seizure**-convulsive movements, post-ictal period
- **Stroke**-focal deficit, usually no LOC
- **Drop attacks**-falls without loss of consciousness

2. R/O EMERGENT CAUSES (10-20%)

History
- **Preceding events**
  - ⇨ During exertion suggests outflow obstruction(e.g. Aortic stensosis)
  - ⇨ Abrupt onset, occurrence while sitting/supine, longer duration suggests cardiac cause
  - ⇨ Syncope after exercise → likely vasovagal
  - ⇨ Syncope during exercise → higher incidence of organic pathology (EM:RAP 2/14)
    - ✓ Work-up: EKG, labs, ECHO?, Holter?
    - ✓ Differential: Arrhythmia, Hypertrophic cardiomyopathy, Arrythmogenic right ventricular dysplasia (ARVD), Long QT syndrome, WPW, Brugada, Heatstroke, Hyponatremia,
- **During**
  - ⇨ Tonic/clonic movements(seizure?), bowel/bladder incontinence (seizure?), fall/trauma as a result of syncope?
- **Post-syncopal**
  - ⇨ Post-ictal state? (Seizure)

Physical Exam
- Vital signs: Persistent hypotension? Bradycardia?
- Evidence of CHF (arrhythmia risk) or murmur suggesting outflow obstruction?
- Abnormal neuro exam?

EKG (Essentials 2012 "5 things to look for in syncope EKG")
- **STEMI:** EKG changes suggesting ischemia, arrhythmias or prolonged intervals
- **Arrhythmia**: SVT, VT/VF, Torsades, bradycardia
- **Brugada syndrome**: RBBB pattern with ST elevations
- **WPW**: delta wave with short PR
- **Long QT syndrome** QTc > 500msec → at risk for Torsades, (medications vs congenital?)
- **HCM**: LVH, LBBB, needle Q waves, high voltage
- **PE**: S1Q3T3; New RBBB, diffuse ST elevation/depression; TWI (anteroseptal and inferior leads)

Labs
- To be considered on clinical situation, although of limited use
- Troponin (MI?),
- Pregnancy/FAST US (ectopic?),
- CBC, stool guaiac (eval for GI bleed-anemia?)
- Glucose

CT Head (EM:RAP 4/13)
- Only indicated if there is a neurologic complaint
- SAH can cause syncope but patients usually have persistent HA or AMS after syncopal event
- Head trauma, neuro deficit, dizziness, sudden/severe HA, anticoagulation (warfarin/clopidogrel)

SYNCOPE

Disposition

- **San Francisco Syncope Rule** (Ann Emerg Med 2004;43:224-32)
  - ⇨ Derivation study (Am J Emerg Med 2005;23:782-6)
    - ✓ **Sensitivity of 96%** and specificity of 62% in predicting a serious outcome in 7 days
    - ✓ Compared to physician judgment, SFSR has potential to decrease admissions by 10% in low risk group and still predict serious outcomes.
  - ⇨ Internal Validation study (Ann Emerg Med. 2006;47:448-454)
    - ✓ Validation study of SFSR was able to predict serious outcomes at 30 days with sensitivity of 98% and decrease admissions by 24%
  - ⇨ External validation study (Ann Emerg Med. 2007;49:420-427)
    - ✓ Cohort of the San Francisco rules, sensitivity and specificity were found to be 89% and 42%, respectively.
- **ACEP Guidelines**
  - ⇨ 2001 Guidelines (Ann Emerg Med 2001;37:771)
    - ✓ Retrospective study showed for level B recs sensitivity and specificity were 100% and 81% respectively.
    - ✓ Level B + C sensitivity and specificity were 100% and 33% respectively, offering no further advantage over level B recs. (Am Heart J 2005;149(5):826-31)
  - ⇨ 2007 Guidelines Level B recommendations (Ann Emerg Med 2007;49:431-444)
    - ✓ Admit patients with syncope and evidence of **heart failure** or **structural heart disease**
    - ✓ Admit patients with syncope and other factors that lead to stratification as high-risk for adverse outcome
      - i. **Older age** and **associated comorbidities** (Different thresholds for age → age is a continuous variable)
      - ii. **Abnormal ECG** (acute ischemia, arrhythmias, or significant conduction abnormalities)
      - iii. **Anemia**: Hct < 30 (if obtained)
      - iv. History or presence of **heart failure**, **coronary artery disease**, or **structural heart disease**
    - ✓ Consider **younger patients** with syncope that is non-exertional, without history or signs of cardiovascular disease, no family history of sudden death, and without comorbidities to be at low risk of adverse events

ROSE: Admit for any of the following:	
B	Bradycardia < 50 at any time BNP > 300 pg/ml
R	Rectal exam with positive fecal occult blood
A	Anemia – Hb < 9g/dL
C	Chest pain in association with episode of syncope
E	ECG with Q wave other than in lead III
S	Saturation (O₂ sat) <94% on room air

- Other Decision Rules:
  - ⇨ ROSE Study (J Am Coll Cardiol 2010;55(8):713)
    - ✓ Admit if any of the ROSE criteria are positive
  - ⇨ OESIL Criteria (Eur Heart J. 2003;24:811-9)
    - ✓ 1) Age > 65 years
    - ✓ 2) Cardiovascular disease in the clinical history
    - ✓ 3) Syncope without prodrome
    - ✓ 4) Abnormal ECG
  - ⇨ Physician judgment (American Journal of Emergency Medicine 2005;23:782–786)
    - ✓ Good at predicting which patients will develop serious outcomes
- Cardiac Monitor: for most patients, monitoring >**24h** unlikely to increase detection of arrhythmias
- Admission work-up (thinking ahead)
  - ⇨ Echo: r/o mechanical causes, CHF
  - ⇨ ETT/Cath: r/o ischemia
  - ⇨ Monitor/Holter/EPS studies → r/o arrhythmia

3. EVAL FOR OTHER CAUSES

- **Vasovagal**: appropriate stimulus upon standing→pallor, dizzy, nausea, diaphoresis, decreased vision
- **Orthostatic syncope**: secondary to volume depletion, meds, autonomic dysfunction
- **Carotid Sinus hypersensitivity**: reflex mediated syncope after stimulation of carotid sinus→ asystole > 3 seconds and/or hypotension
- **Psych**: Panic attacks → consider hyperventilation to provoke

DYSPNEA

1 ABCs

Assess Severity
- ☐ Tripoding
- ☐ AMS
- ☐ Unable to speak
- ☐ Accessory muscle use
- ☐ Retractions
- ☐ Paradoxical breathing?
- ☐ Hypoxia?
- ☐ Hypercapnea?

🖊 Empiric Tx
⇨ IV/O₂/Monitor
⇨ BiPAP? Intubation?
⇨ Advanced airway equipment

2 R/O Critical Cause

Reversible Cause?

🖊 Treatment

Airway Obstruction
- ☐ Stridor
- ☐ Difficulty swallowing

⇨ **Heimlich (complete obstruction)**
⇨ Bronch/Forceps
⇨ Intubation/Cric?

Anaphylaxis
- ☐ Hypotension
- ☐ Airway compromise
- ☐ Acute dyspnea
- ☐ Angioedema
- ☐ Urticaria, pruritis, gen erythema
- ☐ Wheezing, stridor
- ☐ Diarrhea/vomit

⇨ **Epinephrine**
⇨ Bronchodilators
⇨ Antihistamines
⇨ Steroids

Tension Pneumothorax
- ☐ Unilateral absent breath sounds
- ☐ Tension PTX? (JVD, hypotension, deviated trachea)
- ☐ Trauma? Spontaneous PTX?
- ☐ Bedside U/S? CXR

⇨ **Needle decompression**
⇨ Chest Tube

3 Emergent Dx?

	📋 History	🩺 PEX	🩻 CXR	🖊 Treatment
COPD/ Asthma	☐ PMH: COPD/ asthma ☐ Tobacco ☐ H/O intubations ☐ H/O ICU/ hospital admissions	☐ Wheezing ☐ Barrel chest ☐ Pursed lips ☐ Cyanosis	☐ Clear ☐ Infiltrate/ PTX?	⇨ Bronchodilators ⇨ Anticholinergics ⇨ Steroids/MgSO₄ ⇨ Epinephrine ⇨ NPPV
CHF Pulm Edema	☐ CAD risks ☐ Chest pain ☐ Orthopnea ☐ PND ☐ DOE ☐ Med compliance	☐ Rales ☐ JVD ☐ Edema ☐ S3/S4 ☐ New murmur	☐ Pulm edema (interstitial) ☐ Cardiomegaly	⇨ Nitroglycerin ⇨ Furosemide ⇨ Dopamine ⇨ NPPV
Pneumonia	☐ PMH: HIV, COPD ☐ Cough, Sputum ☐ Fever/Chills ☐ Night sweats ☐ +/- Hemoptysis	☐ Fever ☐ Rales ☐ Tachypnea ☐ Hypoxemia	☐ Infiltrate ☐ Airspace/interstitial opacity ☐ Lobar/ consolidation ☐ Pleural effusion	⇨ Antibiotics ⇨ Pulmonary toilet ⇨ Sepsis protocol
Pulmonary Embolus	☐ PE risks? ☐ Pleuritic CP ☐ Acute dyspnea ☐	☐ Clear BS ☐ Calf pain/ swelling ☐ Tachypnea ☐ Tachycardia ☐ Hypoxemia	☐ Usually normal ☐ Hampton's hump ☐ Westermark's sign ☐ Atelectasis	⇨ Anticoagulation ⇨ Thrombolytics?

4 Other Causes?
- ☐ **Acidosis**: Sepsis, DKA, toxins
- ☐ **Neuromuscular**: GBS/MS, CVA/ICH
- ☐ **Mechanical**: Pregnancy, ascites, morbid obesity
- ☐ **Heme**: Anemia, CO poisoning
- ☐ **Psych**: Panic attack

DYSPNEA

GENERAL

- Assess severity of dyspnea, including need for intubation/airway management based on physical examination
- Emergent intubation indicated regardless of cause if severe respiratory distress/arrest
- Consider Critical diagnoses → may be able to cure patient and avert intubation if the underlying cause is corrected (i.e. chest tube insertion, foreign body removal…)
- Then think of emergent diagnoses and begin specific treatment

1. ABCs: EMERGENT INTUBATION?

RAPID SEQUENCE INTUBATION

(CMEdownload UCSF 2012-Simon)(Essentials 2011-Sacchetti)(EM:RAP 2/13-Braude/Levitan)

Indication
- No absolute set criteria → decision to intubate based on physician assessment and comfort
- General Indications:
  - ⇨ Failure of Noninvasive Positive Pressure Ventilation (NPPV)
  - ⇨ Hemodynamic instability
  - ⇨ Patient fatigue
  - ⇨ Acute/progressive respiratory acidosis
  - ⇨ Hypoxia not responsive to supplemental oxygen
  - ⇨ Rapid decline in level of consciousness

RSI Steps
- **Preparation**
  - ⇨ Difficult airway?
    - ✓ Use LEMON law, have back-up devices (LMA, bougie, cricothyrotomy kit) handy, check equipment, have drugs drawn up
    - ✓ Failed airway algorithm: Difficult to intubate? Oxygenate and ventilate? Obtain a surgical airway?
    - ✓ First pass success is goal, complication rate of 47% with second pass
  - ⇨ ET tube size:
    - ✓ Adult → usually 7.5 ETT
    - ✓ Peds → [Age (years)/4] + 4
  - ⇨ Blade:
    - ✓ Adult→usually Mac 4 (varies depending on comfort)

LEMON law
L-Look externally
E-Eval 3-3-2 rule
M-Mallampati
O-Obstruction
N-Neck mobility

- **Pre-oxygenation**
  - ⇨ Goal: establish O_2 reservoir in lungs to prevent desaturation
    - ✓ 100% O_2 for 5 minutes or 8 Vital Capacity breaths
- **Pretreatment**
  - ⇨ Goal: administer drugs to treat adverse effects associated with intubation, **generally not used**
    - ✓ Lidocaine (1.5mg/kg IV) → for ↑ICP or reactive airway disease (controversial)
    - ✓ Fentanyl (3mcg/kg IV) → for ↑HR or ↑BP in ICP, CAD, Aortic dissection, AAA
    - ✓ Atropine (0.02mg/kg IV, minimum 0.1mg) → Have at bedside or consider pretreatment in peds <1yr (controversial)
- **Paralysis** with Induction
  - ⇨ Induction:
    - ✓ **Etomidate** 0.3mg/kg IV
      - i. Onset→20-30sec; Duration→7-14min

Peds Memorize
Weight: 10 + age x 2
ET tube size: ¼ age + 4
Etomidate: 0.3mg/kg
Succinylcholine: 1.5-2 mg/kg
Atropine: 0.02mg/kg (min 0.1mg)
Rocuronium: 1mg/kg
Vecuronium: 0.1-0.3 mg/kg
Blade:
• Age 0 → 0 Miller
• Age 1 → 1 Miller
• Age 2 → 2 Miller

INDUCTION AGENTS

Name/dose	Dose	On/Off	The good	The bad
Etomidate	0.3mg/kg	40s/9m	□ Rapid on/off □ Agent of choice □ BP neutral	□ Adrenal axis suppression with repeat admin (controversial)
Thiopental	3-5mg/kg	40s/10m		□ ↓BP
Propofol	2mg/kg	40s/5m		□ ↓BP □ Storage/Allergy Problems
Ketamine	2mg/kg	60s/30m	□ Good for asthma and penetrating neck trauma (maintains airway if not using paralytic)	□ Can cause psychosis, emergence reaction, laryngospasm
Midazolam	0.07-0.3mg/kg	2m/1h	□ Good for procedural sedation	□ ↓BP □ Usually underdosed

Paralytic Agents					
	Dose	Onset	Duration	Pros	Cons
Depolarizing Succinylcholine	**1.5mg/kg**	10s	9m	Fast on and off	**Contra-indicated in:** ☐ Hyperkalemia ☐ Burns >1d ☐ Denervation Disorder **Adverse effects** ☐ Malignant hyperthermia ☐ Masseter spasm
Nondepolarizing Rocuronium Vecuronium	Roc (1mg/kg) Vec (0.1-0.3 mg/kg)	30s 1min	30-60min 45-60min		☐ Relatively slow ☐ Will not be able to do neuro exam for >30m

  ii. Adverse effects: N/V, myoclonic activity, pain at injection site, adrenal insufficiency (controversial)
- ⇨ Paralysis
  - ✓ Types: Noncompetitive depolarizing (succinylcholine) vs Competitive nondepolarizing (Rocuronium) neuromuscular blockers
  - ✓ **Succinylcholine**
    - i. Type: Noncompetitive Depolarizing
    - ii. Dose: 1.5-2mg/kg IV
    - iii. Onset → 45-60 sec; Duration → 3-5min
    - iv. Contraindications: Hyperkalemia, Hx malignant hyperthermia, Burn>24h, Crush/denervation >7days, Neuromuscular disease
  - ✓ **Rocuronium**,
    - i. Dose: high dose 1mg/kg; Onset → 60sec; Duration → 40-60min
  - ✓ **Vecuronium**
    - i. Dose: 0.1mg/kg vs high dose 0.3mg/kg: Onset → 0-90sec; Duration → 100min
- **Protection and Positioning**
  - ⇨ Avoid BVM (unless hypoxic)
  - ⇨ Sniffing position (unless contraindicated → C-spine)
  - ⇨ External laryngeal manipulation to improve view of epiglottis/cords
- **Placement and Proof**
  - ⇨ EtCO₂, Bilateral breath sounds, pulse oximetry, no gastric sounds, fog in ETT, US?
- **Post-intubation management:**
  - ⇨ Secure tube, sedation, Vent management, CXR, ABG

2. R/O CRITICAL DIAGNOSIS

AIRWAY OBSTRUCTION
(see stridor algorithm)

Assessment
- Partial: Stridor, wheeze, SOB → assess cause and prepare for airway management
- Complete: chest movement without air movement → emergent intubation
- Clear obstruction immediately (complete obstruction)
  - ⇨ Heimlich maneuver (for complete foreign body obstruction)
  - ⇨ Forceps
  - ⇨ Bronchoscopy

ANAPHYLAXIS
(J Allergy Clin Immunol. 2010;126:477) (Guidelines: Resuscitation 2008;77:157)(Essentials 2010-#60)

General
- Acute systemic allergic or hypersensitivity reaction that is rapid and may cause death
- Airway compromise:
  - ⇨ Upper airway → laryngeal edema
  - ⇨ Lower airway → bronchospasm
- Most commonly: Skin manifestations
- Other manifestations: Diarrhea (may be only presenting symptom)
- Cause: Unknown (40%), food (shellfish, peanuts), medication, blood products, latex

Presentation
- Skin: Flushing, urticaria, angioedema
- Eyes: Lacrimation, injection, edema
- Respiratory: Rhinorrhea, stridor, cough, wheeze
- CV: Tachycardia, hypotension, cardiac arrest
- GI: N/V, diarrhea
- CNS: Dizzy, syncope

Anaphylaxis Dx:
☐ Hypotension ☐ Upper airway compromise (stridor) ☐ Lower airway compromise (wheeze) ☐ Persistent GI symptoms

DYSPNEA

Diagnosis (J Allergy Clin Immunol 2006;117:391)

- **Criteria 1**: Acute skin/mucosa illness (hives, pruritis, flushing) + 1 of the following:
  - ⇨ Respiratory compromise (dyspnea, wheeze, bronchospasm, stridor, hypoxia)
  - ⇨ Reduced BP (SBP < 90 or end organ dysfunction → syncope, shock)
- **Criteria 2:** Exposure to **LIKELY** allergen + 2 or more:
  - ⇨ Skin-mucosa involvement
  - ⇨ Respiratory compromise
  - ⇨ Reduced BP
  - ⇨ Persistent GI symptoms (Intestinal anaphylaxis → vomiting, crampy abdominal pain)
- **Criteria 3:** Reduced BP after exposure to **KNOWN** allergen for patient

Treatment:

- General
  - ⇨ Speed of symptom progression determines severity of reaction
  - ⇨ Stop inciting agent (antibiotic, remove venom sac…)
- **Epinephrine**
  - ⇨ First line/Primary treatment for life threatening anaphylaxis!
  - ⇨ Indication:
    - ✓ Laryngeal edema, severe bronchospasm, respiratory arrest, shock.
    - ✓ **NO absolute contraindications to Epi in Anaphylaxis**
    - ✓ Use with caution in CV disease, antidepressants (slow epi metab), recent surgery
  - ⇨ **IM Dosing**:
    - ✓ **Adult**: 0.3-0.5ml of 1:1000 IM
    - ✓ **Peds:** 0.01mg/kg of 1:1000 IM
    - ✓ **IM is route of choice:** IM has shown better absorption and ↑plasma levels vs SC
  - ⇨ **IV Dose**:
    - ✓ 0.1mg IV = 100 mcg IV = 1ml of 1:10,000 (need to dilute to 10 or 100ml→see below!)
    - ✓ Dilution options: go to emrap.tv Episode 92
      - **i.** **Option #1**: add 1ml of 1:10,000 epinephrine solution to 9ml NS →10 ml of 1:100,000 dilution (10mcg/ml) over 5-10 min →10-20mcg/min
      - **ii.** **Option #2:** add 1ml of 1:10,000 (crash cart epi) to 100ml NS (1mcg/ml) and run over 5-10min
      - **iii. Pediatrics:** 0.1mcg/kg/min (diluted to 1:100,000 solution) and titrate to response
  - ⇨ **Epinephrine gtt**
    - ✓ Same dilution as option #2 → (1mcg/ml), to run at 1-4 ml/min (1-4 mcg/min)
    - ✓ Caution in elderly and cardiac disease
- **Oxygen:** 100% O_2
- **IV Fluids:**
  - ⇨ May need large volume if persistently hypotensive
- **Antihistamines**:
  - ⇨ H_1 blocker: Diphenhydramine 25-100 mg IV/SC/PO
  - ⇨ H_2 blocker: Famotidine 20mg IV; Ranitidine 50mg IV or 150 mg po
- **Steroids**: Solumedrol 125 mg IV (2mg/kg)
- Special Case: Patient taking **Beta-blockers**?
  - ⇨ **Glucagon** 1- 3mg IV q 5min
- Special Case: **Cardiac arrest**
  - ⇨ Aggressive fluid resuscitation (4-8L)
  - ⇨ High-dose epinephrine (1mg → 3mg → 5mg)
  - ⇨ Usual care: Antihistamines IV, Steroids IV
  - ⇨ Prolonged CPR (anaphylaxis may resolve)

Disposition

- **Minor allergic reaction** (no hypotension/resp sx)
  - ⇨ Diphenhydramine, Prednisone 40-60mg x 5-7days, H_2 blocker
  - ⇨ Consider observation x 4h?
  - ⇨ Be certain to discharge home with EpiPen x 2
- **Severe Anaphylaxis:** → ICU
- **Anaphylaxis that resolves?**
  - ⇨ Biphasic Reaction? (EM:RAP 3/14-Paper Chase)
    - ✓ Previously, incidence in literature between 3-20% (Journal of Emergency Medicine 2005;28:381)
    - ✓ Grunau et al, (Ann Emerg Med. 2014;63:736)
      - i. Biphasic reaction only occurred in **0.18% of patients**
      - ii. Bouncebacks are possible though (5.25% in 7 days)
    - ✓ Conclusion:
      - i. Biphasic reactions are rare and most anaphylaxis that resolves will unlikely need routine monitoring
      - ii. Consider admission for severe anaphylaxis, even if patient improves
  - ⇨ Consider admission vs observation, depending on severity
  - ⇨ D/C Plan:
    - ✓ Reliable pt?
    - ✓ H_1/H_2, Steroids
    - ✓ EpiPen x 2
    - ✓ Allergist/Immunologist f/u

DYSPNEA

ANGIOEDEMA
(Essentials 2012-Roberts)

General
- Incidence ~ 0.5%
- Almost always secondary to ACE Inhibitors.
- Not related to dose or frequency, can happen any time (even months to years after starting medication)
- Mechanism is bradykinin release (ACE-I inhibits bradykinin breakdown)
- Most commonly seen in African American

Treatment (Am J Card 2012;109:774)
- No proven benefit with Epi, H_1/H_2 blockers, or steroids
- Severe Angioedema
    - ⇨ Consider early intubation in patient with tongue involvement
    - ⇨ Prepare for nasotracheal intubation
    - ⇨ Fiberoptic laryngoscopic intubation (ENT vs anesthesia)
    - ⇨ Sedation: Ketamine
    - ⇨ Anticipate surgical airway
    - ⇨ Consider FFP (C1 esterase deficiency)
        - ✓ 2-3 Units ASAP
        - ✓ Case reports of effectiveness
- Minor lip edema
    - ⇨ Course is unpredictable; observe for 4-6 hours at least, consider admission

TENSION PNEUMOTHORAX
(see Chest trauma algorithm)

Clinical Signs
- Unilateral absent breath sounds
- Beck's triad (JVD, hypotension, deviated trachea)
- Trauma vs Spontaneous PTX?

Diagnosis
- US-look for sliding lung, comet tail
- CXR

Treatment-depends on severity and primary vs secondary
- Immediate needle decompression vs
- Chest tube vs
- Observation (O_2, repeat CXR)

3. EVALUATE FOR EMERGENT DIAGNOSIS

ASTHMA
(EM:RAP: 9/11 & 2/12-Herbert)(CMEDownload: UCSF 2012; Resuscitation 2010-Mallon)

Assess severity of exacerbation (National Heart, Lung, and Blood Institute, 2007) (Chest. 2004;125(3):1081).
- Mild:
    - ⇨ Clinical: Dyspnea only with activity
    - ⇨ FEV_1 or PEF >70% predicted
- Moderate:
    - ⇨ Clinical: Dyspnea interferes/limits activity
    - ⇨ FEV_1 or PEF 40-69% predicted
- Severe:
    - ⇨ Clinical: Dyspnea at rest, interferes with conversation, accessory muscle use, chest retraction
    - ⇨ FEV_1 or PEF <40% predicted
- Life threatening
    - ⇨ Clinical: Too dyspneic to speak, diaphoretic, no air movement, impending intubation
    - ⇨ PEF < 25% predicted

Medication (Emerg Med Clin N Am 2012;30:203)
- **β-agonists**
    - ⇨ MOA:
        - ✓ Potent bronchodilators that act on β-receptors → relax bronchial smooth muscle
    - ⇨ Dosing
        - ✓ Depending on patient severity, can be given as MDI, intermittent nebulizer or continuous nebulizer
        - ✓ Albuterol 2.5-5mg nebulizer q 20min x3 in 1st hour or can use MDI
    - ⇨ Journal club
        - ✓ Cochrane review: (Cochrane Database Syst Rev 2009:CD001115)
            - i. Continuous nebs better than intermittent nebs for preventing hospital admission **(NNT =10)**
- **Anticholinergics**

DYSPNEA

- ⇨ MOA:
  - ✓ Decrease vagally mediated smooth muscle contraction in the airways → bronchodilation
  - ✓ Works synergistically with β-agonists
- ⇨ Dose:
  - ✓ Ipatropium 0.5mg q 20min x 3 in 1st hour or MDI
  - ✓ Usually given concomitant with Albuterol
- ⇨ Journal Club:
  - ✓ Cochrane review: (Cochrane Database Syst Rev 2008:CD000060)
    - i. Anticholinergics decreased hospital admission by 25%
    - ii. **NNT = 12** to prevent hospital admission

- **Steroids**
  - ⇨ Indication:
    - ✓ Moderate or severe asthma
    - ✓ β-agonists do not fully correct the decline in pulmonary function
  - ⇨ Dosing
    - ✓ PO:
      - i. Prednisone 40-60 mg po (1-2 mg/kg)
      - ii. PO preferred and equivalent to IV, if patient is able to tolerate
      - iii. Continue steroids x 5-7 days if d/c
    - ✓ IV:
      - i. Indication: Moderate/severe asthma or not tolerating po
      - ii. Dose: Methylprednisolone 40-125mg IV
    - ✓ IM: IM steroids just as effective as IV (Chest 2004;126(2):362)
  - ⇨ Journal club
    - ✓ Cochrane review: (Cochrane Database Syst Rev 2001;1:CD002178)
      - i. Decreased hospital admission if steroids given within 1 hour of ED presentation
      - ii. Absolute risk reduction 12.5% **(NNT = 8)**

- **Magnesium sulfate**
  - ⇨ MOA:
    - ✓ Inhibits the influx of calcium into smooth muscle cells → causing bronchodilation
  - ⇨ Dosing: $MgSO_4$ 2g IV over 15 min
  - ⇨ Indication
    - ✓ Life-threatening exacerbations or
    - ✓ If the exacerbation remains severe (PEF <40%) after 1 hour of conventional therapy
  - ⇨ Journal club
    - ✓ Cochrane review: (Cochrane Data- base Syst Rev 2009:CD001490)
      - i. $MgSO_4$ significantly improved pulmonary function and ↓ admission rates for severe asthma
    - ✓ Meta-analysis (Ann Emerg Med 2000;36(3):18)
      - i. Improvements seen only in severe asthma exacerbation subgroups
      - ii. Severe asthma: ↓Admission rates and improved pulmonary function (PEFR and FEV_1)

Treatment (aggressiveness depends on severity)

- Mild (Tune up and go home?)
  - ⇨ O_2 for hypoxia, all patients
  - ⇨ β-agonists
    - ✓ Albuterol (2.5-5mg nebulizer q 20min x3 in 1st hour) or MDI
  - ⇨ Anticholinergics
    - ✓ Ipatropium 0.5mg q 20min x3 in 1st hour) or MDI
  - ⇨ Steroids
    - ✓ Prednisone 1-2mg/kg po (Solumedrol if not tolerate PO), continue x 5-7days

- Moderate ("They look kinda bad")
  - ⇨ **Albuterol/Ipatropium** continuous nebulizer
  - ⇨ Steroids: **Solumedrol** 2mg/kg (125mg) IV q6
  - ⇨ **Magnesium sulfate** 2g IV over 15 min

- Severe (**Status Asthmaticus**)
  - ⇨ General: impending intubation, need maximal therapy to prevent intubation because of ↑risk of lung injury with ventilation
  - ⇨ **Moderate therapies** +
  - ⇨ **Epinephrine**
    - ✓ IM: 0.3mg IM or
    - ✓ **Terbutaline** 0.25mg SC q 20min x 2
    - ✓ Caution in elderly, cardiac disease
  - ⇨ **Epinephrine gtt:**
    - ✓ 2.5 mls of 1:10,000 epi in 250mlNS (1mcg/ml) and run over 25 min (10mcg/min)
    - ✓ (see anaphylaxis section for recipe)
  - ⇨ **Epinephrine IV:**
    - ✓ 0.25ml of 1:10,000 and flush (25mcg)
  - ⇨ **Heliox:**
    - ✓ 80:20 or 70:30 helium to oxygen ratio used
    - ✓ Questionable efficacy, worth trying

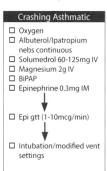

Crashing Asthmatic
- ☐ Oxygen
- ☐ Albuterol/Ipatropium nebs continuous
- ☐ Solumedrol 60-125mg IV
- ☐ Magnesium 2g IV
- ☐ BiPAP
- ☐ Epinephrine 0.3mg IM

- ☐ Epi gtt (1-10mcg/min)

- ☐ Intubation/modified vent settings

- ⇨ **BiPAP**:
    - ✓ Reduces work of breathing and need for intubation
    - ✓ Start low and titrate up: IPAP 7-15, EPAP 3-5
- **Ketamine-** consider sub dissociative dose 0.1-0.5 mg/kg
- **Intubation** (goal is to prevent intubation)
    - ⇨ RSI: ketamine vs etomidate? awake-nasal vs oral intubation
    - ⇨ Most experienced practitioner, patients desaturate rapidly
    - ⇨ Pretreatment with lidocaine to reduce bronchospasm is not proven therapy
- **Ventilator strategies:**
    - ⇨ General
        - ✓ Prolong expiratory time, avoid barotrauma
        - ✓ Do not hyperventilate → breath stacking, barotrauma, ptx, ↓venous return, cardiac arrest
    - ⇨ Settings**:**
        - ✓ **PRVC, RR**: 6-8, **Vt**: 5-7ml/kg; **Insp flow**: 100l/min; **PEEP** : 5; **I:E ratio**: 1:3-4
        - ✓ Keep Pplat <35 and auto-peep <15
    - ⇨ Sedation (ketamine, lorazepam) and paralysis (Vecuronium, but try not to re-paralyze)
    - ⇨ Complications
        - ✓ Barotrauma, PTX, Cardiovascular collapse
        - ✓ **Hypotension/Arrest** → disconnect from vent & push on chest → forced expiration, IVF bolus, bilateral chest tubes?

COPD EXACERBATION

(Global Initiative for Chronic Obstructive Lung Disease (GOLD) 2014 http://www.goldcopd.org.)
(**EM:RAP** 8/12 C3 Project-Mattu) (Emerg Med Clin N Am 2012;30 :223)

General
- Definition: Acute worsening of symptoms including cough, wheeze, SOB, sputum production and fever
- *"Characterized by a worsening of the patient's respiratory symptoms that is beyond normal day-to-day variations and leads to a change in medication"* (GOLD 2014)

Cause
- Cause of exacerbation usually:
    - ⇨ Infection (bacterial, viral, both)
    - ⇨ Airway inflammation from non-infectious source (air pollution, occupational)
    - ⇨ Alternative pathology (PTX, PE, CHF, mucus plug, anxiety/depression, cold)
    - ⇨ Unknown in 1/3 of cases

Severe COPD?
☐ Accessory respiratory muscles
☐ Paradoxical chest wall movements
☐ Worsening/new onset central cyanosis
☐ Development of peripheral edema
☐ Hemodynamic instability
☐ Deteriorated mental status

Diagnosis
- COPD diagnosis:
    - ⇨ Clinical Sx: chronic cough, chronic sputum production, dyspnea at rest or with exertion
    - ⇨ Physical exam: Cyanosis, barrel chest, pursed lip breathing, wheezing, right heart failure
    - ⇨ History of COPD risk factors (exposure to tobacco smoke, occupational dust, and chemicals)
- Acute exacerbation of COPD
    - ⇨ Increasing dyspnea, worsening exercise tolerance, worsening sputum purulence, and increased sputum production in a patient with known or likely COPD

Work-up
- ABG
    - ⇨ Guidelines recommend ABG for mod/severe exacerbation, SaO_2 < 92% follow pH, PO_2 and PCO_2 before and after NPPV/intubation (GOLD 2014)
    - ⇨ Caution with ABGs: painful, associated with complications and often not necessary
- EKG: Rule out ischemia/arrhythmia and evaluate for right heart strain/hypertrophy
- CXR:
    - ⇨ Evaluate for cause, alternative diagnosis and complication (ie PTX) of COPD

Treatment
- Similar to asthma exacerbation (see above)
- **Oxygen**
    - ⇨ Judicious use to keep SaO_2 88-92%
    - ⇨ ↑O_2 causes CO_2 retention and respiratory acidosis → cardiac depression (arrhythmias) and neurologic depression (AMS)
    - ⇨ Increased mortality with high flow O_2 in COPD patients (BMJ. 2010 Oct 18;341:c5462)
        - ✓ Mortality 9% (high flow O_2) vs 4% (O_2 titrated to SaO_2 88-92%)
- **Bronchodilators**
    - ⇨ ß-agonist (Albuterol)
        - ✓ First line therapy (used for the reversible component of COPD)
        - ✓ MDI and nebulizer equivalent efficacy
    - ⇨ Anticholinergics (Ipatropium)
        - ✓ Combination with ß-agonist shown superior to either alone

- **Steroids**
  - ⇨ Improves PaO_2, FEV1, dyspnea improvement and ↓relapse
  - ⇨ Journal club (Cochrane Data- base Syst Rev 2009;1:CD001288)
    - ✓ Cochrane review: Steroid use resulted in decreased treatment failures, shorter hospitalization and improved pulmonary function
    - ✓ **NNT = 10** to avoid treatment failure
- **Antibiotics**
  - ⇨ ↑resolution of symptoms
  - ⇨ Indication: (GOLD 2014)
    - ✓ COPD exacerbation with 3 cardinal symptoms (↑dyspnea, ↑sputum volume, ↑purulence)
    - ✓ Only 2 cardinal symptoms if one of them is ↑purulence
    - ✓ Mechanical ventilation (NPPV/Invasive)
  - ⇨ Antibiotic choice (empiric)
    - ✓ Mild exacerbation: β-lactam, Tetracycline or TMP/SMX
    - ✓ Moderate: β-lactam/ β-lactamase inhibitor
    - ✓ Severe: Fluoroquinolone
  - ⇨ Journal club
    - ✓ Cochrane review (Cochrane Database Syst Rev. 2012;12:CD010257)
    - ✓ Antibiotics reduced treatment failure in severe exacerbations/ICU patients
- **Magnesium sulfate ($MgSO_4$)**
  - ⇨ Improves pulmonary function in severe exacerbations
- **NPPV**
  - ⇨ Benefit: better outcome, ↓intubation rates, ↓mortality rates, ↓hospital stay
  - ⇨ Indications: mod/severe dyspnea, respiratory acidosis, ↓oxygenation,
  - ⇨ Contraindications: respiratory arrest, medically unstable, unable to protect airway, ALOC, ↑secretions, improper fit of mask
  - ⇨ Journal club Cochrane review (Cochrane Database Syst Rev 2004;3)
    - ✓ NPPV resulted in ↓**mortality (NNT = 10)**
    - ✓ Decreased need for **intubation (NNT = 4)**
    - ✓ Reduction in **treatment failure (NNT = 5)**

Mechanical ventilation

- Indications:
  - ⇨ Failed/not tolerate NPPV
  - ⇨ Hypoxia
  - ⇨ Resp failure ($PCO_2 > 60$; pH < 7.25; RR > 35;)
  - ⇨ Respiratory arrest
  - ⇨ Somnolence, AMS
  - ⇨ Other complications (Shock, sepsis, pneumonia, metabolic abnormalities)
- Technique
  - ⇨ Pre-oxygenate to 100%
    - ✓ Pt can desaturate quickly
    - ✓ Use NPPV with increased settings
  - ⇨ Delayed sequence intubation?
    - ✓ Use in pt with AMS/combative and unable to pre-oxygenate
    - ✓ Consider Ketamine for sedation prior to intubation to assist in oxygenation?
  - ⇨ Nasal canula with ↑O_2 flow before and during intubation
  - ⇨ IVF: NS bolus to avoid peri-intubation hypotension
- Ventilator strategy
  - ⇨ Avoid DHI (Dynamic hyperinflation)
    - ✓ COPD pts require prolonged expiratory time to exhale all air
    - ✓ If next breath given too soon before lungs fully evacuated → breath stacking → DHI
    - ✓ DHI causes ↑intra-thoracic pressure → hypotension → obstructive shock → PEA arrest
    - ✓ DHI can also cause barotrauma (PTX, pneumomediastinum, etc.)
  - ⇨ Ventilator settings
    - ✓ **PRVC, RR**: 6-8, **Vt**: 5-7ml/kg; **Insp flow**: 100l/min; **PEEP**:5; **I:E ratio**: 1:3-4
  - ⇨ Permissive hypercapnea
    - ✓ Vent settings lead to ↓ventilation → ↑CO_2 → Acidosis
    - ✓ Can allow pH to go down to 7.15
    - ✓ May need to give supplemental HCO_3 (controversial)
    - ✓ Need adequate sedation to avoid barotrauma and over breathing ventilator
  - ⇨ Measure DHI
    - ✓ Auto-PEEP:
      - i. Elevated alveolar pressure at end of expiration
    - ✓ Plateau pressure
      - i. Airway pressure during inspiratory pause
      - ii. DHI = Plateau pressure > 30 cm
  - ⇨ DHI Treatment (emergent)
    - ✓ Bronchodilators, sedation, ↓RR, ↓TV
    - ✓ **Disconnect from ventilator and manually squeeze chest to decompress**
    - ✓ Check for **tension PTX**

DYSPNEA

CONGESTIVE HEART FAILURE

(CMEDownload Resus 2009-Deblieux)(EM:RAP 4/11-Swadron)
ACC/AHA Guidelines (Circulation. 2013;128(16):e240)
Heart failure society guidelines (J Card Fail. 2010;16(6):e1.)

General
- Causes (acute exacerbation): Arrhythmia, MI, medication non-compliance, PE, pneumonia, pleural effusion, acute valvular emergency

Presentation
- History/Physical
  - ⇨ History: Orthopnea, PND, dyspnea
  - ⇨ Physical: Rales, S3, JVD, increased body weight, pitting edema, wheezing (cardiac asthma), tachycardia, hypotension, new onset murmur (valvular emergency)
- CXR
  - ⇨ Findings
    - ✓ Pulmonary edema, cardiomegaly, Kerley B lines
    - ✓ Cephalization, interstitial edema, alveolar edema (highly specific findings)
  - ⇨ Normal CXR does not exclude acute CHF (Ann Emerg Med. 2006;47:13)
    - ✓ Almost 20% of patients in one series had CHF with a negative CXR (sensitivity 81%)
  - ⇨ Rule out other conditions: Pneumonia, pneumothorax etc.
- EKG
  - ⇨ R/O ischemia, infarction, arrhythmia (e.g. atrial fibrillation), and LVH
- Labs
  - ⇨ Troponin elevated from acute injury/ischemia or increased LV pressures causing demand ischemia
- BNP (Circulation 2002;105:2328)
  - ⇨ BNP < 100 pg/ml essentially rules out CHF
  - ⇨ BNP > 400 pg/ml rules in CHF

Special Case: "Flash" pulmonary edema
- Define: Rapid increase in fluid in pulmonary alveola or interstitium
- Cause: Acute ischemia, hypertensive crisis, acute severe MR, stress induced (takotsubo) cardiomyopathy, bilateral renal artery stenosis (Pickering syndrome)
- Treatment: Similar to Acute CHF, except must treated quicker

Treatment
- **Oxygen**:
  - ⇨ Correct hypoxia
- **Nitrates**
  - ⇨ 1st line therapy→↓**preload**, ↓afterload, ↑CO
  - ⇨ Use: only in hypertensive/normotensive patients
  - ⇨ Nitroglycerin dose:
    - ✓ Mild: **PO, SL**→ 400 mcg
    - ✓ Moderate: 1-2 inches **trans-dermal**
    - ✓ Severe: **IV gtt**→ start at 10mcg/min and **titrate up quickly to 200-250 mcg/min**
  - ⇨ Caution in preload dependent states: RV infarct, PDE-5 inhibitors (Sildenafil)
  - ⇨ Adverse effects: hypotension, headache, tolerance

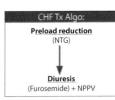

CHF Tx Algo:

Preload reduction
(NTG)

↓

Diuresis
(Furosemide) + NPPV

- **Diuretics**:
  - ⇨ Dose:
    - ✓ Furosemide (20-100 mg IV, equal to or greater than maintenance dose up to 2x maintenance)
  - ⇨ MOA: Decrease preload→ diuretic effect
    - ✓ However pulm edema pts have ↓renal blood flow → leads to delayed effect (30-120min)
    - ✓ Fluid restriction on arrival if hyponatremic (<130 meq/L)
  - ⇨ Caution: severe hypotension, shock
- **Morphine**:
  - ⇨ Use: decrease preload (histamine effect)?, anxiolysis
  - ⇨ Do not use to treat CHF (little evidence, may increase morbidity/mortality)
- **Positive Inotropes**
  - ⇨ Use: avoid if possible (JAMA. 2002;287(12):1541)
    - ✓ Use only for cardiogenic shock or severe hypotension
    - ✓ ?Bridge therapy until cath lab
  - ⇨ Increases incidence of arrhythmias, hypotension, and VT
- **NPPV** (CPAP, BiPAP)
  - ⇨ MOA: ↓preload (increases intrathoracic pressure), ↓Work of breathing (WOB), improves gas exchange, ↓afterload
  - ⇨ Decreases need for intubation, ↓Length of stay (LOS)
  - ⇨ Journal Club: 3CPO Trial (N Engl J Med 2008;359:142)
    - ✓ **No mortality difference** between O_2 and NPPV
    - ✓ NPPV associated with improvement (at 1h) in dyspnea, HR, acidosis, and hypercapnea

DYSPNEA

- **ACE-Inhibitors**
  - MOA: Downregulate RAA system, ↓adrenergic tone, improve LV relaxation→ ↓preload and afterload
  - Use: **Early initiation on ACE-I in CHF not recommended**, avoid in hypotension
  - No good comparisons to nitrates
  - Dose: Captopril 25mg SL (12.5mg if SBP<110) or Enalaprilat 0.625-1.25mg IV Intubation/Vent
  - Indication: Hypoxia SaO$_2$ <90%, unable to tolerate NPPV
- Cardiogenic Shock
  - SBP ≈ 90 → Dobutamine 2-3 mcg/kg/min
  - SBP < 70 → Dopamine (5mcg/kg/min and), if fails → Intra-aortic balloon pump, ultrafiltration, NE gtt

Treatment algorithm
- NTG→ 1st line agent (IV NTG excellent single agent)
- NPPV→ 1st line agent for severe CHF (use early and often)
- Furosemide → 2nd line agent (AFTER preload and afterload reduction)
- ACE-I → 2nd line agent
- Do not use: β-blockers, morphine, Nesiritide

PNEUMONIA

(ACEP: Ann Emerg Med. 2009;54:704-731)(Emerg Med Clin N Am 2012;30:249)

Classical Presentation
- Typical pneumonia
  - Most common organism: S. pneumoniae (60%)
  - Presentation: High fever, rigors, cough with rust-colored sputum, leukocytosis
  - CXR: lobar consolidation
- Atypical pneumonia
  - Organisms: Mycoplasma, Legionella, and Chlamydophila
  - Presentation: more gradual onset, dry cough, well appearing, ambulatory
  - CXR: interstitial pattern

Classification
- **Community Acquired Pneumonia (CAP)**
  - Definition:
    - Acute infection of pulmonary parenchyma, occurring **outside the hospital,** with clinical symptoms accompanied by the presence of an infiltrate on CXR
    - Patient has not been hospitalized or in a nursing home in the previous 14 days
  - Organisms
    - Streptococcus pneumoniae, Mycoplasma pneumoniae, Hemophilus influenzae, Clamydophilia sp, and viruses

Pneumonia classification
☐ **CAP** (Community Acquired Pneumonia)
☐ **HAP** (Hospital Acquired Pneumonia)
☐ **VAP** (Ventilator Associated Pneumonia)
☐ **HCAP** (Health-Care Associated Pneumonia)

- **Hospital Acquired Pneumonia (HAP)**
  - Define
    - New respiratory infection that presents > **48 hours after** hospital admission
  - Organisms
    - Pseudomonas, MRSA, Legionella, Klebsiella, H influenzae, Moraxella catarrhalis
- **Ventilator Associated Pneumonia (VAP)**
  - Define
    - Pneumonia diagnosed > 48 hours after a patient has been **intubated on ventilator** in the ICU
  - Organisms
    - Pseudomonas, MRSA, Legionella, Klebsiella, H influenzae, Moraxella catarrhalis, Acinetobacter
- **Health-Care Associated Pneumonia (HCAP)**
  - Define:
    - Pneumonia in patients **hospitalized for 2 or more days in the previous 90 days**
    - Includes dialysis, chemotherapy, chronic wound care, home IV antibiotics, immunocompromised and patients from nursing home facilities
  - Organisms
    - Pseudomonas, MRSA, Legionella, Klebsiella, H influenzae, Moraxella catarrhalis

Work-up
- Labs (CBC, BMP, lactate etc.)
- Blood Cultures
  - Studies show consistent low sensitivity and results do not alter management
  - ACEP Guidelines: "Do not routinely obtain blood cultures in patients admitted with CAP"
  - IDSA/ATS recommend blood cultures in the following:
    - Admission to the intensive care unit
    - Cavitary infiltrates
    - Leukopenia
    - Chronic severe liver disease
    - Asplenia
    - Pleural effusion
    - A positive pneumococcal urinary antigen test
    - Active alcohol abuse

- Sputum culture (Clinical Infectious Diseases 2007; 44:S27–72)
  - ⇨ Recommended in:
    - ✓ ICU admission;
    - ✓ Failure of outpatient antibiotic management
    - ✓ Cavitary infiltrates
    - ✓ Active alcohol abuse
    - ✓ Severe obstructive or structural lung disease
    - ✓ Positive Legionella urinary antigen test (UAT)
    - ✓ Positive pneumococcal UAT
    - ✓ Pleural effusion
- CXR
  - ⇨ Standard used to make diagnosis of pneumonia and r/o other pathology

Predictors:
- CURB 65 (Thorax 2003;58:377)
  - ⇨ Criteria:
    - ✓ Confusion, Uremia (BUN>20), RR>30, ↓BP (SBP<90 or DBP<60), Age>65
  - ⇨ Management:
    - ✓ 0-1: Outpatient management
    - ✓ 2: Inpatient care
    - ✓ >3: ICU care
- PSI Score (Pneumonia Severity Index) (NEJM 1997;336:243)
  - ⇨ Uses 2 step process for assigning risk and prognosis
- CURB-65 vs PSI
  - ⇨ Equivalent in predicting mortality
- SMART COP (Clinical Infectious Diseases 2008;47:375)
  - ⇨ Assessment tool to help predict need for ICU/pressors
- ATS Guidelines
  - ⇨ Admit to ICU for **1 Major or 3 Minor criteria:**
  - ⇨ Major criteria:
    - ✓ Intubated
    - ✓ Septic Shock requiring vasopressors
  - ⇨ Minor criteria:
    - ✓ Hypoxia: $PaO_2/FiO_2 < 250$
    - ✓ Hypothermia (Temp <36°C)
    - ✓ RR > 30
    - ✓ BUN > 20 mg/dl
    - ✓ Hypotension requiring aggressive fluids
    - ✓ Confusion
    - ✓ Thrombocytopenia
    - ✓ Leukopenia
    - ✓ Multilobar infiltrates

CURB-65
☐ **C**onfusion
☐ **U**remia (BUN>20)
☐ **RR**>30
☐ ↓**B**P (SBP<90 or DBP<60)
☐ **A**ge>**65**

NPPV (Noninvasive Positive Pressure Ventilation)
- Conflicting evidence in regards to the usefulness of NPPV in pneumonia
- ATS/IDSA recommend trial of NPPV

Antibiotics (Clinical Infectious Diseases 2007; 44:S27–72)
- Empiric antibiotics based on pneumonia classification, severity of illness and most likely organisms
- Outpatient
  - ⇨ Healthy, no risk factors:
    - ✓ Macrolide or
    - ✓ Doxycycline
  - ⇨ Comorbidity:
    - ✓ Respiratory fluoroquinolone or
    - ✓ β-lactam plus macrolide
- Inpatient Ward
    - ✓ Respiratory fluoroquinolone or
    - ✓ β-lactam plus macrolide
- Inpatient ICU
  - ⇨ Minimum treatment:
    - ✓ β-lactam plus macrolide
  - ⇨ Antipseudomonal coverage:
    - ✓ Antipseudomonal β-lactam (piperacillin-tazobactam, cefepime, imipenem, or meropenem) plus either
      - i. Ciprofloxacin or levofloxacin (750-mg dose) or
      - ii. Aminoglycoside and azithromycin or
      - iii. Aminoglycoside and a respiratory fluoroquinolone
  - ⇨ CA-MRSA coverage (consider)
    - ✓ Add vancomycin or linezolid

DYSPNEA

PULMONARY EMBOLUS

(EM:RAP 6/13-Tabas,Arora)(Essentials 2011/2013-Kline)(CMEDownload UCSF High Risk 2013-Tabas)
ACEP Guidelines 2011 (Ann Emerg Med. 2011;57:628-652)

PE: WORK-UP

History and Physical
- **Risk factors**
  - ⇨ Classic risk factors: Family history, Cancer, CHF, history of DVT/PE, Estrogen/Pregnancy, Abdominal/Pelvic Surgery, LE paralysis/trauma/immobility, Obesity
  - ⇨ Strongest Risk factors: (Ann Emerg Med. 2010;55:307)
    - ✓ History of venous thromboembolism
    - ✓ History of thrombophilia
    - ✓ Unilateral lower-extremity swelling
    - ✓ Recent surgery
    - ✓ Estrogen use
    - ✓ Hypoxia: oxygen saturation less than 95%
    - ✓ Active cancer
- **Signs/Sx**
  - ⇨ Consider PE in any patient that presents with: pleuritic CP, dyspnea, or syncope
  - ⇨ Classic: Dyspnea, pleuritic chest pain, leg swelling, tachypnea, syncope
  - ⇨ Common sx: clinical impression alone → sens 85% spec 51% (Ann Intern Med. 2011;155(7):448.)

Initial testing
- **EKG** (Am J Cardiol. 1991;68(17):1723.)
  - ⇨ Useful if provides alternate diagnosis
  - ⇨ Nonspecific: non-specific ST -T wave abnormality (most common), sinus tachycardia (30%), S1Q3T3 (classic but non-specific)
  - ⇨ Concerning for PE: Inverted T-waves right precordial leads
- **CXR**
  - ⇨ Atelectasis/effusion/elevated HD; cardiomegaly, normal (10-20%)
  - ⇨ Classic: Hampton's hump, Westermark's sign
- **ABG**: A-a gradient (Stein, Chest 1991)
  - ⇨ Normal O_2 sat/A-a gradient does not exclude PE
  - ⇨ ↓O_2 sat and ↑A-a gradient in absence of alternate diagnosis (COPD, Pneumonia) increases suspicion
- **D-dimer**
  - ⇨ Indication: Low risk pre-test probability patient
  - ⇨ High sensitivity D-dimer can be used to also rule-out moderate risk patients
  - ⇨ Negative result + Low risk patient → excludes PE
  - ⇨ Positive result → requires further testing

Diagnostic Tests
- **V/Q** (PIOPED I JAMA 1990;263(20):2753)
  - ⇨ **Normal** → 98% sensitive and **near normal** → 97% sensitivity to exclude PE
  - ⇨ High probability has 85-90% PPV
  - ⇨ **Indeterminate** results not helpful in excluding PE → need further imaging
- **CT** (PIOPED II NEJM 2006;354(22):2317)
  - ⇨ CTA (sensitivity 83%; specificity 96%)
  - ⇨ CTA-CTV (sensitivity 90%; specificity 95%)
  - ⇨ Probability of PE varies depending on patients pre-test probability of PE (low, intermediate, high)
  - ⇨ At least as good as VQ (JAMA. 2007;298(23):2743.)
  - ⇨ Similar radiation to V/Q
- **Lower Extremity U/S** (Ann Intern Med. 1997;126(10):775.)
  - ⇨ DVT only present in approx 30% of pts with PE, operator dependent
- **Echocardiography** (Arch Intern Med. 2005;165(15):1777.)
  - ⇨ Look for signs of RV strain, ↑RV size, ↓RV function, tricuspid regurgitation, interventricular septal bowing
  - ⇨ Not sensitive, but rapid info, more helpful in massive PE

Clinical algorithms
- Gestalt
  - ⇨ Multiple decision rules (Well's, Geneva, Wicki, Charlotte and ACEP recommendations) → perform similar to provider's clinical gestalt (Thromb Haemost 2000;83(3):416)
  - ⇨ Clinical gestalt performed better than clinical decision rules in this study (Wells and revised Geneva score) (Ann Emerg Med 2013;62:117)
- **Wells' Criteria** (Ann Intern Med 2001;135(2):98)
  - ⇨ See chart

Wells' Clinical Probability Score			
Criteria	Points	Score	Probability
Other dx less likely than PE	3	Low (<2 points)	3.6%
Suspect DVT	3		
Immobile/surgery prior 4 wks	1.5	Moderate (2-6 points)	20.5%
HR>100	1.5		
Prior DVT/PE	1.5	High (>6 points)	66.7%
Hemoptysis	1		
Cancer	1		

46

DYSPNEA

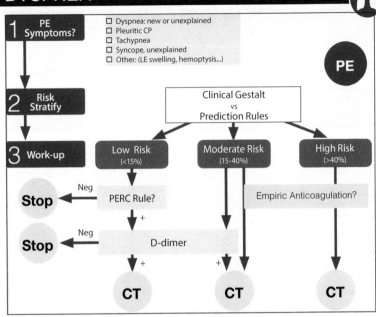

- **PERC Rule** (Pulmonary Embolism Rule-out Criteria) (J Thromb Haemost 2004;2:1247)
  - ⇨ When to use
    - ✓ Use in patient that is low risk as determined by the clinician's gestalt
    - ✓ Rule consists of eight clinical criteria (see chart)
  - ⇨ Evidence
    - ✓ Sensitivity of 96% (low risk pt) and 100% (very low risk pt)
    - ✓ False negative rate of: **Low clinical gestalt + PERC(-) = <2%**
  - ⇨ PERC Review/meta-analysis (Ann Emerg Med 2012;59:517)
    - ✓ Consistent high sensitivity and negative LR
    - ✓ Sensitivity of 97% to rule-out PE in patients with low pre-test probability

PERC Rule
☐ Age < 50 years
☐ Pulse < 100 bpm
☐ SaO2 > 94%
☐ No unilateral leg swelling
☐ No hemoptysis
☐ No recent trauma or surgery
☐ No prior PE or DVT
☐ No hormone use

- **Summary**: Combining Clinical probability, D-dimer and CT (JAMA 2006;295(2):172)
  - ⇨ Low probability + D-dimer (-) → no further testing (0.5% PE risk)
  - ⇨ Low probability + D-dimer (+) → need further work-up (CT PA, V/Q…)
  - ⇨ High Probability + CT PA (-)→ ? further testing if ↑clinical suspicion (1.3% PE risk overall)

PE: THE APPROACH
(EM:RAP 6/13-Tabas)

1) Consider diagnosis in:
- Patient with **dyspnea, pleuritic chest pain** or **tachypnea** without alternate diagnosis (JAMA 2003;290(21):2849)
  - ⇨ Absence of above sx have sensitivity of **97%** in excluding PE (if all 3 absent → PE very unlikely)
  - ⇨ Also consider PE in patient that presents with **unexplained syncope** (Circulation 1997;96:882)

2) Risk Stratify
- Stratify into <u>low</u>, <u>intermediate</u> and <u>high</u> risks using:
  - ⇨ Clinical findings: Risk factors, signs/symptoms, and alternate diagnosis?
  - ⇨ Prediction rules (Well's, Geneva, Wicki, Charlotte etc.)
  - ⇨ ACEP: Level B evidence to use PERC rule in low pretest patients (Ann Emerg Med 2011;57:628)
  - ⇨ Gestalt: combining above factors
    - ✓ Shown to be just as sensitive as algorithms for detecting PE (JAMA 2003;290(21):2849)

DYSPNEA

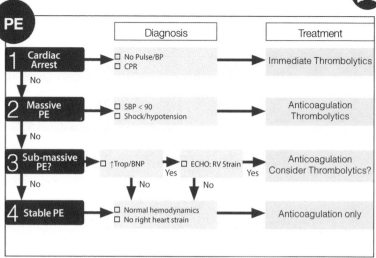

3) Diagnostic tests
- Order appropriate **diagnostic testing** based on risk
  - ⇨ Very low risk (0-2% risk) → no further work-up
  - ⇨ Low risk (2-15% risk) → D-dimer then CT if positive
  - ⇨ Moderate risk (15-35% risk) → CT (some advocate D-dimer is useful in moderate risk patients)
  - ⇨ High risk (>35% risk) → CT
4) Post-test probability?
  - ⇨ Consider further imaging (Angiography? MRI?) and empiric anticoagulation in high risk patients with negative initial work-up based on above negative predictive value of CT

PE Special Case: Pregnancy

(NEJM 2008;359:2025) (EM:RAP 12/10 "CP in Pregnancy"-Kline)

D-dimer (low risk patient)
- Evidence (Ann Intern Med 2007;147:165)
  - ⇨ Negative D-dimer in 1st or 2nd trimester has sensitivity of 100% and NPV of 100%
- Test result
  - ⇨ Positive → not helpful, continue work-up (?utility because d-dimer normally elevated in pregnancy→positive ≈ 70%)
  - ⇨ Negative → PE excluded

PE in pregnancy
1. Rule out other causes (CXR etc.)
2. D-dimer +/- LE US
3. V/Q (1/2 dose Q) vs CTPA

Lower extremity Bilateral U/S
- Consider empirically in all patients vs only if having symptoms?
- Positive → treat for PE
- Negative → continue work-up

CT vs V/Q scan (Radiation exposure)
- Low-dose radiation is defined as < 5Rads (50,000uGy)
  - ⇨ Teratogenicity risk → none
  - ⇨ Oncogenic risk → 1.2-2.4RR

V/Q (100-400uGy)
- Can do only the perfusion portion (Q) and use 1/2 dose
- Omit Ventilation portion (V) if pt has normal CXR
- Cancer risk (V/Q associated with higher risk of childhood cancer)

CTPA (3-131uGy) (Radiology 2002;224:487)
- Mother: 35,000uGy direct exposure to mother's chest
  - ⇨ Increased risk of breast CA (lifetime risk is up to 13% greater with CTPA than with V/Q)
- Fetus: Radiation dose to fetus based on trimester:
  - ⇨ 1st trimester→ 3-20 uGy
  - ⇨ 2nd trimester → 8-75 uGy
  - ⇨ 3rd trimester→ 50-130 uGy

48

DYSPNEA

Conclusion:
- CTPA has less radiation exposure than V/Q to fetus, better sensitivity, and gives more information
- Radiation dose delivered to mother is higher with CTPA
- Consider V/Q with only perfusion study? 1/2 dose perfusion?

An approach
1. Rule out other causes (CXR etc...)
2. Start with D-dimer +/- lower extremity US then
3. V/Q (Perfusion only with 1/2 dose) vs CT PA?

PE: TREATMENT

General (N Engl J Med 2008;359:2804-13)
- Anticoagulation
  - ⇨ Stops clot progression, endogenous fibrinolysis
  - Immediate parenteral anticoagulation + oral anticoagulants for minimum of 3-6 months
- LMWH vs UFH
  - ⇨ LMWH has less bleeding and better outcomes vs UFH

Heparin, Unfractionated (UFH)
- Dose: Loading 5000 Units IV (80Units/kg) + 1280 Units/h (18Units/kg/h)
- Goal PTT: 46-70 sec (1.5 to 2.5x control)
- Indication: (ESC Guidelines-European Heart Journal 2008;29:2276)
  - ⇨ "High risk-Massive PE", ↑bleeding risk, severe renal dysfunction
  - ⇨ **Otherwise-all patients should be treated with LMWH**

LMW Heparin
- Contraindications: severe obesity, renal failure (need dose adjustment), wt<40kg
- Dose:
  - ⇨ 1 mg/kg SQ q 12h or 1.5 mg/kg daily
  - ⇨ If creatinine clearance is <30 ml/min→ reduce enoxaparin dose to 1 mg/kg once daily or use UFH
- Evidence (Ann Intern Med 2004;140:175)
  - ⇨ LMWH is at least as safe and effective as UFH
  - ⇨ Greater ease of use vs UFH
  - ⇨ Better safety profile vs UFH
  - ⇨ Conclusion: Use LMWH unless contraindication present

Rivaroxaban: (N Engl J Med 2012;366:1287)
- Oral factor Xa inhibitor. Very limited evidence.
- Non-inferior to warfarin

Thrombolytics (Am J Emerg Med 2009;27:84-95)
- Dosing
  - ⇨ Tenecteplase: 30-50mg IV bolus
  - ⇨ Alteplase: 100mg IV over 2 hours (accelerated regimen: 0.6mg/kg over 15min)
  - ⇨ Cardiac arrest: bolus some part of dose, up to 50mg IV bolus?
  - ⇨ Give UFH/LMWH concomitantly to ensure unopposed fibrinolysis (no new clots forming)
- Adverse effect: ↑Bleed risk
  - ⇨ <50 yo: 1% risk of bleed
  - ⇨ 50-70yo: 2-3% risk of bleed
  - ⇨ >70yo: >5% risk of bleed

Prognosis
- Overall mortality 1-4%
- Elevated troponin → mortality increased to 19%-23% (Circulation 2007;116:427)
- Elevated BNP + elevated troponin: mortality 38% (Am J Cardiol 2005;96:303)
- Syncope presentation → 14.4% mortality (Circulation 1997;96:882)
- Cardiac arrest mortality 66-95%

PE: PRESENTATIONS
(Review-Am J of Emergency Medicine 2009;27:84) (Essentials 2013-J Kline)

Cardiac arrest
- Mortality 66-95%
- Thrombolytics improve ROSC and may improve survival
- Dose: Alteplase 50mg IV bolus (multiple dosing regimens)

Massive PE
- Define: SBP<90 (any single reading), cardiogenic shock
- Mortality 22-65%
- Thrombolytics
  - ⇨ Multiple studies show trend towards improved mortality (J Thromb Thrombolysis 1995;2:227)
  - ⇨ Thrombolysis recommended if accepting increased risk of bleeding
  - ⇨ ↓**Mortality**: Reduced the risk of death or recurrent PE by 55% (9.4% vs 19%) (Circulation 2004;110:744)
  - ⇨ NNT = 10

Journal Club: Thrombolytics for sub-massive PE

Multiple studies show:
- ↓Pulmonary art pressures & improved RV function with thrombolytics

Goldhaber 1993 (Lancet 1993;341:507)
- Heparin only group: 2 fatal and 3 non-fatal recurrent PEs
- Heparin + t-PA: No recurrent PEs

Konstantinides 1997 (Circulation 1997;96:882)
- ↓Mortality (11.1% → 4.7%)
- ↓recurrent PE (18.7% → 7.7%)

Konstantinides 2002 (NEJM 2002;347:1143)
- No difference in mortality (3.4% vs 2.2%)

MOPETT (Am J Cardiol 2013;111:273)
- 1/2 dose thrombolytics were given to "moderate PE"
- No difference in mortality or recurrent PE
- Thrombolytics improved post-PE pulmonary hypertension

TOPCOAT (J Thromb Haemost 2014;12:459)
- No difference in mortality at 90 days
- Improved QOL: At 90 days, 37% of placebo and 15% of tenecteplase patients had at least one adverse outcome

PEITHO (N Engl J Med 2014;370:1402)
- **Mortality**: No difference in 30d mortality (3.2% placebo vs 2.4% tenecteplase)
- ↑**Major bleeding** with tenecteplase (11.5% vs 2.4%)
- ↑**Hemorrhagic stroke** with tenecteplase (2% vs 0.2%)
- ↓**Hemodynamic decompensation** with tenecteplase (5% vs 1.6%)

- Guidelines
  - ⇨ **ACCP**: "For patients with evidence of hemodynamic compromise, we recommend use of thrombolytic therapy unless there are major contraindications (Grade 1B)" (Chest 2008;133:454S-545S)
  - ⇨ **European Society of Cardiology** "...thrombolytic therapy is the first-line treatment in patients with high-risk PE presenting with cardiogenic shock and/or persistent arterial hypotension, with very few absolute contraindications" (European Heart Journal 2008;29:2276)
- Conclusion (N Engl J Med 2008;359:2804-13)
  - ⇨ Thrombolysis indicated for patients with Massive PE (unless absolute contraindications)

Submassive PE
- Define: Stable hemodynamics with RV dysfunction
  - ⇨ ↑Troponin, ↑BNP, US (loss of inspiratory collapse of IVC)
  - ⇨ EKG: complete/incomplete RBBB, $S_1Q_3T_3$, TWI V_1-V_3
  - ⇨ ECHO (↑RV diameter, paradoxical septal wall motion, RV free wall hypokinesis)
- Thrombolytics for sub-massive PE:
  - ⇨ Guidelines
    - ✓ **ACCP: "In selected high-risk patients without hypotension who are judged to have a low risk of bleeding, we suggest administration of thrombolytic therapy (Grade 2B)"** (Chest 2008;133:454S-545S)
  - ⇨ Conclusion: Uncertain benefit, determine on case by case basis

Syncope (Circulation 1997;96:882)
- Patients with syncope have:
  - ⇨ ↑ Pulmonary artery obstruction
  - ⇨ ↓Cardiac Index (CI) <2.5 L/min/m^2
  - ⇨ Hypoxia (arterial pO_2 below 60 mm Hg)
  - ⇨ Cardiac arrest (24% vs 1%).
  - ⇨ 94% of the patients with syncope had cor pulmonale and 76% were hypotensive on presentation
- Increased mortality: The most significant baseline clinical characteristic associated with mortality was syncope, with a mortality rate of 14.4% for patients with syncope compared to 7.8% for patients without

Stable PE
- Normal hemodynamics, Stable
  - ⇨ Thrombolytics had no benefit in patients with stable hemodynamics and normal RV function
  - ⇨ Bleeding rate approx 1% (less bleeding vs t-PA in stroke)

Disposition:
- Admit for at least 24 h because of ↑rate of complications and recurrence

Drug	Dose	Onset	Duration	Peds	The Good	The Bad	Also...
NO Nitrous Oxide	50-66% N₂O/O₂ inhalational	3-5 min 2-3 min	3-5 min 15-20 min	Same	• Amnesia • Analgesia • Anxiolysis	• Vomiting • Accumulates • ↑ Cerebral blood flow • Unpredictable • Abuse potential	• Great for abscesses • Patient-controlled delivery • Contraindicated in pregnancy (inhibits folate metabolism) • Contraindicated in pulmonary HTN
Midazolam [Versed] (Benzodiazepine)	0.03-0.1 mg/kg IV 0.1 mg/kg IM	3-5 min IV 15-30 min IM	30-60 min IV 1-2 hr IM	0.5 mg/kg PO/PR 0.1 mg/kg IV/IM 0.2 mg/kg IN Onset: • 20-30 min PO/PR • 1 min IV • 5-10 min IM • 5 min nasal	• Decent amnesia & anxiolysis • Reversal: flumazenil • Can be given IV, IM, PO, PR, IN	• No analgesia – give with opioid • Respiratory depression • Hypotension • Disinhibition/paradoxical agitation	Retrograde amnesia 20-30 min
Fentanyl (Opioid)	1-3 mcg/kg IV Can be titrated up to 5 mcg/kg	<1 min	30-60 min	1-2 mcg/kg IV	• Minimal histamine release (less hypotension and respiratory depression) • Analgesia • Quick onset • Reversible with naloxone	• No amnesia • Minimal sedation • Rigid chest syndrome with rapid push and high doses	Accumulates in fat and muscle leading to potential for prolonged effects with large doses
Methohexital [Brevital] (Barbiturate)	1-1.5 mg/kg IV	<1 min	<10 min	1 mg/kg IV Onset: seconds Duration: 10-90 min	• Amnesia • Anxiolysis	• Hypotension • Laryngospasm • Respiratory depression • No analgesia	3 syringe method (in case of laryngospasm) • Syringe 1: Dose pt • Syringe 2: Re-dose pt (1/2 initial dose) • Syringe 3: Laryngospasm tx (Full dose)

Drug	Dose	Onset	Duration	Peds	The Good	The Bad	Also...
Ketamine (PCP derivative, dissociative anesthetic)	1-2 mg/kg IV 4-5 mg/kg IM	1-3 min IV 5-20 min IM	10-15 min 30-60 min IM	IV • Onset: 1-2 min • Duration: 10 min IM • Onset: 3-5 min • Duration: 30-45 min	• Analgesia • Amnesia • Maintains airway reflexes • Minimal CV depression/hypotension • No pain perception • IM, IV, PO, PR, SQ • Bronchodilation	• Sympathomimetic • ↑ICP (myth) • ↑IOP (controversial, do not use in glaucoma) • ↑BP • Emesis • Laryngospasm • Emergence Reaction • ↑Muscle tone • Patient still moves • Hypersalivation	**Contraindications** • Infants <3 mo • ↑IOP or ICP, ↑BP • Severe CAD • Psychosis • Tracheal surgery **Emergence Rxn** • Minimize stimulation • Consider Midazolam for tx/prophylaxis **Hypersalivation:** • Atropine 0.01 mg/kg or • Glycopyrrolate 0.004 mg/kg **Laryngospasm:** • Airway manipulation, BVM • RSI and Intubation
Etomidate (Non-barb/benzo→ GABA receptors)	0.1-0.2 mg/kg IV Re-dose: by 0.1 mg/kg every 2 min, if needed	30-60 sec	5-10 min	0.1-0.3 mg/kg IV Onset: seconds Duration: minutes	• Quick on-off • No histamine release • Minimal CV/respiratory effect • +/- Amnesia	• Myoclonus (up to 20% pts) • Nausea/vomiting • Adrenal axis inhibition • No analgesia	
Propofol (Sedative-hypnotic)	Initial: 1 mg/kg IV Redose: 0.5 mg/kg every 3 min, as needed	<1 min	3-5 min	1-2 mg/kg IV Onset: seconds Duration: minutes	• Quick on/off • Antiemetic • Amnesia • Anticonvulsant • ↓ICP and IOP	• Burns going in • Hypotension • Respiratory depression/apnea • No analgesia	• Contraindicated if egg or soybean allergy • Always have a line running NS to offset potential hypotension • Potentiates all other agents that may be on board (opiate, benzo, barb, TCA, phenothiazines)

PROCEDURAL SEDATION & ANALGESIA

General
- Procedural sedation is a spectrum
- Goal for ED procedural sedation is deep sedation.
- Always be prepared to deal with the patient at a deeper level of sedation than that which you originally intended

	Minimal Sedation (anxiolysis)	Moderate Sedation	*Deep Sedation	General Anesthesia
Responsiveness	Normal response to verbal stimulation	Purposeful response to verbal or tactile stimulation	Purposeful response after repeated or painful stimulation	Unarousable even with painful stimulus
Airway	Unaffected	No intervention required	Intervention may be required	Intervention often required
Spontaneous Ventilation	Unaffected	Adequate	May be inadequate	Frequently inadequate
Cardiovascular Function	Unaffected	Usually maintained	Usually maintained	May be impaired

Indications
- Laceration repair
- Large abscess I&D
- Cardioversion
- Joint/fracture reduction
- Diagnostic radiology
- Endoscopy
- Outside the box: LP, chest tube, foreign body removal, multi-system trauma

PATIENT ASSESSMENT

Pre-procedure Assessment/Patient Evaluation
- History of reactions to anesthesia/previous sedation experiences
- PMH (esp. cardiovascular or pulmonary disease)
- Pregnancy status
- Meds/Allergies (esp. egg/soybean for propofol)
- Airway assessment – body habitus, loose teeth, dentures, Mallampati, LEMON, etc.
- ASA classification
- Last PO intake/Fasting status (ACEP Policy Ann Emerg Med. 2014;63:247)
  - ⇨ **"Do not delay procedural sedation** in adults or pediatrics in the ED based on fasting time."
  - ⇨ "Preprocedural fasting for any duration **has not demonstrated a reduction in the risk of emesis or aspiration** when administering procedural sedation and analgesia. "
- Also:
  - ⇨ Informed consent
  - ⇨ Discussion with MD performing procedure about length of time anticipated, molding of cast, etc.
  - ⇨ Prep any family members about what to expect – (e.g. nystagmus in ketamine)

(ASA) Physical Status Classification System	
ASA I	Healthy patient without systemic disease
ASA II	Patient with mild systemic disease
ASA III	Patient with severe systemic disease
ASA IV	Patient with severe systemic disease that is a constant threat to life
ASA V	Moribund patient who cannot survive without surgery

Mallampati Classification

Mallampati I	Mallampati II	Mallampati III	Mallampati IV
Soft palate, uvula, fauces, pillars visible	Soft palate, uvula, fauces visible	Soft palate, base of uvula visible	Hard palate only visible

PROCEDURAL SEDATION

LEMON Law (Emerg Med J 2005;22,99-102.)
- **L:** Look externally for any signs of predicted difficult airway (facial trauma, large incisors, macroglossia, etc.)
- **E:** Evaluate the 3-3-2 Rule: Inter-incisor distance (3 fingers), Hyoid-mental distance (3 fingers), thyroid to floor of mouth (2 fingers)
- **M:** Mallampati Score
- **O:** Obstruction? (e.g. epiglottitis, PTA, trauma)
- **N:** Neck Mobility (chin to chest, extend, c-collar?)

Things to have at the Bedside
- RT, Pharmacy, Nursing (recorder, monitor)
- IV access/IV fluids
- O_2 Non-rebreather mask
- Suction
- Monitoring equipment – BP, pulse ox, cardiac, capnography
- Basic airway equipment – oral/nasal airways, non-rebreather, BVM
- Advanced airway equipment – intubation equipment, rescue airway equipment
- Defibrillator
- Extra drugs (more than calculated if needed for higher dose or prolonged procedure)
- Saline flushes
- Reversal agents if available

Discharge Criteria
- CV function and airway satisfactory and stable
- Baseline level of consciousness
- Patient can talk, walk, sit up (age appropriate)
- Tolerating oral fluids
- Has a responsible adult to go home with

ABDOMINAL PAIN: GENERAL

1 Initial Resuscitation

- ABCs
- IV/O₂/Monitor
- Resuscitation: IVF/PRBCs?
- Surgery consult?

2 Critical Condition?

📋 H & P 🩺

🖊 Critical Action

AAA

- Usually asymptomatic until rupture
- Acute epigastric & back pain
- Wide pulsatile abd mass
- Syncope, shock
- **Renal colic mimic** (back pain, hematuria)
- **Diverticulitis mimic** (LLQ pain, guaiac+ stools)
- **Risk factors** (age, male, HTN, smoking, CAD/PVD, Famhx)

Stable
⇨ CT Scan

Unstable
⇨ Bedside U/S
⇨ Surgery C/S
⇨ OR

Ruptured Ectopic

See Pregnant VB Algorithm

Mesenteric Ischemia

- **Risk factors:** elderly, etiology specific (see text)
- Sudden abdominal pain, poorly localized **out of proportion to exam** (visceral pain)
- N/V/D
- GI bleeding (SMA supplies R colon)
- Late: peritoneal signs
- Subacute: gradual development vague abdominal S/Sx

⇨ **Labs:** Met acidosis, ↑WBC, ↑Hb, ↑amylase, guaiac +, ↑LDH, ↑Lactate
⇨ CT A/P vs Angiography
⇨ IVF/ABx/anticoag
⇨ Papaverine?
⇨ Surgery C/S

Bowel Perforation

- Sudden onset sharp, severe abdominal pain
- Peritoneal signs: rigidity, rebound, guarding
- Motionless, +distress

⇨ Upright CXR: free air
⇨ CT?
⇨ Antibiotics
⇨ NG suction
⇨ Surgery C/S

Bowel Obstruction

- Colicky abdominal pain
- Abdominal distention
- Vomiting (bilious, feculent)
- Obstipation/Constipation

⇨ AAS: obstructive pattern, air/fluid levels
⇨ IVF/Decompression (NG)
⇨ CT? Antibiotics?
⇨ Surgery consult

Referred Pain

- Myocardial Infarction
- Aortic dissection
- Pneumonia-lower lobe
- Pulmonary Embolism

⇨ EKG
⇨ CXR
⇨ Further testing as needed

3 Focused Evaluation

Upper AP
See Upper Abdominal Pain Algorithm

Lower AP
See Lower Abdominal Pain Algorithm

Pelvic Pain
See Pelvic Pain Algorithm

ABDOMINAL PAIN: GENERAL

1. GENERAL APPROACH/RESUSCITATION:

(CMEDownload:UCSF High Risk 2009-Snoey)

- If patient unstable, begin with ABCs, fluid resuscitation and blood transfusion if necessary. Stabilize before diagnosis if necessary
- Then always consider life-threatening causes of abdominal pain → most can be ruled out by age, history, and physical alone
- Further evaluate by location (quadrant) and character of pain (peritoneal, referred, visceral) and associated symptoms

2. CRITICAL DIAGNOSIS

AAA

(Essentials 2012-"AAA The Great Masquerader")

Clinical

- Common Presentation
  - ⇨ Usually asymptomatic until rupture
  - ⇨ Acute epigastric & back pain
  - ⇨ Wide pulsatile abdominal mass (JAMA 1999;281:77-82)
    - ✓ The only physical exam maneuver of demonstrated value is abdominal palpation to detect abnormal widening of aortic pulsation →Sensitivity 76% for AAAs greater than 5cm
  - ⇨ Shock
- Uncommon Presentations
  - ⇨ Syncope (5% of ruptured AAA)
  - ⇨ Renal colic mimic (back pain, hematuria)
  - ⇨ Diverticulitis mimic (LLQ pain, guaiac pos stools)
  - ⇨ Neuropathy
    - ✓ Retroperitoneal rupture → compressive neuropathy to femoral/ obturator nerve → ant thigh pain/numbness & weak knee flex/hip extension)
  - ⇨ Unexplained ecchymosis
    - ✓ Blue toe syndrome (embolism from AAA)
  - ⇨ Fistula (Aorto-caval or aorto-enteric fistulas)
    - ✓ GI bleed in patient with AAA or AAA repair is Aorto-Enteric Fistula (until proven otherwise)
- Risk factors (age, male, HTN, smoking, CAD/PVD, Fam hx)

Size	Risk of rupture
<4cm	0%
4-5cm	0.5-5%
5-6cm	3-15%
6-7cm	10-20%
7-8cm	20-40%
>8cm	30-50%

Work-up

- **ED U/S** (J Emerg Med 2005;29:455-460)
  - ⇨ Sensitivity 0.94 and specificity of 1
  - ⇨ ED physicians can accurately determine the presence of AAA as well as the maximal aortic diameter
  - ⇨ Use for an unstable patient that can't go to CT
  - ⇨ Use to look for alternate diagnosis
- CT scan
  - ⇨ Best study for **stable** AAA → measure size and extent

Disposition options

- Risk of rupture increases as size increases (watchful waiting vs surgical repair) (J Vasc Surg 2009;50(4 Suppl):S2)
- Incidental AAA <5cm
  - ⇨ Observation vs home, close follow-up (discuss with surgery)
  - ⇨ No improved survival seen with repair of small aneurysms < 5.5cm
- **Incidental AAA>5cm**
  - ⇨ Admit
  - ⇨ Surgical eval → OR (unless high risk)
- **AAA + unexplained symptoms**
  - ⇨ Surgery consult + monitored bed or the OR
  - ⇨ Blood pressure control (β-blocker + Nipride vs Labetalol)
- **Ruptured AAA**
  - ⇨ OR (fatal if not treated surgically)
  - ⇨ Resuscitation
    - ✓ Large bore IVs, IVF, T&C 6 Units PRBCs
    - ✓ Permissive hypotension: ↑BP may lead to loss of retroperitoneal tamponade effect and increased bleeding
  - ⇨ Poor prognostic factors: hypotension, ↓hematocrit, advanced age
  - ⇨ Improved survival seen in patients taken to OR soon after ED arrival vs delayed. (Arch Surg 2003;138:898-901)
- **Indications for OR** (J Vasc Surg. 2009;50(4 Suppl):S2)
  - ⇨ Ruptured AAA is uniformly fatal if not treated surgically
  - ⇨ Rupture, symptomatic, rapid expansion, or asymptomatic > 5.5cm
  - ⇨ Operative mortality: Ruptured → 80%; Elective repair → 2-6%

ABDOMINAL PAIN: GENERAL

ACUTE MESENTERIC ISCHEMIA

(Arch Intern Med. 2004;164:1054-1062, Gastroenterology 2000;118:951-968)
(Essentials 2012: "There is a Clot in the Gut")

Etiology
- **SMA embolism** (50 percent)
  - ⇨ Embolism from dislodged thrombus in LV, LA, A-fib, or heart valves → impacted 3-10cm from SMA origin
  - ⇨ Classic Triad
    - ✓ Pain out of proportion to exam
    - ✓ Gut emptying (vomiting/diarrhea)
    - ✓ Underlying cardiac disease
  - ⇨ 1/3 of patients have had a previous embolic event
- **SMA thrombosis** (15 to 25 percent)
  - ⇨ "ACS of the Gut"
  - ⇨ Chronic SMA plaque acutely thromboses at origin of SMA
  - ⇨ H/O chronic mesenteric ischemia (intestinal angina) → postprandial pain, weight loss, "food fear", early satiety
  - ⇨ Risk factor: smoking, CAD risks
- **Mesenteric venous thrombosis** (5 percent)
  - ⇨ Clinical: Less acute, 1/2 have personal/family h/o VTE
  - ⇨ Risk factors: hypercoagulable states (hx DVT/PE, malignancy), portal HTN, visceral infections, perforated viscus, pancreatitis
  - ⇨ Bowel wall edema → systemic hypovolemia & hemoconcetration → arterial flow impeded → venous capillary congestion and bowel infarction
- **Non-occlusive ischemia- NOMI** (20 to 30 percent)
  - ⇨ Low flow state from cardiac failure, sepsis, cocaine, digoxin, dialysis, vasopressors

Work-up
- Consider in elderly patients with abdominal pain disproportionate to exam
- Labs:
  - ⇨ Non-specific and occur late, once bowel necrosis has occurred
  - ⇨ ↑Lactate: late sign, not diagnostic but predictive of mortality? (Am Surg 1998;64:611-16)
- Xray
  - ⇨ Plain films: used to exclude other causes of abdominal pain
- CT A/P
  - ⇨ Findings
    - ✓ Focal/segmental bowel wall thickening, thumb printing, mesenteric v. thrombus
    - ✓ Non-enhancement of arteries
    - ✓ Pneumatosis, portal venous gas
- Angiography: definitive study, diagnostic and therapeutic

Treatment
- Mortality 70-90% overall → diagnosis prior to infarction is strongest predictor of survival
- Resuscitation → IVF, management of arrhythmias/CHF, correction of acidosis
- **Antibiotics** (treat bacterial translocation)
- **Anticoagulation** (Heparin) → arterial & venous thrombosis/embolism
- **Thrombolysis** → arterial embolism
- **Vasodilation** (Papaverine) → NOMI
- **IR**: Vasodilator/stent therapy, thrombectomy/embolectomy
- **Surgery**: Arterial bypass, resection of necrotic bowel

BOWEL OBSTRUCTION

Causes (Rosen's Emergency Medicine: Chapter 90, Disorders of the Small Intestine)
- Intrinsic: Congenital, inflammatory, neoplasm, intussusception, hematoma
- Extrinsic: Hernias, adhesions (most common), volvulus, mass
- Intraluminal: Foreign body, gallstones, bezoars

Clinical
- Colicky abdominal pain
- Abdominal distention
- Vomiting (bilious, feculent)
- Obstipation/Constipation

Work-up
- Acute abdominal series (AAS): obstructive pattern, air/fluid (A/F) levels
- CT AP

ABDOMINAL PAIN: GENERAL

Complications
- Hypovolemia → intestinal ischemia → infarction → peritonitis and sepsis

Treatment
- Non-operative trial
  - ⇨ Up to 75% with partial SBO and 35-50% complete SBO resolve with IVF and bowel decompression alone
- Early surgery
  - ⇨ Signs of strangulation (fever, peritonitis)
  - ⇨ De novo obstruction (no h/o abdominal surg/adhesions) → unlikely to respond to conservative treatment

INTESTINAL PERFORATION

Clinical
- Sudden onset sharp, severe abdominal pain
- Peritoneal signs: rigidity, rebound, guarding
- Motionless, +distress

Work-up
- Upright CXR → free air under diaphragm
- CT AP

Treatment
- Antibiotics
- Surgery Consult → OR

3. FOCUSED EVALUATION

RUQ/Epigastric Pain (see Abdominal Pain-Upper algorithm)

Lower Abdominal Pain (see Abdominal Pain-Lower algorithm)

Pelvic Pain (see Pelvic pain algorithm)

ABDOMINAL PAIN: UPPER

1. Resuscitation R/O Critical Dx

- ☐ AAA
- ☐ Mesenteric Ischemia
- ☐ Perforation
- ☐ SBO
- ☐ Ectopic pregnancy

→ See General Abdominal Pain Algorithm

2. Emergent GI Cause?

📋 H & P 🩺   ✏️ Critical Action

B I L I A R Y   T R A C T

Biliary Colic

- ☐ **Episodic** RUQ/epigastric pain
- ☐ Precipitated by meals/fatty foods
- ☐ +/- RUQ tender, afebrile, nausea
- ☐ Consider Cholecystisitis?

⇨ U/S
⇨ Pain control (opiates)
⇨ Cholecystectomy (outpatient)

Cholecystitis

- ☐ Continuous RUQ/epigastric pain
- ☐ RUQ tender, **+ Murphy's**
- ☐ N/V, fever
- ☐ ↑WBC, mild ↑LFTs

⇨ U/S
⇨ Pain control/IVF
⇨ Antibiotics
⇨ Surgery consult → OR

Choledocho-lithiasis

- ☐ ↑**LFTs** (AP, T. Bili, AST/ALT)

Gallstone Pancreatitis

- ☐ ↑Amylase, ↑lipase

⇨ Cholecystitis +
⇨ Cholangiogram
⇨ ERCP, papillotomy
⇨ Ascend cholangitis: Resusc, ABx

Ascending Cholangitis

- ☐ **Charcot's triad** (RUQ pain, fever, jaundice)-70%
- ☐ **Reynold's pentad** (triad + AMS + shock)

Pancreatitis

- ☐ H/O EtOH/gallstones (see above)
- ☐ Epigastric pain radiate to back
- ☐ N/V/fever, +/- jaundice
- ☐ Abd tender/guarding
- ☐ Cullen's, Gray Turner's sign
- ☐ ↑amylase, ↑lipase, ↓Ca (tetany)

⇨ Resuscitation
⇨ NPO/IVF/NG?
⇨ U/S → r/o gallstones
⇨ CT?
⇨ Pain control
⇨ ABx?

PUD/GERD Gastritis

- ☐ **GERD:** heartburn, atypical angina, water brash, cough
- ☐ **Gastritis:** asymptomatic vs epigastric pain, N/V, anorexia
- ☐ **PUD:** epigastric pain relieved (duodenal) or worsened by food (gastric), back pain & ↑lipase (posterior perf)

⇨ Lifestyle Δ
⇨ Stop precipitants (NSAIDS/EtOH)
⇨ Antacid/H₂ blocker/PPI
⇨ H. Pylori treatment
⇨ Complications?

3. Other Causes

- ☐ Acute hepatitis
- ☐ Liver abscess
- ☐ Appendicitis
- ☐ Splenic infarct/aneurysm (L sided pain)
- ☐ MI
- ☐ Lower lobe pneumonia

ABDOMINAL PAIN: UPPER

1. RESUSCITATION & R/O CRITICAL DX

General
- Work-up for upper abdominal pain begins with resuscitation and exclusion of critical dx
  - ⇨ See General abdominal pain algorithm
- Then, through a detailed history and physical, consider all the causes of upper abdominal pain (see below)
- The differential may then come down to Gallstone etiology vs Gastritis/PUD → will need further imaging based on suspicion (US abdomen)

Resuscitate
  - ⇨ IV/O₂/Monitor, IV Fluids, Labs as needed, pregnancy test

R/O Critical diagnoses:
  - ⇨ AAA, Mesenteric Ischemia, Perforation, SBO, ectopic pregnancy

2. EMERGENT GI CAUSES

BILIARY TRACT DISEASE
(EM:RAP 2/08-Sheppard) (Gastroenterol Clin Nam 2003:32;1145-1168)

General:
- The goal is to find the location of the stone and its associated complications→ Is it still in the gallbladder (symptomatic cholelithiasis), in the cystic duct (cholecystitis), or in the CBD (choledocholithiasis, gallstone pancreatitis, ascending cholangitis)???

CHOLELITHIASIS
- Prevalence of 10% in US, usually asymptomatic (symptoms develop in 2%/yr)

BILIARY COLIC
- Symptomatic cholelithiasis → obstruction of cystic duct by gallstones
- Clinical:
  - ⇨ Episodic pain in RUQ, minutes to hours, resolves spontaneously
  - ⇨ Precipitated by meals/fatty foods
- Treatment: Recurrent biliary colic → pain control, elective outpatient cholecystectomy

CHOLECYSTITIS
- Clinical (vs biliary colic, may be difficult to distinguish)
  - ⇨ Pain longer in duration (>6 hours), localizes to RUQ, ↑N/V/F
  - ⇨ Murphy's sign:
    - ✓ Localized peritonitis over gallbladder → arrest of inspiration on gallbladder palpation,
    - ✓ Highest LR+ of PE/lab values
    - ✓ Diminished in elderly
- Course
  - ⇨ 1/3 will worsen → complications (cholangitis, perforation)
  - ⇨ 1/2 will improve spontaneously (7-10days)
- Laboratory: ↑WBC, mild ↑LFTs
- Radiology
  - ⇨ RUQ U/S (sensitivity 84-97%, specificity up to 100%)
  - ⇨ Findings: Gallstones, pericholecystic fluid, gallbladder wall thickening (>3mm), sonographic Murphy's
- HIDA scan: non-visualization of contrast in gallbladder (cholecystitis) or intestine (choledocholithiasis)
- Treatment
  - ⇨ NPO/IVF/Abx (broad spectrum)
  - ⇨ Semi-urgent Cholecystectomy, laparoscopic (at 24-48h) with CBD exploration or ERCP if CBD stone of concern
- Complications: gallbladder perforation, emphysematous cholecystitis, gangrenous cholecystitis, cholangitis, gallstone ileus

Ransom's criteria	
At diagnosis	At 48 hours
Age>55	Hct↓>10%
WBC>16,000	↑BUN>5
Glucose>200	Base deficit>4
AST>250	Ca<8
LDH>350	PaO2<60
	Fluid sequest >6L

CHOLEDOCHOLITHIASIS
- Define: Gallstone lodged in common bile duct
- Clinical: similar presentation to cholecystitis except elevated LFTs (↑Alk Phos, ↑T. Bili)
- Radiology: RUQ U/S
  - ⇨ Dilated CBD (>6mm)
  - ⇨ Common bile duct stone?
- ERCP
  - ⇨ Diagnose and treat common duct stones (with sphincterectomy)
  - ⇨ R/O other causes of obstruction (tumors…)

GALLSTONE PANCREATITIS
- Elevated amylase, lipase
- ERCP to decompress biliary tree

Ascending cholangitis

- CBD obstruction causing infection proximal to obstruction → sepsis (↑mortality)
- Charcot's triad (RUQ pain, fever, jaundice)
- Reynold's pentad (Charcot + hypotension + AMS)
- Tx
  - ⇨ Conservative (NPO, IVF, broad-spectrum Abx → elective ERCP at resolution)
  - ⇨ If failure of conservative tx (15%) → emergent surgery (Percutaneous vs ERCP)

ACUTE PANCREATITIS

(Emerg Med Clin N Am 2003;21:873-907)

Etiology:

- Gallstones (35%), Alcohol (30%)
- Idiopathic (10%), ERCP complications (4%), Tumors, Drugs (furosemide, sulfa, thiazides, valproate, tetracyclines…), infection (viral, mycoplasma), blunt trauma (1.5%), scorpion, hypercalcemia, elevated triglycerides

Clinical

- Epigastric pain radiating to back
- N/V/fever, +/- jaundice
- Abd tender/guarding, Cullen's (peri-umbilical ecchymosis), Gray Turner's (flank bruising)

Diagnosis:

- Lipase
  - ⇨ Levels peak (12-36h), duration (2 weeks)
  - ⇨ Test of choice, better sensitivity and specificity over amylase → lipase level 3x normal, more specific
  - ⇨ If high suspicion for pancreatitis and lipase negative → CT scan
  - ⇨ Level of lipase not predictive of severity of pancreatitis
- Amylase
  - ⇨ Less specific, duration (1 week)
  - ⇨ Not used: many false+ and false-
  - ⇨ Many sources: bowel, uterus, pancreas Amylase: level 3x normal, not specific,
- CT A/P
  - ⇨ Unsure of diagnosis (high index of suspicion and lipase low)
    - ✓ Will see acute and chronic changes on CT
  - ⇨ Rule out surgical issues
  - ⇨ Staging system (Balthazar) → help stage and predict which patients will develop severe complication: necrotizing pancreatitis (Radiology 1994;193(2):297)
- RUQ U/S → diagnose gallstone pancreatitis

Treatment

- Resuscitation
  - ⇨ NPO/bowel rest/IVF/NG suction
  - ⇨ Fluid resuscitation (up to 10L/day → maintain adequate UOP)
- Antibiotics
  - ⇨ Meta-analysis → prophylactic antibiotics for necrotizing pancreatitis decreased sepsis and mortality
  - ⇨ Save for sickest pts → Imipenem/meropenem (Ann Surg. 2006;243(2):154)
- Necrotizing Pancreatitis
  - ⇨ Antibiotics (Imipenem), CT A/P, Urgent surgical consultation, ICU
  - ⇨ Fluid collections → CT or U/S guided drainage
  - ⇨ Infected pancreatic collections → benefit from early surgery
- Gallstone Pancreatitis
  - ⇨ RUQ US to diagnose
  - ⇨ MRCP if not sure of obstructive etiology
  - ⇨ Treatment: ERCP (but may cause pancreatitis)

Complications

- #### Necrotizing Pancreatitis
  - ⇨ Pancreatitis → necrosis/liquefaction of tissue → local/systemic complications
  - ⇨ Greatest life-threatening complication of pancreatitis (mortality up to 50%)
  - ⇨ Predisposes to sepsis, multi-organ failure and death
  - ⇨ Predictive factors:
    - ✓ Hemorrhage? (Gray-Turner, Cullen's → delayed 48h),
    - ✓ Pancreatic enzymes (low levels more consistent with necrosis),
    - ✓ ↑Severity of pancreatitis (↑Ranson's)
      - i. Hemoconcentration: Hct >47% at 48h has high sensitivity and may need CT early in course (Am J Gastroenterol 1998;93:2130-4)
  - ⇨ Treatment
    - ✓ Antibiotics (Imipenem), CT A/P, Urgent surgical consultation, ICU
    - ✓ Fluid collections → CT or U/S guided drainage
    - ✓ Infected pancreatic collections → benefit from early surgery

- Sepsis
  - ⇨ Responsible for most mortality associated with AP
  - ⇨ See Sepsis algorithm
- Pseudocyst
  - ⇨ Drainage → >6cm after 6 wks observation, or causing sx (abd pain, gastric outlet obstruction, biliary obstruction)
- Other
  - ⇨ ↓Ca, ↑glucose, ↑TG, GI hemorrhage, ascites, pleural effusion, ARDS, renal failure

GASTRITIS/GERD/PUD

General:
- If patient stable → often considered default diagnosis when work-up negative and excluded life-threats (MI, perforation…)
- Empiric therapy given with abdomen re-check

Clinical
- **GERD**: Heartburn, atypical angina, water brash, cough
- **Gastritis**: Asymptomatic vs epigastric pain, N/V, anorexia
- **PUD**: Epigastric pain relieved (duodenal) or worsened (gastric) by food; back pain & ↑lipase (post perf)

Treatment
- Lifestyle Δ (↑Head of bed), stop precipitants (NSAIDS/EtOH)
- H. Pylori treatment, antacid/H_2 blocker/PPI

Complications:
- **Peptic Ulcer Disease:**
  - ⇨ Hemorrhage, Perforation, Intractable pain, Obstruction
  - ⇨ Posterior perforation → may present like pancreatitis (back pain, ↑enzymes, vomiting…)

3. OTHER CAUSES
- Consider other causes above and below the area of tenderness
  - ⇨ Acute hepatitis, liver abscess, appendicitis, splenic infarct/aneurysm (L sided pain), MI, lower lobe pneumonia

ABDOMINAL PAIN: LOWER

1 Resuscitation R/O Critical Dx

- ☐ AAA
- ☐ Mesenteric Ischemia
- ☐ Perforation
- ☐ SBO
- ☐ Ectopic pregnancy

→ See General Abdominal Pain Algorithm

2 Emergent Cause?

📋 H & P   💉 Critical Action

RLQ R/O Appendicitis

- ☐ Periumbilical colicky pain
- ☐ Migration to right iliac fossa → constant & sharp
- ☐ Anorexia, nausea, constipation/diarrhea
- ☐ Vomiting (perf → peritonitis?)
- ☐ Localized peritoneal irritation (Mc Burney's point)
- ☐ Other: Rovsing's, Psoas and obturator signs
- ☐ Fever, tachycardia, ↑WBC, ↑CRP

⇨ Resuscitation
⇨ Antibiotics
⇨ Labs
⇨ U/S vs CT?
⇨ Surgery C/S

LLQ R/O Diverticulitis

- ☐ Hypogastric pain migrates to LLQ (93-100%)
- ☐ Fever, ↑WBC
- ☐ Diarrhea, guaiac + stools

⇨ Empiric Tx?
⇨ Labs?
⇨ CT
⇨ ABx/liquid diet

GU Causes

See LBP algorithm
- ☐ Cystitis/Pyelonephritis
- ☐ Nephrolithiasis
- ☐ Testicular etiology (torsion, epididymitis...)

⇨ UA
⇨ CT
⇨ U/S?
⇨ ABx

Gyn Causes

See Pelvic Pain algorithm
- ☐ Ectopic pregnancy
- ☐ Torsion
- ☐ PID/TOA
- ☐ Cyst/Mittleschmirtz
- ☐ Fibroids

⇨ Pregnancy
⇨ UA/U dip
⇨ U/S?

3 Other GI Causes

IBD (UC & Crohn's)

- ☐ RLQ pain → terminal ileitis?
- ☐ Diarrhea, guaiac +
- ☐ IBD flare vs complication?
- ☐ Complication: Obstruction, Perforation, Abscess, Toxic megacolon?

Colitis

- ☐ Ischemic vs infectious vs inflammatory
- ☐ Gastroenteritis?
- ☐ N/V/D
- ☐ Guaiac + stools

⇨ IVF
⇨ Antimotility agents
⇨ ABx?
⇨ See Diarrhea algorithm

4 Appy/Tics Mimics

- ☐ Mesenteric adenitis (dx of exclusion)
- ☐ Typhlitis
- ☐ Intussusception
- ☐ Ileocecitis
- ☐ Omental infarct
- ☐ Epiploic appendigitis (L>R)
- ☐ Spigelian hernia

ABDOMINAL PAIN: LOWER

1. Resuscitation & R/O Critical Dx

(Essentials 2012 "Appy 2012 Style")(EM:RAP 12/11 "RLQ Pain in the Pregnant Pt")

General
- Work-up for lower abdominal pain begins with resuscitation and exclusion of critical dx
  - ⇨ See General abdominal pain algorithm
  - ⇨ AAA, Mesenteric Ischemia, Perforation, SBO, ectopic pregnancy
- Then, through a detailed history and physical, consider all the causes of lower abdominal pain
- Rule out GU causes (pyelonephritis vs kidney stone) if possible with UA
- The differential may then come down to GI (appendicitis, diverticulitis) vs pelvic etiology (in females) → will need further imaging based on suspicion (CT A/P vs pelvic ultrasound)

Resuscitate
- IV/O$_2$/Monitor, IV Fluids, Labs as needed, pregnancy test

R/O Critical diagnoses:
- AAA, Mesenteric Ischemia, Perforation, SBO, ectopic pregnancy

2. R/O Emergent Causes

APPENDICITIS

(BMJ 2006;333:530-4) (ACEP Guidelines: Ann Emerg Med. 2010;55:71-116) (Essentials 2013 "Appy/Tics")

Clinical Presentation
- General
  - ⇨ Abdominal pain
    - ✓ Periumbilical colicky pain
    - ✓ Migration to right iliac fossa → constant & sharp
    - ✓ Localized peritoneal irritation (**McBurney's point**)
    - ✓ **Rovsing's** (palpation in LLQ elicits pain in RLQ)
    - ✓ **Psoas** (passive extension of thigh or active flexion of hip → pain → retrocecal appendicitis)
    - ✓ **Obturator** signs (flexion and internal rotation of hip → pain)
  - ⇨ Anorexia, nausea/vomiting constipation/diarrhea
  - ⇨ Fever, tachycardia, ↑WBC, ↑CRP
- Strongest predictors of appendicitis (Meta-analysis Brit J Surg 2004;91:28-37)
  - ⇨ Inflammatory response variables (PMN, WBC, CRP)
  - ⇨ Peritoneal irritation (rebound, percussion tenderness, guarding, rigidity)
  - ⇨ Migration of pain (epigastric/periumbilical → RLQ)
- Patients at extremes of age may have non-specific sx → diagnostic difficulty

Appy triad
☐ Inflammatory markers
☐ Peritoneal irritation
☐ Migration of pain

Work-up (Ann Intern Med 2004;141:537-46)
- Ultrasound
  - ⇨ Aperistaltic and non-compressible structure > 6mm
  - ⇨ Sensitivity 86%; Specificity 81%
- CT
  - ⇨ Abnormal appendix, calcified appendicolith + periappendiceal inflammation or diameter >6mm
  - ⇨ Sensitivity 94%; Specificity 95%

Treatment
- Resuscitation
  - ⇨ Large bore IV, IVF
- Pain control
  - ⇨ Opiate administration has no significant association with management errors (JAMA 2006;296:1764-1774)
- Antibiotics
  - ⇨ Broad spectrum, empiric
  - ⇨ ↓Incidence of postoperative wound infection and intra-abdominal abscess formation (Cochrane Database Syst Rev 2005;(3):CD001439)
  - ⇨ Antibiotics alone for treatment? (Lancet. 2011:377(9777):1573)
    - ✓ Spontaneous resolution can also occur
    - ✓ 1 year recurrence rate with antibiotics as sole therapy → 15%, most within 10 days
- Surgery
  - ⇨ Risk of rupture: 0-36h → <2%;
  - ⇨ Each ensuing 12h period after 36h → 5%
  - ⇨ Timing (Arch Surg 2006;141:504-7)
    - ✓ No significant difference between early (<12h after presentation) and later (12-24h) appendectomy

ABDOMINAL PAIN: LOWER

DIVERTICULITIS

Clinical Presentation
- Presents like appendicitis, but of the LLQ
- Hypogastric pain migrates to LLQ (93-100%)
- Fever, ↑WBC
- Diarrhea, guaiac + stools

Work-up (Am J Roentgenol 2002;178:1313-8)
- Empiric treatment?
  - ⇨ No imaging studies needed if diagnosis is clear-cut → can begin empiric treatment
- CT
  - ⇨ Sensitivity 69-95%, Specificity 75-100%
  - ⇨ Use for uncertain diagnosis, exclude other causes of abdominal pain, r/o diverticular complications, or clinical deterioration
  - ⇨ Findings: bowel wall thickening (96%), fat stranding (95%), detects complications (free air, abscess, phlegmons, cancer)
- Ultrasound?
  - ⇨ Sensitivity 84%, Specificity 93%
  - ⇨ R/O AAA, hypoechoic bowel wall thickening, diverticula, abscess, hypoechoic around bowel wall

Complications (Emerg Med Clin N Am 2003;21:937-969)
- Abscess
  - ⇨ Can lead to fistula formation, sepsis
- Free perforation, peritonitis
  - ⇨ Rupture of diverticular abscess → acute surgical abdomen
  - ⇨ ↑ In elderly and immunosuppressed, high mortality (6-25%)
- Fistula
  - ⇨ Fistula between colon and surrounding structures → colovesicular, colovaginal, colocutaneous, coloenteric
  - ⇨ Colovesicular most common (dysuria, pyuria, pneumaturia, fecaluria)
- Obstruction
  - ⇨ Uncommon-2% of cases
  - ⇨ May cause SBO when loops of bowel entangled in peridiverticular adhesions

Treatment
- **Outpatient**
  - ⇨ Indication: Mild sx, tolerating oral fluids, well appearing(Am Fam Physician 2005;72(7):1229)
  - ⇨ Antibiotics, 7-10days (amox/clav, TMP/SMX, cipro/metronidazole)
  - ⇨ Liquid diet, may consider no abx in extremely well appearing pts (Br J Surg 2012;99(4):532)
  - ⇨ If no improvement in 2-3 days → consider peridiverticular disease (reassessment & admission?)
- **Inpatient**
  - ⇨ Indication: Severe sx requiring narcotics, unable to tolerate oral fluids, elderly, comorbid illnesses, ill/septic, no home support or f/u
  - ⇨ IV antibiotics (gram negative/anaerobes), bowel rest
  - ⇨ Laparotomy? → generalized peritonitis, sepsis, visceral perforation, clinical deterioration

PYELONEPHRITIS
(See LBP Algorithm)

NEPHROLITHIASIS
(See LBP Algorithm)

TORSION/PID/TOA
(See Pelvic Pain Algorithm)

ACUTE SCROTUM
(See Acute Scrotum Algorithm)

ABDOMINAL PAIN: LOWER

3. OTHER CAUSES

IBD

Clinical Presentation
- RLQ pain → terminal ileitis?
- Diffuse abdominal pain, diarrhea, guaiac +

Complications
- May be difficult to distinguish "flare" from an acute complication → consider further diagnostic imaging
- TOXIC MEGACOLON
  - ⇨ Define: Lethal complication of IBD or infectious colitis → total or segmental non-obstructive colonic dilatation plus systemic toxicity
  - ⇨ Clinical: abrupt onset bloody diarrhea, fever, ↑WBC, tachy, third space losses, ill appearing, abdominal distension → perforation (peritoneal signs may be masked by steroids)
  - ⇨ Tx: Resuscitation, blood transfusion, broad spectrum antibiotics, corticosteroids, +/- immunosuppressants, bowel rest and bowel decompression
  - ⇨ Surgery: indicated if no improvement on medical therapy (subtotal colectomy with end-ileostomy)
- Hemorrhage: (CD > UC) → Resuscitation, blood transfusion, surgery consult (bowel resection?)
- Other: Obstruction, Perforation, Abscess

COLITIS

Etiology
- Ischemic vs infectious vs inflammatory
- Mesenteric Ischemia (see General Abdominal Pain algorithm)

Clinical Presentation
- Gastroenteritis?
- N/V/D
- Guaiac + stools

4. OTHER APPY MIMICS
- Mesenteric adenitis (dx of exclusion)
- Typhlitis
- Intussusception
- Ileocecitis
- Omental infarct
- Epiploic appendigitis (L>R)
- Spigelian hernia

DIARRHEA

1 Hydration Status

- □ ABCs
- □ IV/O2/Monitor/IVF → NS bolus
- □ Evaluate hydration status (tachy, ↓BP, ↓UOP, orthostatic, mucous membranes, skin turgor)

2 Inflammatory vs Toxigenic

	Toxigenic	Inflammatory
Timing	□ **Sudden onset** (incubation 2-12h) □ Duration 10-24h	□ **Gradual onset** (incubation 1-3 days) □ Duration 1-7days
Symptoms	□ Non-toxic, afebrile, benign abdomen	□ Toxic, febrile, systemic sx □ Severe abdominal pain
Stool	□ Large, watery, frequent	□ Small, frequent □ +Blood, +WBC, O&P

3 Specific Cause?

PMH
- □ Cirrhosis: Vibrio vulnificus
- □ AIDS: Cryptosporidium, Isospora
- □ Sickle cell: Salmonella
- □ Achlorhydria: Salmonella
- □ Transplant hx: CMV

Exposure
- □ HUS: Shigella, EHEC
- □ Reiter's: Salmonella, Shigella, Campylobacter, Yersinia
- □ Peritoneal Sx: C. diff, EHEC

Other Sx
- □ Day Care: Shigella, Camp, Rota, C.diff.
- □ Hospital/Abx: C.diff
- □ Pool: Giardia, Cryptosporid, Shigella
- □ Travel: Enterotoxigenic E. Coli, Cholera (rice water diarrhea)
- □ Oral/anal sex: STD
- □ Farm animals: Yersinia (pseudoappy)

- □ Poultry: Campylobacter, Salmonella
- □ Shellfish: Vibrio
- □ Cheese: Listeria
- □ Hamburger: E. Coli
- □ Rice: B. cereus
- □ Canned food: C. perfringens
- □ Fresh berries: Cyclospora
- □ Reptile: Salmonella
- □ Well water: Aeromonas

4 Treatment

Rehydrate Treat Sx
- ⇨ Fluids: IV vs PO
- ⇨ Solids
- ⇨ Antimotility agents

Antibiotics
- ⇨ **Toxigenic**: not indicated unless Traveler's (E. coli)
- ⇨ **Inflammatory**-(indicated if systemic illness, febrile, toxic)
- ⇨ Cipro 500 bid x 3-7d
- ⇨ Bactrim DS 1 bid

Specific Tx
- ⇨ **Salmonella**: Tx prolongs carrier state unless typhoid, Sickle cell disease, immunocomp
- ⇨ **Shigella**: Tx all
- ⇨ **Campylobacter**: Erythromycin
- ⇨ **C. diff**: stop offending Rx?, Flagyl/Vanco PO
- ⇨ **Entamoeba**: Flagyl

Dispo

Consider Admit:
- ⇨ Age extremes (<3 mos)
- ⇨ Not tolerating PO
- ⇨ Immunocompromised
- ⇨ Toxic/Severe dehydration
- ⇨ Co-morbid dz

ACUTE SCROTUM

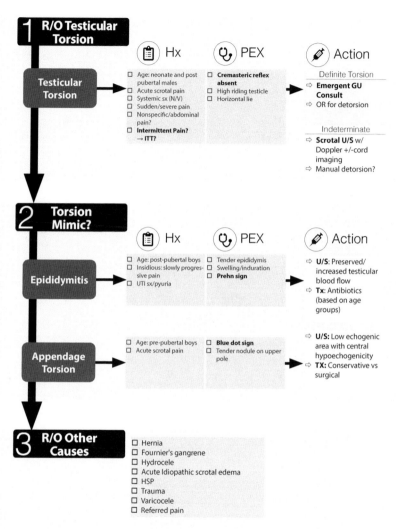

1 R/O Testicular Torsion

Testicular Torsion

Hx
- Age: neonate and post pubertal males
- Acute scrotal pain
- Systemic sx (N/V)
- Sudden/severe pain
- Nonspecific/abdominal pain?
- **Intermittent Pain?** → ITT?

PEX
- **Cremasteric reflex absent**
- High riding testicle
- Horizontal lie

Action

Definite Torsion
⇨ **Emergent GU Consult**
⇨ OR for detorsion

Indeterminate
⇨ **Scrotal U/S w/ Doppler +/-cord imaging**
⇨ Manual detorsion?

2 Torsion Mimic?

Epididymitis

Hx
- Age: post-pubertal boys
- Insidious: slowly progressive pain
- UTI sx/pyuria

PEX
- Tender epididymis
- Swelling/induration
- **Prehn sign**

Action
⇨ **U/S**: Preserved/increased testicular blood flow
⇨ **Tx**: Antibiotics (based on age groups)

Appendage Torsion

- Age: pre-pubertal boys
- Acute scrotal pain

- **Blue dot sign**
- Tender nodule on upper pole

⇨ **U/S**: Low echogenic area with central hypoechogenicity
⇨ **TX**: Conservative vs surgical

3 R/O Other Causes

- Hernia
- Fournier's gangrene
- Hydrocele
- Acute Idiopathic scrotal edema
- HSP
- Trauma
- Varicocele
- Referred pain

ACUTE SCROTUM

GENERAL

(CMEDownload 6/11-Tamkin)(EM:RAP 12/11-Herbert)(EM Clinics NA 2011;29:469)

- The general approach to acute scrotal pain is to work-up the patient for **testicular torsion** by first risk stratifying them based on age group, history and physical.
    - ⇨ Based on the patient's pre-test probability → call GU emergently or obtain testicular U/S.
- The U/S will also help in the evaluation of other serious causes of testicular pain such as appendage torsion and epididymitis.
- The etiology of acute scrotal pain varies among different age groups, the most common being: (Journal of Pediatric Surgery 1995;30(2):277-82)
    - ⇨ 0-1yo: Testicular torsion
    - ⇨ 3-13 yo: Appendage torsion
    - ⇨ >13 yo: Epididymitis

1. R/O TESTICULAR TORSION

TESTICULAR TORSION

History
- **Age**
    - ⇨ Torsion can occur at any age, and up to 39% of cases occur in adulthood (J Urol 1990;143:62)
    - ⇨ Adults with torsion may have a lower salvage rate (likely because of the severity of cord twisting) (J Urol 2002;167:2109)
- Presentation
    - ⇨ Acute scrotal pain-Sudden/severe pain
    - ⇨ Systemic sx (N/V)
    - ⇨ Nonspecific/abdominal pain?
- **Pitfall:** Intermittent Testicular Torsion (torsion-detorsion)
    - ⇨ ITT should be considered in patients who present with **recurrent, rapid onset, severe pain** with spontaneous resolution.
    - ⇨ Hyperperfusion of testis can occur after detorsion or intermittent torsion and give a false diagnosis of epididymitis on U/S.
    - ⇨ **Whirlpool sign** (caused by twisting of the spermatic cord) on spermatic cord imaging can help identify these patients along with horizontal lie of the testis (J Ultrasound Med 2006;25:563-574)
    - ⇨ **Horizontal lie** of testis is the only physical exam finding significantly associated with bell clapper deformity (Spec 100%) (J Urology 2005;174:1532-35)
    - ⇨ GU should be contacted if intermittent torsion suspected for future surgical fixation to prevent future pain and infarction.

Physical Exam
- **Cremaster reflex** (J Urol 1984;132(1):89-90)
    - ⇨ Most sensitive physical exam finding is the cremasteric reflex (sensitivity100%) in one series of 245 patients
    - ⇨ If you see scrotum rising when you stroke the inner thigh → less likely there is torsion (other series have confirmed these findings)
    - ⇨ Disclaimer: Cannot rely solely on presence of reflex, must interpret in context of other clinical findings.
    - ⇨ Absence of cremasteric reflex is meaningless, kids normally lack this reflex.
- High riding testicle
- Horizontal lie

Salvage rates for Torsion (Am Fam Physician 2006;74:1739-43)
- <6 hours: 90-100%
- 12-24 hours: 36-50%
- >24 hours: 0-10%

Diagnostic work up
- Based on **pre-test probability** of torsion
    - ⇨ **Definite Torsion: GU C/S for emergent eval, especially if <4hours**
    - ⇨ Indeterminate: U/S +/- GU consulting
- Color Doppler U/S
    - ⇨ Sensitivity and specificity to diagnose torsion across multiple studies are 85-100% and 75-100%, respectively. (J Urol 2004;172:1692-1695)
    - ⇨ U/S is not perfect in ruling-out torsion and multiple studies have shown false negatives → must look for intra-testicular (not peripheral) flow
    - ⇨ **Pitfall:** Emergent surgical exploration should still be considered for those at high risk for torsion despite negative U/S

ACUTE SCROTUM

- **Cord Imaging**:
  - ⇨ Rotated spermatic cord **"whirlpool sign"** is a highly sensitive and specific sign for torsion, especially when vascular flow is present on Doppler U/S.
- **Manual detorsion**
  - ⇨ Procedure: Detorse from inside to out → like opening a book
  - ⇨ 30-80% success rate (Go to **emrap.tv** Episode 6 for demonstration)
  - ⇨ If successful, relief of ischemia can convert a urologic emergency into an elective surgical procedure and will salvage the testes

2. R/O TORSION MIMICS

EPIDIDYMITIS

Clinical Presentation
- Age: post-pubertal boys
- Insidious onset: slowly progressive pain
- UTI sx/pyuria
- Tender epididymis with swelling/induration
- Prehn sign (physical lifting of the testicles relieves the pain of epididymitis but not pain caused by testicular torsion)

Etiology
- Varies by age groups
  - ⇨ Pre-pubertal: Chemical irritation secondary to reflux of sterile urine (STD? → child abuse?)
  - ⇨ Young males: STD
  - ⇨ Older male: STD vs urinary pathogens (reflux from BPH)
- **Special Case**: Child with Epididymitis? (J Urol. 1987;138:1100-3)
  - ⇨ Will need GU follow up for upper tract imaging and VCUG because of the known association with urinary tract pathology

Work-up
- Urine GC/Chlamydia
- US-shows preserved/increased testicular blood flow

Treatment (based on age group)
- Empiric antibiotics to cover most likely etiology (STD vs urinary pathogens)
- Children: Antibiotics against coliforms
- Adults: GC/Chlamydia +/- coliforms

APPENDAGE TORSION

Clinical Presentation
- Age: pre-pubertal boys
- Acute scrotal pain
- Physical exam: Blue dot sign, tender nodule on upper pole

Work up
- Clinical diagnosis
- US- Low echogenic area with central hypoechogenicity

Treatment
- Conservative: Rest, ice, anti-inflammatories → slow recovery and pain may last weeks to months
- Surgical: excision of appendix testes → not necessary but is safe and pts can resume activity in days

3. R/O OTHER CAUSES

- Hernia
- Fournier's gangrene
- Hydrocele
- Acute Idiopathic scrotal edema
- HSP
- Trauma
- Varicocele
- Referred pain (nephrolithiasis, appy etc...)

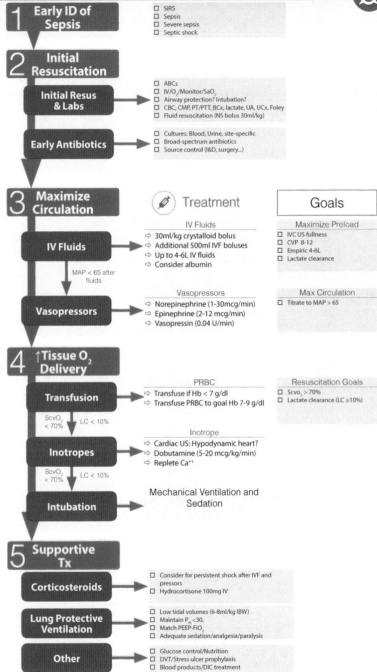

SEPSIS

1 Early ID of Sepsis
- ☐ SIRS
- ☐ Sepsis
- ☐ Severe sepsis
- ☐ Septic shock

2 Initial Resuscitation

Initial Resus & Labs
- ☐ ABCs
- ☐ IV/O$_2$/Monitor/SaO$_2$
- ☐ Airway protection? Intubation?
- ☐ CBC, CMP, PT/PTT, BCx, lactate, UA, UCx, Foley
- ☐ Fluid resuscitation (NS bolus 30ml/kg)

Early Antibiotics
- ☐ Cultures: Blood, Urine, site-specific
- ☐ Broad-spectrum antibiotics
- ☐ Source control (I&D, surgery...)

3 Maximize Circulation

🖊 Treatment

IV Fluids
- ⇨ 30ml/kg crystalloid bolus
- ⇨ Additional 500ml IVF boluses
- ⇨ Up to 4-6L IV fluids
- ⇨ Consider albumin

IV Fluids

MAP < 65 after fluids

Vasopressors
- ⇨ Norepinephrine (1-30mcg/min)
- ⇨ Epinephrine (2-12 mcg/min)
- ⇨ Vasopressin (0.04 U/min)

Vasopressors

Goals

Maximize Preload
- ☐ IVC US fullness
- ☐ CVP 8-12
- ☐ Empiric 4-6L
- ☐ Lactate clearance

Max Circulation
- ☐ Titrate to MAP > 65

4 ↑Tissue O$_2$ Delivery

PRBC
- ⇨ Transfuse if Hb < 7 g/dl
- ⇨ Transfuse PRBC to goal Hb 7-9 g/dl

Transfusion

Resuscitation Goals
- ☐ Scvo$_2$ > 70%
- ☐ Lactate clearance (LC ≥10%)

ScvO$_2$ < 70%   LC < 10%

Inotrope
- ⇨ Cardiac US: Hypodynamic heart?
- ⇨ Dobutamine (5-20 mcg/kg/min)
- ⇨ Replete Ca^{++}

Inotropes

ScvO$_2$ < 70%   LC < 10%

Intubation

Mechanical Ventilation and Sedation

5 Supportive Tx

Corticosteroids
- ☐ Consider for persistent shock after IVF and pressors
- ☐ Hydrocortisone 100mg IV

Lung Protective Ventilation
- ☐ Low tidal volumes (6-8ml/kg IBW)
- ☐ Maintain P$_{pl}$ <30,
- ☐ Match PEEP-FiO$_2$
- ☐ Adequate sedation/analgesia/paralysis

Other
- ☐ Glucose control/Nutrition
- ☐ DVT/Stress ulcer prophylaxis
- ☐ Blood products/DIC treatment

SEPSIS

1. EARLY ID OF SEPSIS

DEFINITIONS

(EM:RAP 6/13-Swadron)(EM:RAP 10/12-Weingart)(Surviving Sepsis Campaign Crit Care Med 2013; 41:580–637)
(NEJM 2006;355:1699-1713) (Crit Care Med 1992;20:864-74)

SIRS (Systemic Inflammatory Response Syndrome)
- Inflammatory response to a non-infectious insult (pancreatitis, burn, surgery...)
    - ☐ Temperature (<36 or >38°C)
    - ☐ Tachycardia (HR >90)
    - ☐ Tachypnea (RR>20 or $PaCO_2$<32)
    - ☐ WBC (>12,000, <4,000 or >10%bands)

Sepsis (Crit Care Med 2013;41:580-637)
- Systemic, deleterious inflammatory response to infection
- Diagnosis: Infection (documented or suspected) and some of the following
    - ⇨ General variables
        - ☐ Fever (> 38.3°C)
        - ☐ Hypothermia (core temperature < 36°C)
        - ☐ Heart rate > 90
        - ☐ Tachypnea
        - ☐ Altered mental status
        - ☐ Significant edema or positive fluid balance (> 20 mL/kg over 24 hr)
        - ☐ Hyperglycemia (plasma glucose > 140mg/dL in the absence of diabetes)
    - ⇨ Inflammatory variables
        - ☐ Leukocytosis (WBC count > 12,000)
        - ☐ Leukopenia (WBC count < 4000)
        - ☐ Normal WBC count with greater than 10% immature forms (bands)
        - ☐ Plasma C-reactive protein more than two standard deviations (sd) above the normal value
        - ☐ Plasma procalcitonin more than two standard deviations (sd) above the normal value
    - ⇨ Hemodynamic variables
        - ☐ Arterial hypotension (SBP < 90mm Hg, MAP < 70mm Hg, or an SBP decrease > 40mm Hg in adults or less than two sd below normal for age)
    - ⇨ Organ dysfunction variables
        - ☐ Arterial hypoxemia (PaO_2/FiO_2 < 300)
        - ☐ Acute oliguria (urine output < 0.5 mL/kg/hr for at least 2 hrs despite adequate fluid resuscitation)
        - ☐ Creatinine increase > 0.5mg/dL
        - ☐ Coagulation abnormalities (INR > 1.5 or aPTT > 60 s)
        - ☐ Ileus (absent bowel sounds)
        - ☐ Thrombocytopenia (platelet count < 100,000)
        - ☐ Hyperbilirubinemia (plasma total bilirubin > 4mg/dL)
    - ⇨ Tissue perfusion variables
        - ☐ Hyperlactatemia (↑Lactate)
        - ☐ Decreased capillary refill or mottling

Sepsis induced hypotension
- ☐ SBP < 90 mm Hg or MAP < 70 mm Hg or
- ☐ SBP decrease > 40mm Hg in the absence of other causes of hypotension.

Severe sepsis
- Sepsis + organ dysfunction
- Definition: Sepsis induced tissue hypoperfusion or organ dysfunction with any of the following thought to be due to the infection
    - ☐ Sepsis-induced hypotension
    - ☐ Lactate above upper limits of laboratory normal
    - ☐ Urine output <0.5 mL/kg/hr for more than two hours despite adequate fluid resuscitation
    - ☐ Acute lung injury with PaO_2/FIO_2 <250 in the absence of pneumonia as infection source
    - ☐ Acute lung injury with PaO_2/FIO_2 <200 in the presence of pneumonia as infection source
    - ☐ Creatinine >2 mg/dL
    - ☐ Bilirubin >4 mg/dL
    - ☐ Platelet count <100,000
    - ☐ Coagulopathy (INR >1.5)
- Mortality rate: 25-30%

Septic shock:
- Mortality rate: 40-70%
    - ☐ Severe sepsis + hypotension, not responsive to fluid resuscitation
    - ☐ Sepsis induced hypotension persisting despite adequate fluid resuscitation (30ml/kg)

SEPSIS

2. INITIAL RESUSCITATION

(Surviving Sepsis Campaign Crit Care Med 2013; 41:580–637)

Initial Resuscitation
- ABCs/ IV/O$_2$/Monitor/SaO$_2$
- Labs: CBC, CMP, PT/PTT, BCx x 2, lactate, UA, UCx, Foley
- Fluid resuscitation (30ml/kg NS bolus to start)
- Early broad spectrum antibiotics
- Consider central line +/- CVP monitoring

Oxygenation
- Goal: maximize O$_2$ delivery to tissue
- Supplemental oxygen for all patients
- Consider Intubation?
  - ⇨ Altered mental status and unable to protect airway
  - ⇨ Persistent hypoxia despite (SaO$_2$ <90%) despite O$_2$ supplementation (non-rebreather mask)
  - ⇨ Severe hypotension/shock
  - ⇨ Respiratory failure

Goals
☐ CVP 8–12 mm Hg
☐ MAP ≥ 65 mm Hg
☐ Urine output ≥ 0.5 mL/kg/hr
☐ Superior vena cava oxygenation saturation (ScvO$_2$) 70% or mixed venous oxygen saturation (SvO$_2$) 65%

Antibiotics
☐ Blood cultures prior to antibiotics   ☐ Antibiotics within 1 hour of diagnosis

Target
☐ Target: Normalizing lactate (in patients with elevated lactate)

Early Antimicrobials (Crit Care Med 2013;41:580-637)
- Blood Cultures
  - ⇨ 2 sets, at least one peripheral and one via each vascular device
  - ⇨ Cultures before antibiotics if no significant delay (>45 min)
  - ⇨ Cultures from other sites (CSF, Urine, body fluids) should also be obtained before antibiotics if no delay
- Antibiotics
  - ⇨ Begin broad-spectrum empiric antibiotics within **one hour** of diagnosis of sepsis to cover likely source and pathogens
  - ⇨ Each hour delay in antibiotics is associated with a measurable increase in mortality

Source control
- Evaluate patient for focus of infection amenable to source control (abscess drainage, debridement, device removal etc..)
- Look for cause of infection that can be surgically controlled (peritonitis, cholangitis, intestinal infarction, necrotizing soft tissue infection etc.)
- If intravascular access devices are a possible source, they should be removed promptly after other vascular access has been established

3. MAXIMIZE CIRCULATION

(Severe Sepsis & Septic Shock)
(Surviving Sepsis Campaign Crit Care Med 2013; 41:580–637)

Fluids (Preload)
- Crystalloids
  - ⇨ Initial fluid of choice
  - ⇨ Initial fluid challenge: 30ml/kg (2-3L) bolus
  - ⇨ Additional fluid in boluses (500ml) and reassess after each bolus
- Goal (maximize preload)
  - ⇨ Goal → No additional stroke volume from more fluids
  - ⇨ **Empiric IV fluids:** Begin with 30ml/kg bolus and continue up to 4-6 L (goal MAP>65)
  - ⇨ **IVC US:** Fluid bolus until there is ↓ change in size of IVC with respiration
  - ⇨ **CVP monitoring:** Fluid bolus until goal CVP >10 (CVP>14 in intubated pts)
  - ⇨ ProCESS trial showed no benefit to using invasive monitoring and CVP measurements (N Engl J Med 2014; 370:1683)
  - ⇨ Caution:
    - ✓ Cardiogenic pulmonary edema
    - ✓ Non-Cardiogenic pulmonary edema (ARDS) → more fluid worsens prognosis
- Albumin
  - ⇨ Indication: Patient has already received a substantial amount of crystalloid (4-6L) → use albumin to help prevent third spacing
  - ⇨ Dose: 500cc bolus of 5% albumin (or a dose of 25% albumin)

MAP formula
MAP= (2xDBP + SBP)/3

⇨ Journal club
- ✓ Meta-analysis (Crit Care Med 2011; 39:386–391)
  - i. Use of albumin solutions for the resuscitation of patients with sepsis was associated with lower mortality compared with other fluid resuscitation regimens.
- ✓ SAFE study (N Engl J Med 2004;350:2247)
  - i. Similar outcomes for saline and albumin
- ✓ ALBIOS Trial (N Engl J Med 2014; 370:1412)
  - i. No improved survival at 28 and 90 days when with albumin added to crystalloid

Vasopressors

- Indication: MAP <65 after **adequate fluid loading**
- Goal: Target MAP > 65 mmHg

Vasopressors
Ensure that patient is adequately hydrated before starting vasopressors

  ⇨ Supplemental endpoints: BP, regional/global perfusion, urine output, mental status, lactate
- **Norepinephrine** (Levophed-NE)
  - ⇨ First line drug of choice
  - ⇨ Dose:
    - ✓ Start: 0.5-1 mcg/min (up to 30mcg/min in refractory shock)
  - ⇨ Increases MAP due to its vasoconstrictive effects, with little change in heart rate and less increase in stroke volume compared with dopamine
  - ⇨ NE vs Dopamine (N Engl J Med 2010;362:779)
    - ✓ No overall difference in mortality (52.5% vs 48.5%; p= 0.10)
    - ✓ Increased rate of arrhythmias with Dopamine (24.1% vs 12.4%)
    - ✓ Increased mortality in patients with cardiogenic shock with Dopamine
- **Epinephrine**
  - ⇨ 2nd line agent to be added to or substituted for NE
  - ⇨ Dose: 2-10 mcg/min IV
- **Vasopressin**
  - ⇨ Dose:
    - ✓ 0.04 U/min IV
    - ✓ Can be added to NE with the intent of raising MAP to target or decreasing NE dosage
  - ⇨ Not recommended as single agent
- Dopamine
  - ⇨ Alternative to NE only in highly selective patients
  - ⇨ Dose:
    - ✓ Low-dose: 1-5 mcg/kg/minute, increased renal blood flow and urine output
    - ✓ Intermediate-dose: 5-15 mcg/kg/min: ↑ renal blood flow, heart rate, cardiac contractility, and CO
    - ✓ High-dose: >15 mcg/kg/min alpha-adrenergic effects predominate, vasoconstriction, increased BP
- Phenylephrine
  - ⇨ Not recommended except in certain circumstances:
    - ✓ Patient at risk for arrhythmias (NE is associated with serious arrhythmias)
    - ✓ Cardiac output is known to be high and blood pressure persistently low
    - ✓ Salvage therapy when combined inotrope/vasopressor drugs and low-dose vasopressin have failed to achieve the MAP target
    - ✓ No Central line: can be given peripherally temporarily
  - ⇨ Dose:
    - ✓ 40-60 mcg/min IV (Start 100-180 mcg/min IV until BP stable)

4. MAXIMIZE TISSUE O_2 DELIVERY

Resuscitation end points:

- Vital sign endpoints (MAP, BP, HR etc...) are **not sufficient** to gauge adequacy of resuscitation and tissue hypoxia
- Patients resuscitated to normal VS may continue to have tissue hypoxia as evidenced by decreased lactate clearance and persistently low $ScvO_2$ (Am J Emerg Med 1996;14(2):218)
- **Goals of resuscitation:**
  - ☐ Superior vena cava oxygenation saturation ($ScvO_2$) > 70%
  - ☐ Lactate clearance (LC) ≥10%

Lactate clearance (LC)

- Goal: lactate clearance by at least 10%
- Lactate as predictor of **mortality**

Lactate Clearance (LC)
Lactate clearance can be used in place of $ScvO_2$ to measure adequacy of resuscitation

  - ⇨ Mortality rates increase as lactate increases (Ann Emerg Med. 2005;45:524)
  - ⇨ As lactate increases from 2 to 8 mg/dL, mortality increases from 10-90% (Crit Care Med 1992;20:80)
- Lactate clearance (↓ lactate ≥ 10%)
  - ⇨ Alternative to $ScvO_2$ (JAMA 2010;303:739):
    - ✓ Lactate clearance may be **acceptable alternative** to $ScvO_2$ in determining tissue perfusion
    - ✓ Lactate clearance of at least 10% over ≥ 2 hours (adequate tissue oxygen delivery) produces a similar short-term survival rate as a protocol using $ScvO_2$ monitoring.

⇨ Mortality
  ✓ The Shock Society (Shock 2009;32:35-3)
    i. Mortality was **60% for lactate non-clearance** versus 19% for lactate clearance
    ii. Lactate non-clearance was an **independent predictor of death** (OR= 4.9)
    iii. ScvO₂ optimization did not reliably exclude lactate non-clearance
  ✓ Nguyen et. al (Crit Care Med 2004;32:1637)
    i. Lactate clearance had a significant **inverse relationship with mortality**
    ii. There was an approximately 11% decrease likelihood of mortality for each 10% increase in lactate clearance
  ✓ Each **10% increase** in repeat lactate values was associated with a **9.4% increase** in the odds of hospital death (Ann Am Thorac Soc 2013;10:466)

IVF
- Patient may require additional IV fluids (NS bolus)
- Reassess using CVP or US as applicable

Inotropic Support
- Dobutamine
  ⇨ Bedside ECHO/US: Hypodynamic heart?
  ⇨ Trial of dobutamine for
    ✓ Persistent hypoperfusion (with normal MAP and adequate intravascular volume)
    ✓ Myocardial dysfunction
  ⇨ Dose: up 5-20 mcg/kg/min
- Calcium: replete Ca if low

Blood Products
- Indication: Red blood cell transfusion if hemoglobin concentration decreases to < 7.0 g/dL
- Target a hemoglobin concentration of 7.0 to 9.0 g/dL
- Increases O₂ delivery to tissues

Mechanical Ventilation/Intubation
- Decrease work of breathing and pulmonary metabolic load

5. SUPPORTIVE THERAPY

Corticosteroids
- Indication:
  ⇨ Unable to restore hemodynamic stability with IV fluid resuscitation and vasopressors
- Dose: Hydrocortisone 100mg q8h (200-300mg/d)
- Evidence
  ⇨ ACTH Stimulation test (not recommended)
    ✓ Low cortisol → cortisol levels < 15mcg/dl
    ✓ "Non-responder" or "inadequate adrenal reserve"→ cortisol levels rise less than 9 mcg/dl to corti-cotropin stim test (250 mcg ACTH stim test)
    ✓ Option: Check cortisol level before test and 30, 60 min after test
  ⇨ French trial ((JAMA 2002;288:862-871)
    ✓ **All patient mortality decreased with hydrocortisone (61% vs 55%)**
    ✓ Mortality benefit was in "**non-responders**" in septic shock (63% vs 53%)
    ✓ No mortality benefit in "responders"
    ✓ Conclusion: Survival benefit is seen in patients with adrenal suppression and are non-responders to ACTH stimulation test
  ⇨ Meta-analysis (BMJ 2004;329:480)
    ✓ Overall, randomized controlled trials show that **short-course, high-dose** steroids do not improve survival in severe sepsis
    ✓ **Low dose** (HCT<300mg/d) and **longer duration** of treatment (≥5days) improves hemodynamics, reduces time on vasopressor, and reduces 28 day mortality
  ⇨ CORTICUS trial (NEJM 2008;358:111-24)
    ✓ Hydrocortisone showed no mortality benefit for patients in septic shock, even for patients with "inadequate adrenal reserve"
    ✓ Hydrocortisone group → shock was reversed more quickly than in the placebo group (2-3 days)
    ✓ Hydrocortisone group → more episodes of superinfection, including new sepsis and septic shock

Lung protective ventilation (NEJM 2000;342:1301-1308)
- Avoid high tidal volumes and high plateau pressures in ALI/ARDS

Anticipated PEEP settings at various FIO2 requirements													
(N Engl J Med 2000; 342:1301)													
F₁O₂	0.3	0.4	0.4	0.5	0.5	0.6	0.7	0.7	0.7	0.8	0.9	0.9	0.9	1.0
PEEP	5	5	8	8	10	10	10	12	14	14	14	16	18	20-24

SEPSIS

- ARDS-Net protocol:
  - ⇨ 9% decrease in all-cause mortality in patients with **Vt 6-8ml/kg** (vs 12ml/kg) while aiming for a **plateau pressure of <30 cm H$_2$O**
  - ⇨ **Assist-control** Mode ventilation
  - ⇨ Match **PEEP to FiO$_2$** requirements
  - ⇨ Maintain **SaO$_2$ 88-95%**
  - ⇨ Permissive hypercapnea (allowing PCO$_2$ to increase above normal) can be tolerated to minimize Vt and P$_{PL}$

Glucose Control
- Protocolized approach if glucose > 180mg/dl to **target upper glucose of < 180 mg/dl**
- NICE-SUGAR Trial (N Engl J Med 2009;360:1283)
  - ⇨ **Conventional** glucose control (<180 mg/dl) resulted in lower mortality vs **Intensive** glucose control (81-108 mg/dl) (Mortality 27.5% vs 24.9%; p=0.02)
  - ⇨ Intensive glucose control protocol also resulted in more episodes of hypoglycemia
- Oral feedings as tolerated

Bicarbonate
- Bicarbonate not recommended for pH > 7.15
- No evidence supports the use of bicarbonate therapy in the treatment of hypoperfusion induced lactic acidemia associated with sepsis

Other Modalities
- DVT prophylaxis
- Stress ulcer prophylaxis
- Sedation/analgesia/paralysis
- DIC treatment
- Nutrition

PROTOCOLS

Early Goal Directed Therapy
- References: (EGDT - NEJM 2001;345:1368-77) (SAFE Study - NEJM 2004;350:2247-56)(Crit Care Med. 2013 41(2):580)
- General
  - ⇨ Goal oriented manipulation of cardiac preload, afterload and contractility to achieve a balance between oxygen delivery and oxygen demand
  - ⇨ Resuscitation to EGDT goals in first six hours decreased in-hospital mortality and mortality at 28 and 60 days
  - ⇨ Equipment: Central venous catheter capable of measuring central venous oxygen saturation (ScvO$_2$ and A-Line)
- Maximize Circulation (MAP>65)
  - ⇨ **Fluid bolus (NS)**
    - ✓ Goal CVP 8-12 (12-15 for mechanical ventilation) or urine output >0.5ml/kg/hr
    - ✓ 500-mL bolus of crystalloid every 30 minutes to achieve a CVP of 8-12 mm Hg
  - ⇨ **Vasopressors** (NEJM 2010;362:779-789)
    - ✓ Indication: fluid challenge fails to restore blood pressure and adequate perfusion (MAP<65)
    - ✓ Goal: Vasopressors or vasodilators to achieve MAP 65 mm Hg or SBP 90 mm Hg
    - ✓ Recommendation: Norepinephrine (first line agent) or Dopamine
    - ✓ Epinephrine should be used as second line agent in conjunction with NE if still need BP support
    - ✓ Vasopressin can be used as a low-dose background agent (0.04 Units/min) in conjunction with a vasopressor.
    - ✓ Inotropic therapy (Dobutamine) if adequate MAP/fluid resuscitation but ongoing hypoperfusion
- Maximize Oxygenation (Goal ScvO$_2$>70%)
  - ⇨ PRBC Transfusion to Hct>30%
  - ⇨ Inotropic agent (Dobutamine) to maximum dose of 20 mcg/kg/min
  - ⇨ Mechanical ventilation & Sedation

ProCESS (N Engl J Med 2014; 370:1683)
- Study protocol
  - ⇨ RCT compared 3 arms of trial:
    - ✓ EGDT targets (ScvO2, CVP, MAP, UOP; ; central access required) vs
    - ✓ A protocol that used some of the EGDT targets (MAP, UOP; protocol-based standard therapy; central access not required) vs
    - ✓ Usual care (no protocol used to direct fluid management)
- Results
  - ⇨ **No mortality difference** in the three groups (21 versus 18 versus 19 percent)
  - ⇨ **No significant benefit of the mandated use of central venous catheterization and central hemodynamic monitoring** in all patients

ALTERED MENTAL STATUS

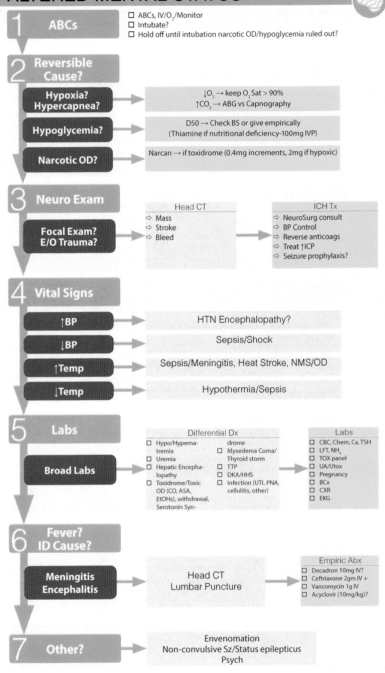

1 ABCs
- ☐ ABCs, IV/O₂/Monitor
- ☐ Intubate?
- ☐ Hold off until intubation narcotic OD/hypoglycemia ruled out?

2 Reversible Cause?

Hypoxia? Hypercapnea?
→ ↓O₂ → keep O₂ Sat > 90%
↑CO₂ → ABG vs Capnography

Hypoglycemia?
→ D50 → Check BS or give empirically
(Thiamine if nutritional deficiency-100mg IVP)

Narcotic OD?
→ Narcan → if toxidrome (0.4mg increments, 2mg if hypoxic)

3 Neuro Exam

Focal Exam? E/O Trauma?

Head CT
⇨ Mass
⇨ Stroke
⇨ Bleed

ICH Tx
⇨ NeuroSurg consult
⇨ BP Control
⇨ Reverse anticoags
⇨ Treat ↑ICP
⇨ Seizure prophylaxis?

4 Vital Signs

↑BP → HTN Encephalopathy?

↓BP → Sepsis/Shock

↑Temp → Sepsis/Meningitis, Heat Stroke, NMS/OD

↓Temp → Hypothermia/Sepsis

5 Labs

Broad Labs

Differential Dx
- ☐ Hypo/Hyperna-tremia
- ☐ Uremia
- ☐ Hepatic Encepha-lopathy
- ☐ Toxidrome/Toxic OD (CO, ASA, EtOHs), withdrawal, Serotonin Syn-drome
- ☐ Myxedema Coma/Thyroid storm
- ☐ TTP
- ☐ DKA/HHS
- ☐ Infection (UTI, PNA, cellulitis, other)

Labs
- ☐ CBC, Chem, Ca, TSH
- ☐ LFT, NH₄
- ☐ TOX panel
- ☐ UA/Utox
- ☐ Pregnancy
- ☐ BCx
- ☐ CXR
- ☐ EKG

6 Fever? ID Cause?

Meningitis Encephalitis
→ Head CT
Lumbar Puncture

Empiric Abx
- ☐ Decadron 10mg IV?
- ☐ Ceftriaxone 2gm IV +
- ☐ Vancomycin 1g IV
- ☐ Acyclovir (10mg/kg)?

7 Other?
→ Envenomation
Non-convulsive Sz/Status epilepticus
Psych

ALTERED MENTAL STATUS

1. ABCs
(EM:RAP 8/06 & 9/06 "Altered mental status; an approach part 1 & 2" – Swadron)
- If patient unstable, begin with ABCs and resuscitate as needed before a diagnosis is determined.
- Patient may require airway protection (ETT) because of altered level of consciousness.
    - ⇨ GCS < 8 and no gag reflex?
    - ⇨ Perform neuro exam prior to intubation
- However, ensure narcotic overdose or hypoglycemia not present, as administration of Narcan/D50 will rapidly reverse cause and preclude need for intubation

2. Rapidly Reversible Causes
- Rule out **Hypoxia:**
    - ⇨ Check SaO_2 or ABG → give supplemental O_2
- Rule out **CO_2 narcosis:** COPD patient given excessive O_2?
    - ⇨ Check ABG or capnography
    - ⇨ ↓O_2, NPPV trial, treat COPD
- Rule out **Hypoglycemia**:
    - ⇨ Check blood sugar or give D50 empirically
    - ⇨ Glucagon IM if no IV access (slow onset of action)
    - ⇨ OK to give D50 before thiamine (JAMA 1998;279:583-4)
    - ⇨ Early thiamine administration essential for treatment of Wernicke's encephalopathy (alcoholics)
- Rule out **Narcotic OD**:
    - ⇨ Give Narcan empirically?
    - ⇨ Dose: 0.4mg increments, 2mg if hypoxic
    - ⇨ Naloxone may also transiently improve valproic acid, tramadol, clonidine, captopril, and EtOH intoxication
        (Ann Emerg Med 1994;12:650-660)

3. Neuro Exam

HEMORRHAGIC STROKE
(Emerg Med Clin N Am 2012;30(3):771-94)
(EM:RAP 9/10 "American Stroke Association ICB Guidelines" – Herbert)

General
- SAH (see Headache algorithm)
- Intraparenchymal
    - ⇨ Causes: hypertension, AVMs (can also be SAH), trauma, anticoagulants

Symptoms
- Sudden onset HA, vomiting, ↑BP, AMS/coma, focal neuro deficits, +/- seizure
    - ⇨ May not present with any of these symptoms
    - ⇨ Can present similar to ischemic stroke (focal neuro symptoms)
- Can start as agitation/lethargy → progress to stupor/coma quickly
- Assess GCS and pupils (blown/nonreactive, anisocoria, pinpoint)
- Cheyne-Stokes respirations with large ICH → herniation
- Herniation → arrhythmias (sinus arrhythmias, PVCs, VTach)

ICH Checklist
☐ BP Control
☐ Reverse anticoags
☐ Treat ↑ICP
☐ Seizure prophylaxis?
☐ Fever/hyperglycemia
☐ Vent drain/surgery

Diagnosis
- CT Brain
    - ⇨ Rapid and readily available
    - ⇨ Eval for hematoma location, extension to the ventricular system, surrounding edema, mass effect, and midline shift
    - ⇨ Can miss very small hemorrhagic strokes
- CT angiography
    - ⇨ Use
        - ✓ R/O a vascular cause for ICH (ie aneurysm, AVM)
        - ✓ R/O active bleeding/hematoma expansion (spot sign - active extravasation of contrast)
    - ⇨ Gaining traction in early diagnosis to show vascular abnormalities → up to 15% change in acute manage-ment (Am J Neuroradiol 2009;30:1213-1221)
- MRI
    - ⇨ Equivalent to CT for detection of acute ICH (JAMA 2004;292:1823)

Management
- Airway
    - ⇨ Monitor airway closely
        - ✓ Quickly expanding hemorrhage → herniation → compromised airway
    - ⇨ Complete neuro exam (including rectal tone) before RSI/Intubation
    - ⇨ Consider Propofol for sedation post-intubation
        - ✓ Short half-life for frequent neuro checks
        - ✓ Decreases intracranial pressure

ALTERED MENTAL STATUS

- **BP control**: AHA/ASA guidelines (Stroke 2010;41(9):2108-2129)
  - ⇨ Decreases hemorrhage expansion, questionable mortality benefit (Lancet Neurol 2008;7:391-99)
  - ⇨ BP Control:
    - ✓ SBP>200 or MAP>150
      - i. Aggressive continuous IV Rx (do not reduce >20%)
    - ✓ SBP>180 or MAP>150 **w/ ↑ICP**
      - ii. Intermittent/continuous IV Rx for CPP>60
    - ✓ SBP>180 or MAP>150 **w/o ↑ICP**
      - iii. Modest BP reduction, IV Rx to MAP 110, **target BP 160/90**
  - ⇨ Can use various IV Rx including **Nicardipine**, Labetolol, Esmolol, Hydralazine etc.
  - ⇨ Journal Club
    - ✓ Two studies (ATTACH 2007 and INTERACT 2008) showed aggressive BP lowering likely safe but did not show improvement in morbidity/mortality
    - ✓ Interact 2 (N Engl J Med 2013;368:2355)
      - i. No difference in death or disability in patients with intensive (SBP<140) vs guideline based lowering (SBP<180)
- **Anticoagulation reversal**
  - ⇨ Warfarin: (CHEST 2012; 141(2)(Suppl):e152S–e184S) (EM:RAP 12/13- Arora)
    - ✓ FFP
      - i. 15cc/kg begins working immediately
      - ii. Use if PCC not readily available
    - ✓ Vitamin K
      - i. 10mg IV over 30 min (prevents anaphylactoid rxn)
      - ii. Begins working at 4 hours, full effect at 24h
    - ✓ 4-factor Prothrombin Complex Concentrate (PCC)
      - i. Contains Factor II, VII, IX, X and some benefits over FFP (Neurocrit Care 2010;12:403-413)
      - ii. VS FFP: PCC has a smaller volume, higher concentration of factors, complete reversal, only one dose in 24h, no need for thawing

Elevated INR (Chest 2012)		
INR	Bleeding	Action
Any INR	**Serious/life threatening bleeding**	☐ Hold warfarin ☐ Vitamin K 5-10mg IV ☐ PCC 25-50 U/kg ☐ Repeat INR 30min post infusion ☐ FFP if PCC not available

  - ⇨ Clopidogrel/ASA:
    - ✓ Platelet transfusion
    - ✓ dDAVP 0.3mcg/kg IV?
  - ⇨ Heparin:
    - ✓ Protamine sulfate 20mg/min
  - ⇨ Factor Xa/thrombin inhibitors:
    - ✓ Factor Xa inhibitors (apixaban and rivaroxaban); direct thrombin inhibitor (dabigatran)
    - ✓ No reversal agent; stop immediately, supportive/symptomatic treatment

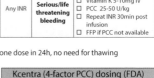

Kcentra (4-factor PCC) dosing (FDA)			
Pre-treatment INR:	2-4	4-6	>6
Dose of 4-PCC (U/kg)	25	35	50
Max dose:	2500	3500	5000

- **Increased ICP**
  - ⇨ Elevate HOB to 30°, elevate bedrails (fall safety), NPO
  - ⇨ Analgesia for pain, sedation
  - ⇨ Hyperventilation
    - ✓ If ventilated → PCO_2 35mmHg (do not over-ventilate)
    - ✓ Limited time of efficacy (6-12h)
  - ⇨ Normal Saline for maintenance (hypotonic fluids contraindicated)
  - ⇨ Medical treatment
    - ✓ Indication: If mental status deterioration, e/o increasing ICP/herniation
    - ✓ Mannitol 0.25-1g IV
      - i. Adverse effects: hypotension, dehydration
    - ✓ Hypertonic saline (HS)
      - i. Dose: 250 ml of 3% over 30 min
      - ii. HS vs mannitol: better outcomes, no hypotension
  - ⇨ Paralysis
  - ⇨ ICP monitoring indications with external ventricular drain (AHA/ASA Guidelines):
    - ✓ GCS ≤ 8
    - ✓ Clinical evidence of transtentorial herniation
    - ✓ Significant IVH or hydrocephalus
  - ⇨ Hematoma evacuation indications (emergent Neurosurgical consultation):
    - ✓ Cerebellar hemorrhage with neurological deterioration
    - ✓ Brainstem compression
    - ✓ Hydrocephalus from ventricular obstruction
- **Fever/hyperglycemia**: treatment → decreased mortality (Lancet 2011;378:1699-1706)
- **Seizure prophylaxis**
  - ⇨ Keppra vs Phenytoin? (per neurosurgery consult?)
  - ⇨ Not recommended to be used prophylactically by AHA/ASA unless clinical seizure or EEG evidence with mental status change

ALTERED MENTAL STATUS

4. Vitals

HYPERTENSIVE ENCEPHALOPATHY
(EM:RAP 2/12 "Hypertension" – Weingart) (Ann Emerg Med 2003 Apr;41(4):513--29)

Definition
- Presence of signs and/or symptoms of cerebral edema caused by severe and/or sudden rises in BP
- Failure of cerebral auto-regulation
- MAP 150 → failure of autoregulation, endothelial dysfunction and vasogenic edema, micro-hemorrhages
- If not treated → leads to coma and death

Symptoms
- Headache
- Mental status changes (confusion → lethargy → coma)
- Visual changes (cortical blindness, scotoma, hemianopsia)
- Rare: seizures, focal neuro deficits, papilledema

Differential Diagnosis
- Ingestion/withdrawal, uremia, ICH, CVA

Management
- Fluid resuscitation
  - ⇨ Usually volume depleted 2/2 pressure induced natriuresis
- BP reduction: **Decrease BP by 25% in first 2 hours**
  - ⇨ 1st hour: decrease BP by 10-15%
  - ⇨ 2nd hour: decrease BP by an additional 10%
  - ⇨ If BP reduction >40% → at risk for neurologic event!!!
- Medication route:
  - ⇨ IV titratable medication should be used
  - ⇨ SL, transdermal, oral route should not be used → can cause precipitous decline that can not be reversed
- Dosing
  - ⇨ Nicardipine gtt (5-15 mg/h)
  - ⇨ Labetalol 20mg IV
  - ⇨ Fenoldopam
  - ⇨ **Not recommended**: Clonidine (CNS depressant effects), diuretcs (volume depleted already), Hydralazine (can give sharp decline in BP; OK for eclampsia), Nitroprusside (linked to ↑ICP, CN toxicity), Enalapril

SEPSIS
(see Sepsis algorithm)

HYPOTHERMIA
(see Hypothermia algorithm)

5. Labs

HYPONATREMIA
(EM:RAP 3/2006 "Electrolyte Emergencies" – Slovis) (Emerg Med Clin N Am 2014;32:379)

Definition
- Excess free H_2O relative to Na → serum Na < 135 mEq/L

Symptoms
- Neurologic spectrum 2/2 water shift in cells:
- Fatigue → lethargy → AMS (usually starting <120 mEq/L) → seizure → coma

Diagnosis (NEJM 2000;342:1581-89)
1. Hypovolemic? → check volume status (mucous membranes, skin turgor, pitting edema, BUN/Cr, U/S IVC, etc)
2. Calculate plasma osmolality: 2[Na+] + [Glucose]/18 + [BUN]/2.8 + [Ethanol]/4.6
3. Calculate osmolar gap: calculated osmolality - measured osmolality
4. Differential:
   - ⇨ **Hypotonic** (<280 mOsm/kg): most common type of hyponatremia
     - ✓ *Hypovolemic*
       - i. Extra-renal Na loss: (↓UNa)
         - a. Diarrhea, vomiting (pancreatitis), inadequate intake, blood loss, excessive sweating (marathon runners), "third spacing" fluid sequestration
       - ii. Renal Na loss: (↑UNa)
         - a. Diuretics (loop, thiazides), ACE inhibitors, adrenal insufficiency, osmotic diuresis

ALTERED MENTAL STATUS

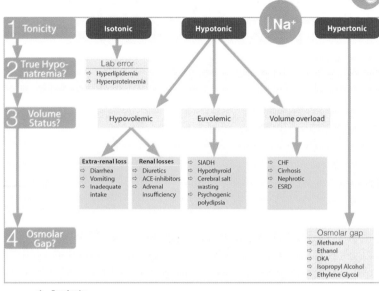

- ✓ **Euvolemic**:
    - i. SIADH (malignancy?), hypothyroid (check TSH), adrenal insufficiency (↑K), psychogenic polydipsia, beer potomania/"tea & toast" diet, cerebral salt wasting (trauma, stroke)
- ✓ **Hypervolemic**:
    - i. CHF, cirrhosis, nephrotic syndrome, ESRD
- ⇨ **Isotonic**: usually lab "error" 2/2 hyperlipidemia, hyperproteinemia
- ⇨ **Hypertonic** (>295 mOsm/kg): unaccounted solute
    - ✓ Glucose: every 100mg/dL > 100mg/dL → ↓[Na^+] by 1.6 mEq/L
    - ✓ Toxic Alcohols (EtOH, ethylene glycol, isopropyl alcohol, methanol)
        - i. Calculate osmolal gap (measured - calculated) if suspected: normal<10

Management

- Hypertonic saline 3%
    - ⇨ Indication: Seizure, AMS, Coma
    - ⇨ Dose: **100 ml 3% saline**, may repeat every 10 min until symptoms resolve
- Rate of correction
    - ⇨ **0.5 to 1 mEq/L/h** or a total of **10 to 12 mEq/L per 24 hours**
    - ⇨ Rapid correction ok?:
        - ✓ AMS/seizure/coma/focal neuro (use hypertonic saline)
        - ✓ Hyponatremia <12-24 hours
        - ✓ Max: Rise of 6mEq in first 6 hours in severely symptomatic patients
- Adverse effects
    - ⇨ Over rapid correction
        - ✓ Consider DDAVP and free water replacement
    - ⇨ Central pontine myelinolysis
        - ✓ Caused by too rapid correction of Na/osmolality
        - ✓ Symptoms: AMS, dysphagia, seizures → locked-in state
- Free H_2O restriction
- Electrolyte replacement
    - ⇨ Watch for concurrent hypokalemia and hypophosphatemia
- Specific treatment
    - ⇨ Hypovolemic
        - ✓ IV NS: repletes volume and Na
    - ⇨ Euvolemic
        - ✓ **No IV NS**: will worsen SIADH
        - ✓ Free H_2O restriction <1L/day
        - ✓ Treat underling cause
    - ⇨ Hypervolemic
        - ✓ Free H_2O restriction <1L/day + diuresis (monitor possible resulting electrolyte disturbances)

Hypertonic saline
☐ Use for AMS, seizure, coma
☐ Dose: 3% saline 100mls, repeat q 10min
☐ Rate of Na correction: 0.5 mEq/L/h

ALTERED MENTAL STATUS

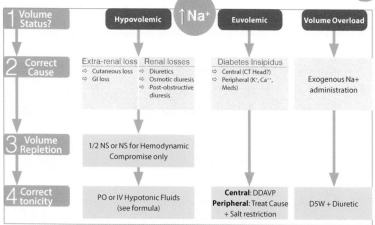

1 Volume Status?	Hypovolemic ↑Na⁺		Euvolemic	Volume Overload
2 Correct Cause	Extra-renal loss ⇨ Cutaneous loss ⇨ GI loss	Renal losses ⇨ Diuretics ⇨ Osmotic diuresis ⇨ Post-obstructive diuresis	Diabetes Insipidus ⇨ Central (CT Head?) ⇨ Peripheral (K⁺, Ca⁺⁺, Meds)	Exogenous Na+ administration
3 Volume Repletion	1/2 NS or NS for Hemodynamic Compromise only			
4 Correct tonicity	PO or IV Hypotonic Fluids (see formula)		**Central**: DDAVP **Peripheral**: Treat Cause + Salt restriction	D5W + Diuretic

HYPERNATREMIA

(NEJM 2000;342:1493-99) (**EM:RAP** 3/2006 "Electrolyte Emergencies" – Slovis)

Definition
- By definition dehydration: free H_2O deficit (excess loss and inadequate intake) → serum Na>145 mEq/L
  - ⇨ Often seen in elderly patients with dementia (unable to perform ADLs) → decreased H_2O intake
  - ⇨ Few symptoms until Na > 160

Diagnosis
- Check fluid status (mucous membranes, skin turgor, pitting edema, BUN/Cr, U/S IVC, etc)
  - ⇨ Hypovolemic
    - ✓ Renal losses: diuretics, osmotic diuresis (hyperglycemia, mannitol, urea), postobstructive diuresis
    - ✓ Non-renal losses:
      - i. Cutaneous loss: Insensible loss →burns, fever, sweating
      - ii. GI loss: diarrhea (osmotic, lactulose), vomiting
  - ⇨ Euvolemic
    - ✓ Diabetes Insipidus (DI)
      - i. Central: trauma, post-op, tumor, hemorrhage/stroke, infection
      - ii. Nephrogenic: Hypercalcemia, hypokalemia, drugs (demeclocycline, lithium)
  - ⇨ Hypervolemic
    - ✓ Post-resus NaHCO₃ administration or hypertonic saline

Management
- Hypovolemic or unstable
  - ⇨ Begin with volume resuscitation: NS
- Calculate free H_2O deficit (mdcalc.com)
  - ⇨ Free H_2O deficit = TBW* x (Na/140 – 1)
    - ✓ *TBW = 0.60 x ideal body weight (IBW), (x 0.85 if female or age>60)
  - ⇨ Half free water deficit should be given in first 12-24h
  - ⇨ Do not correct >12 mEq/L/day unless hypernatremia <12-24 hours, otherwise→cerebral edema
- If can tolerate PO → PO free water
- Hypervolemic → D5W + diuretic
- DI
  - ⇨ Central: DDAVP 1-2mcg IV q12h
  - ⇨ Nephrogenic: treat underlying condition

ALTERED MENTAL STATUS

UREMIC ENCEPHALOPATHY

Symptoms
- AMS: lethargy, irritability, hallucinations, rambling speech, seizure
- Tremor, myoclonus, asterixis
- May have transient focal weakness

Diagnosis
- Markedly elevated BUN in setting of renal failure (specific toxins not identified)
- Other complications:
  - ⇨ Pericarditis/pericardial effusion (EKG/US)
  - ⇨ Ileus
  - ⇨ Coagulopathy (impaired platelet function → DDAVP 0.3mcg/kg IV)
  - ⇨ Impaired immunity (opportunistic infections)
- Be aware of other concomitant electrolyte abnormalities that will be present with renal failure
- Dialysis dysequilibrium syndrome
  - ⇨ Neurologic symptoms that affect dialysis patients when first started on dialysis (cerebral edema?)

Emergent Dialysis
☐ A: Acidosis
☐ E: Electrolytes ($\uparrow K^+$)
☐ I: Intoxication (OD)
☐ O: Overload, fluid
☐ U: Uremia

Management
- Emergent hemodialysis (see table of indications- AEIOU)
- Reverses with dialysis with lag time of 1-2 days

HEPATIC ENCEPHALOPATHY

(Am J Gas 2001;96:1968-76)

Definition
- Multifactorial: results from impaired toxic metabolite clearance usually in setting of liver failure
- In cirrhotics: diagnosis of exclusion! Rule out all other critical diagnoses

Symptoms
- Grade I: Changes in behavior, mild confusion, slurred speech, disordered sleep
- Grade II: Lethargy, moderate confusion
- Grade III: Marked confusion (stupor), incoherent speech, sleeping but arousable
- Grade IV: Unresponsive to pain, gross disorientation → coma

Diagnosis
- Mostly clinical (asterixis)
  - ⇨ In altered patient not able to comply with exam: bend knees/hips with feet flat on bed, let legs fall to side → asterixis with legs flapping at hip
  - ⇨ Asterixis can be absent in grades 0, 3, 4
- Ammonia level (Am J Med 2003;114:188-93) (N Engl J Med. 1985;313(14):865)
  - ⇨ **Normal ammonia does not exclude diagnosis** and does not correlate well with level of encephalopathy

Management
- Lactulose 60cc PO if can comply, or per NGT
  - ⇨ Titrate to 3-4 BMs/day
  - ⇨ Should see clinical improvement within hours
- Neomycin (po or NG)

MYXEDEMA COMA

(EM:RAP 3/10 "Severe Hypothyroidism" – Lopresti)(EM Clinics NA 2014;32:303)

General
- Often seen during winter months in elderly women who are undiagnosed or undertreated hypothyroidism
- Definition: Decompensated hypothyroidism + vascular collapse

Symptoms
- AMS (can be subtle), hypothermia, hypotension, bradycardia, dry skin, ↓DTRs
- Pre-tibial myxedema: "Dough-like" non-pitting edema
- Rarely: edematous or comatose
- Most patients have "decompensated hypothyroidism" and not full myxedema coma

Myxedema Pearls
☐ Always give hydrocortisone prior to T4!
☐ Check cortisol level prior to T4
☐ Do not give T3 empirically
☐ Do not rapidly rewarm
☐ Vasopressors may worsen hypotension

Causes
- Can be precipitated by **infection**
- Hypothyroid patients dependent on vasoconstriction for heat → infection/ sepsis causes vasodilation → cardiovascular collapse
- Other precipitants: CHF, trauma, drugs (esp. opioids), or cold exposure

Diagnosis
- ↑TSH and ↓↓T4, hyponatremia, leukopenia, delayed DTR

ALTERED MENTAL STATUS

Management
- **Hydrocortisone**
  - ⇨ Dose: 100mg IV (q8h) **before IV T4**
  - ⇨ Adrenal dysfunction may accompany myxedema coma (Schmidt's syndrome)
  - ⇨ Check cortisol level prior to T4
- T4 will increase metabolism → deplete cortisol stores
- **T4**
  - ⇨ If suspected in right clinical setting, treat empirically with **T4 500mcg IV** until thyroid tests result
  - ⇨ **Do not give T3 empirically!** (T4 safe to give without TSH results)
  - ⇨ Give hydrocortisone prior to T4
  - ⇨ Restores approx half thyroid stores with one dose, but takes hours to days to manifest effect
- **IV Fluids**:
  - ⇨ Treat hypotension with IVF
  - ⇨ Vasopressors may have paradoxical effect → worsen hypotension
- Rapid reversal of hypothermia → decompensation
  - ⇨ Vasodilation in a patient with decreased cardiac output will cause hypotension
  - ⇨ Treat hypothermia with passive rewarming measures only (not active)
- Treat underlying cause
  - ⇨ Labs, Sepsis work-up, LP to r/o meningitis, CT head, EKG, ECHO?
  - ⇨ Empiric antibiotics

THYROID STORM

(EM:RAP 6/10 "Hyperthyroidism" – Lopresti) (Emerg Med Clin NA 2014;32:277)

General
- Uncommon in ages <15 years.
- More common in women (10x more likely)
- Can be 2/2 Graves' disease, toxic multinodular goiter, etc.
- Mortality: 100% without treatment, 20-50% with treatment

> **Thyroid Storm Pearls**
> ☐ Do not use PTU in first trimester pregnancy→use Methimazole
> ☐ Give Iodine only after Thioamides (1 hour)
> ☐ Avoid aggressive cooling measures→decompensation

Symptoms
- Essential: fever, tachycardia (SVT, Afib), **AMS**
- Other: tremor, ↑DTRs, sweating
- Like myxedema coma, precipitating event (infection/sepsis, trauma, surgery) causes decompensation
- Pts are dependent on vasodilation to release heat → precipitating event → catecholamine surge → insufficient vasodilation

Diagnosis
- Diagnosis subtle/difficult in elderly as decreased response to hyperthyroid state
- ↓↓TSH and ↑↑T4, normocytic anemia, thrombocytopenia, leukopenia, hypocalcemia
- Evidence of hyperthyroidism: proptosis, goiter, thin hair, ↑DTR, CHF/A-fib
- Point scale with specific criteria (Endocrinol Metab Clin North Am 1993;22(2):263)

Management
- (see PDR for updated dosing recommendations)
- β-**blocker**
  - ⇨ MOA: controls signs/symptoms of adrenergic surge, ↓peripheral T4 → T3 conversion
  - ⇨ Propranolol 3-5mg IV for goal HR 90-100
    - ✓ Can give in 1mg IV doses q5-10min until goal HR achieved
    - ✓ Preferred route is IV for appropriate titration, if vitals deteriorate → hold further doses
    - ✓ Propranolol gtt: 3-5mg/h
  - ⇨ Treats the high-output CHF with good response
- **Thioamides**
  - ⇨ MOA: blocks synthesis of new T4/T3
  - ⇨ PTU 100-150mg PO q8h
    - ✓ MOA: decrease T4 synthesis and ↓peripheral T4 → T3 conversion
    - ✓ Do not use in pregnancy → crosses placenta
    - ✓ Black box warning: liver failure/death
  - ⇨ Methimazole 5-20mg po q8h
    - ✓ Less hepatotoxic, ok to use in pregnancy
- **Iodine solution**
  - ⇨ MOA: blocks release of thyroid hormone
  - ⇨ SSKI 10 drops PO q6h
  - ⇨ Start 1 hour **after** methimazole or PTU
- **Glucocorticoids**
  - ⇨ MOA: blocks T4 → T3 conversion, treats concomitant adrenal insufficiency
  - ⇨ Dexamethasone 4mg IV q6h

ALTERED MENTAL STATUS

- Fluid overload?
  - ⇨ High output heart failure → likely respond to β-blockade
  - ⇨ Paradoxically need cautious IVF (3-5L) and β-blockade in acute setting
  - ⇨ Diuresis/aggressive cooling measures can cause decompensation → not indicated
- Treat underlying **cause/complications**
  - ⇨ May empirically treat for infection/sepsis → antibiotics/cultures
  - ⇨ Dehydration: may require 3-5L
  - ⇨ Atrial fibrillation: most spontaneously convert with β-blockade
  - ⇨ Hyperthermia:
    - ✓ Avoid aggressive cooling → will worsen vasoconstriction and shivering → ↑Temp
    - ✓ Treat with: Thorazine 25mg IV, Demerol 25mg IV

TTP

(J Emerg Med 2012;43(3):538-44) (EM:RAP 3/13 "The Paper Chase: TTP Update 2013" – Arora)

General
- Occurs 2x as often in women (usually previously healthy)
- Can be associated with certain drugs: clopidogrel, quinine, chemotherapy
- Pathophysiology:
  - ⇨ IgG rxn to ADAMTS13 → large uncleaved vWF multimers → platelet aggregation → thrombus/MAHA/etc
- Mortality: Untreated 100%; With treatment 10-20%

TTP Pentad
☐ **F**ever
☐ **A**nemia
☐ **T**hrombocytopenia
☐ **R**enal Failure
☐ **N**eurologic dysfunction

Symptoms
- Only 40% manifest all of TTP "pentad" (below)
- ~75% manifest MAHA, thrombocytopenia, neuro deficit
- Vague symptoms: abdominal pain, nausea, vomiting, weakness
- Risk factors: Obese, African American, female, rheumatologic diseases, HIV, clopidogrel

Diagnosis
- "FAT RN" mnemonic
  - ⇨ **F**ever
  - ⇨ **A**nemia (MAHA) Micro Angiopathic Hemolytic Anemia – **schistocytes** on peripheral smear
  - ⇨ **T**hrombocytopenia
  - ⇨ **R**enal failure (50-75%)
  - ⇨ **N**eurologic dysfunction (50-70%) - most common: **AMS**, seizure, stroke mimic
- If suspect TTP: Order peripheral smear to look for schistocytes
- Unexplained thrombocytopenia + MAHA → sufficient for dx
- Normal coags/D-dimer, LDH, ↓↓haptoglobin
- Differential: DIC, HUS (peds), preeclampsia/HELLP syndrome (pregnant)

Management
- **Plasmapheresis**
  - ⇨ Emergent!
  - ⇨ Superior to plasma infusion and decreases mortality (NEJM 1991;325:393-7)
  - ⇨ Begin empiric treatment: Thrombocytopenia + MAHA + no alternate cause
- No platelet transfusion
  - ⇨ Possibly worsens aggregation (controversial)
  - ⇨ Use only for life-threatening hemorrhage, ICH
  - ⇨ Uncertain if true harm from platelet transfusion (Transfusion 2009;49:873-87)
- High dose steroids
  - ⇨ Methylprednisolone 10mg/kg/d (start empirically)
  - ⇨ Superior to low dose steroids (Methylpred 1mg/kg/d) (Ann Hematol 2010;89:591-6)
- FFP
  - ⇨ 10U/24h period (provides active ADAMST13)
  - ⇨ May give while awaiting plasmapharesis
- Aspirin (once platelet level >50,000)
- Supportive therapy:
  - ⇨ Anticonvulsants (seizures), anti-hypertensinves (renal failure), PRBC (severe anemia)
- If febrile → LP (if platelets >50,000) and start empiric antibiotics

ALTERED MENTAL STATUS

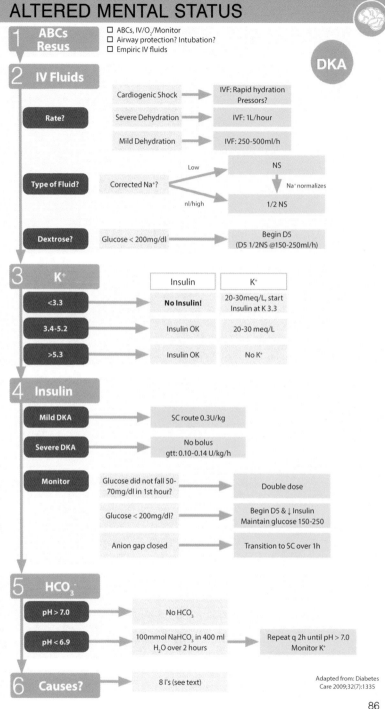

1 ABCs Resus
- ☐ ABCs, IV/O₂/Monitor
- ☐ Airway protection? Intubation?
- ☐ Empiric IV fluids

DKA

2 IV Fluids

Rate?

Cardiogenic Shock	IVF: Rapid hydration / Pressors?
Severe Dehydration	IVF: 1L/hour
Mild Dehydration	IVF: 250-500ml/h

Type of Fluid?

Corrected Na⁺? — Low → NS — Na⁺ normalizes → 1/2 NS
Corrected Na⁺? — nl/high → 1/2 NS

Dextrose?

Glucose < 200mg/dl → Begin D5 (D5 1/2NS @150-250ml/h)

3 K⁺

	Insulin	K⁺
<3.3	No Insulin!	20-30meq/L, start Insulin at K 3.3
3.4-5.2	Insulin OK	20-30 meq/L
>5.3	Insulin OK	No K⁺

4 Insulin

Mild DKA	SC route 0.3U/kg
Severe DKA	No bolus / gtt: 0.10-0.14 U/kg/h

Monitor

Glucose did not fall 50-70mg/dl in 1st hour?	Double dose
Glucose < 200mg/dl?	Begin D5 & ↓ Insulin / Maintain glucose 150-250
Anion gap closed	Transition to SC over 1h

5 HCO₃⁻

pH > 7.0	No HCO₃	
pH < 6.9	100mmol NaHCO₃ in 400 ml H₂O over 2 hours	Repeat q 2h until pH > 7.0 / Monitor K⁺

6 Causes? → 8 I's (see text)

Adapted from: Diabetes Care 2009;32(7):1335

86

ALTERED MENTAL STATUS

DKA

(EM:RAP 5/13 & 3/13)(Essentials 2010-Arora)(Diabetes Care 2009;32(7):1335)

Presentation
- 3Ps-Polyuria, Polydipsia, Polyphagia
- Non-specific sx:
  - ⇨ Weakness, vomiting, abdominal pain, blurry vision
- PEX:
  - ⇨ Acetone smell
  - ⇨ Dehydration/tachycardia/hypotension/shock
  - ⇨ Kussmaul's respiration (deep/labored breathing 2/2 acidosis)

DKA Diagnosis
☐ **D**-Diabetes, BS>250
☐ **K**-Ketones in urine/serum
☐ **A**-Acidosis-pH<7.3, HCO3<18

Diagnosis
- DKA diagnostic criteria:
  - ⇨ **Hyperglycemia**: serum glucose >250 mg/d
  - ⇨ **Acidosis**: arterial pH <7.3, anion gap >10, serum bicarbonate <18 mEq/l
  - ⇨ **Ketosis**: ketonuria or ketonemia
    - ✓ Serum beta-OH-butyrate is the preferred method for measuring ketonemia

Causes (The 8 I's)
- **Infection** (UTI, pneumonia, gastroenteritis, pancreatitis) in 40-50%
- **Infarction** (ACS, MI)
- **Infraction** (patient noncompliance with therapy)
- **Infant** (pregnancy)
- **Ischemic** (CVA)
- **Illegal** (alcohol, drug abuse/cocaine abuse)
- **Iatrogenic** (prescription drug interactions, e.g. steroids)
- **Idiopathic** new onset type 1 diabetes or other cause)

Treatment
- Initial Resuscitation
  - ⇨ Altered sensorium based on level of combination of hyperosmolarity and acidosis (Diabetes Care 2010;33:1837–1839)
  - ⇨ Start with 2L IV NS empiric before labs
- IV Fluids
  - ⇨ Start with 2L IV NS bolus
  - ⇨ Fluid deficit about 100ml/kg (7-8L deficit) 2/2 glucose osmotic diuresis
  - ⇨ Can decrease glucose to 300 with IV fluids
- Sodium
  - ⇨ Falsely lowered level 2/2 hyperglycemia
  - ⇨ Correction: Add 1.6 to Na for every 100 over 100 in glucose level
  - ⇨ Corrects with IV Fluids
  - ⇨ 1/2NS: Switch to 1/2 NS when Na normalizes
- Insulin
  - ⇨ MOA: Stops ketogenesis and breakdown of fatty acids
  - ⇨ **Caution: Hypokalemia**
    - ✓ Prevalence 5.6% (3 out of 54 patients with hypokalemia)(Am J Emerg Med. 2012;30(3): 481)
    - ✓ Do not start insulin until you check potassium → if patient hypokalemic, can drop K even more → arrhythmia
    - ✓ Hold insulin until K>3.3
  - ⇨ Dose: Start 0.1 U/kg/h gtt
    - ✓ Do not need bolus → insulin bolus not associated with any benefit to patients (J Emerg Med 2010;38(4):422)
    - ✓ Priming dose of insulin unnecessary if dosing adequately (Diabetes Care 2008;31(11):2081)
    - ✓ Bolus option dosing: bolus 0.1 U/kg; gtt: 0.1 U/kg/h
  - ⇨ Monitor
    - ✓ If glucose **not decrease by 50mg/dl in first hour** → double rate or SQ insulin bolus
    - ✓ If BS >1000, rapid correction puts patient at risk for cerebral edema
    - ✓ Glucose reaches **200mg/dl**:
      - i. Reduce Insulin gtt to 0.02-0.05 U/kg/hr or
      - ii. Rapid acting insulin 0.1 U/kg SC every 2 hours
    - ✓ Anion **gap closed**
      - i. Goal: Resolution of acidosis/ketosis (not euglycemia) → **do not stop insulin until anion gap closed**
      - ii. Transition dose SQ insulin (5 Units per 50 over 150-max 20)
      - iii. D/C insulin gtt one hour after SQ dose
  - ⇨ Dextrose: When glucose is < 200 mg/dl, **add D5** to replacement fluids
    - ✓ Allows continued insulin administration until ketonemia is controlled while at the same time avoiding hypoglycemia

DKA Severity			
	Mild	Moderate	Severe
Serum pH	7.25-7.30	7.00-7.24	< 7.0
Serum HCO3	15-18	10-15	<10
Mental status	Alert	Drowsy	Coma

- Potassium
  - ⇨ Total body potassium deficit (average deficit 3-5 meq/kg)
  - ⇨ May see relative hyperkalemia because of acidosis
  - ⇨ Repletion: PO (if able to tolerate) and IV
  - ⇨ **Do not start insulin until potassium is > 3.3**
- HCO_3
  - ⇨ Controversial, recommended by ADA for pH<7.0
  - ⇨ Retrospective studies show no improvement in outcome (Crit Care Med 1999;27:2690)
  - ⇨ No prospective randomized studies concerning the use of bicarbonate in DKA with pH values <6.9 have been reported (Diabetes Care 2002;25:2113–2114)
- Other Electrolytes
  - ⇨ Mg → depleted 2/2 osmotic diuresis, ok to replete
  - ⇨ Phos → may precipitously drop with treatment of DKA, must replete
- Monitoring
  - ⇨ Glucose q 1 hour
  - ⇨ pH and electrolytes q 2-4h
    - ✓ ABG not needed, VBG is adequate for monitoring (Emerg Med J 2006;23(8):622)

Complications

- Hypoglycemia- 2/2 overzealous DKA treatment
- Hyperglycemia-2/2 undertreatment
- Hypokalemia
  - ⇨ Caused by insulin tx, correction of acidosis and volume expansion
- Return of DKA (Must bridge with SQ insulin dose)
- Hyperchloremia
- Cerebral Edema (EM:RAP 1/14-Arora/Menchine)
  - ⇨ Prognosis: mortality (20-50%), 1/3 survivors in vegetative state
  - ⇨ Risk factors: age < 5, new onset DM
  - ⇨ Symptoms: Depressed LOC/AMS, pupillary changes, seizures
  - ⇨ Treatment
    - ✓ Mannitol 1-2 gm/kg
    - ✓ Consider: Intubation, decadron, hypertonic saline (5-10ml/kg)

Journal Club: Cerebral edema in DKA

Risk Factors For Cerebral Edema In Children With Diabetic Ketoacidosis
(N Engl J Med 2001;344:264-9)
- Retrospective trial
- 6977 DKA cases → 61 cases of cerebral edema
- No relation between IVF rate and cerebral edema
- Cerebral edema associated with increased BUN

Subclinical Cerebral Edema in DKA (Pediatrics 2013;131:e73–e80)
- Prospective RCT trial
- Tested different IVF rates for MRI evidence of cerebral edema
- **Conclusion: Rate of IVF administration did not affect rate of subclinical cerebral edema**

ALTERED MENTAL STATUS

6. Infectious

Meningitis
(see Headache algorithm)

Encephalitis
(Lancet 2002;359:507-13) (EM:RAP 11/05 "Meningioencephalitis" – Benson)

General
- Inflammation of the brain, usually from viral infection (HSV, HHV, EBV, VZV, Arbovirus, etc)
- Can be in conjunction with meningitis, myelitis or mimic brain abscess, toxins, vasculitis

Symptoms
- Similar to meningitis (see Meningitis algorithm)
  - ⇨ Triad: Fever, HA, AMS but triad not always present
  - ⇨ AMS almost universal: hallucinations, bizarre behavior, dysphasia, **seizures**
- HSV Encephalitis: (temporal lobe) aphasia, anosmia, temporal lobe seizures

Encephalitis Triad
☐ Fever
☐ Headache
☐ ALOC

Diagnosis
- Triad: Fever, AMS, CSF pleocytosis w/ negative GS
- CT
  - ⇨ HSV encephalitis: hypodense lesions in temporal lobe
  - ⇨ If suspect abscess: CT w/ contrast
- LP
  - ⇨ Elevated WBC and protein
    - ✓ ↑WBC: exclusively mononuclear in viral encephalitis
    - ✓ ↑Protein: nonspecific→vasculitis, demyelinating disease, meningitis, bacterial infxn
  - ⇨ Viral PCR/ELISA? (hold extra tube of CSF in lab)
  - ⇨ May have completely normal CSF (3-5%)
- EEG for HSV encephalitis has characteristic findings
  - ⇨ Periodic high voltage spike wave from temporal regions and slow wave complexes at 2-3s intervals

Management
- Supportive care
- Abx pre/empiric treatment?
- HSV suspected and gram stain (-)
  - ⇨ Acyclovir 10mg/kg IV empiric

7. Other

Non-Convulsive Status Epilepticus
(Emerg Med Clin N Am 2011;29:65-72)

General
- Two types
  - ⇨ Absence (ASE) or complex partial (CPSE): confusion, abnormal behavior
  - ⇨ Subtle (SSE): postictal/comatose → subtle signs (facial/hand twitching)
- More common than is thought (Q J Med 1987;62:117-126)
  - ⇨ Causes: vascular, trauma, metabolic, mass/tumor
- All have AMS which can vary: mild confusion → → Coma

Symptoms
- Varying presentations, suspect in postictal person whose mental status does not improve
- AMS
  - ⇨ Functional: slow mentation, confusion, psychosis, unresponsiveness
  - ⇨ Motor: bizarre gross movements, twitches
  - ⇨ Automatisms: mimicry, verbal, lip smacking, finger picking

Diagnosis
- Three clues
  - ⇨ Abrupt onset
  - ⇨ Fluctuating mental status
  - ⇨ Subtle clinical signs: i.e. eye fluttering, automatisms, tonic eye deviation
- DX: EEG

Management
  - ⇨ If cannot obtain EEG in ER, treat empirically (see Seizure algorithm)
  - ⇨ Treat while continuously monitoring on EEG for titration (with neurology consult)
  - ⇨ Rx: Benzodiazepines and barbiturates

WEAKNESS

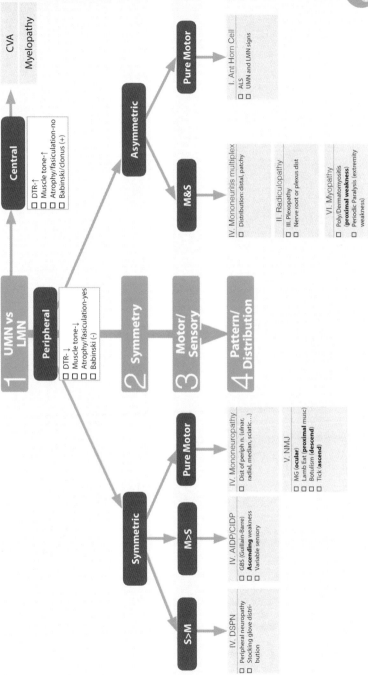

1 UMN vs LMN

Central
- ☐ DTR-↑
- ☐ Muscle tone-↑
- ☐ Atrophy/fasiculation-no
- ☐ Babinski/clonus (+)

- CVA
- Myelopathy

Peripheral
- ☐ DTR- ↓
- ☐ Muscle tone-↓
- ☐ Atrophy/fasiculation-yes
- ☐ Babinski (-)

2 Symmetry

3 Motor/Sensory

4 Pattern/Distribution

Asymmetric

Pure Motor

I. Ant Horn Cell
- ☐ ALS
- ☐ UMN and LMN signs

M&S

IV. Mononeuritis multiplex
- ☐ Distribution: distal, patchy

II. Radiculopathy
- ☐ III. Plexopathy
- ☐ Nerve root or plexus dist

VI. Myopathy
- ☐ Poly/Dermatomyositis (**proximal weakness**)
- ☐ Periodic Paralysis (extremity weakness)

Symmetric

S>M

IV. DSPN
- ☐ Peripheral neuropathy
- ☐ Stocking glove distribution

M>S

IV. AIDP/CIDP
- ☐ GBS (Guillain-Barre) **Ascending** weakness
- ☐ Variable sensory

Pure Motor

IV. Mononeuropathy
- ☐ Dist of periph n. (ulnar, radial, median, sciatic...)

V. NMJ
- ☐ MG (**ocular**)
- ☐ Lamb Eat (**proximal musc**)
- ☐ Botulism (**descend**)
- ☐ Tick (**ascend**)

(+) = "Positive (LMN) type sx" = excitation or increased activity in nervous system
(-) = "Negative (LMN) type sx" = deficit or decreased activity in nervous system

	Symmetry	Motor	Sensory	Pattern/Dist	Other
I. Anterior Horn Cell (ALS)	Asymmetric	(+): fasciculations/cramps; (-): weakness/atrophy	0	Distal; Patchy, asymmetric	☐ UMN (↑reflexes, spastic, hypertonia) signs and; ☐ LMN signs; ☐ Manage airway if in respiratory distress
II. Nerve root (Radiculopathy)	Asymmetric	(+): fasciculations/cramps; (-): weakness/atrophy	(+) pain; (-) paresthesia/hyp/anesthesia	Distal & Proximal; Nerve root distribution	☐ DDx: Cord compression vs systemic disease; ☐ Physical therapy, NSAIDs
III. Plexus (Plexopathy)	Asymmetric	(+): fasciculations/cramps; (-): weakness/atrophy	(+) pain; (-) paresthesia/hyp/anesthesia	Distal & Proximal	☐ Sx of radiculopathy, but not in same distribution (may involve multiple nerve roots/distributions); ☐ e.g. Brachial plexus
IV. Peripheral Nerve (Neuropathy)					
AIDP/CIDP (GBS)	Symmetric	(-): weakness; motor sx predominate	Variable	Distal to proximal (ascending weakness)	☐ DTR(-); ☐ Autonomic sx: hypotension; ☐ Resp sx: intubate at FVC 10-12ml/kg; ☐ MF (Miller Fisher) variant: weakness begins in cranial nerves, descends; ☐ Tx: IVIG
DSPN (Distal Symmetric Polyneuropathy)	Symmetric	(-): weakness; dorsiflex big toe → foot drop → steppage gait	Sensory sx predominate: initial (+) then (-) sx	Distal; Stocking glove distribution, ascending	☐ DDx: DANG THERAPIST; ☐ DM, Amyloid, Nutritional: B12, Guillain-Barre, Toxic, Hereditary, HIV, Endocrine, Recurring Alcohol, Pb (lead), Idiopathic, Sarcoidosis, Thyroid, Lyme
Mononeuropathy	Asymmetric	(+): fasciculations/cramps; (-): weakness/atrophy	(+) pain; (-) paresthesia/hyp/anesthesia	Distal; Distribution of peripheral nerve	☐ 2/2 compression of peripheral nerve; ☐ e.g. radial, median, ulnar, sciatic, lat fem cut
Mononeuritis multiplex	Asymmetric	(+): fasciculations/cramps; (-): weakness/atrophy	(+) pain; (-) paresthesia/hyp/anesthesia	Distal; Patchy, unorganized distribution	☐ DDx: vasculitis, DM, neoplastic, infectious, sarcoid/rheum, Lyme, HIV, amyloid, jellyfish, dapsone

WEEKNESS

{+} = "Positive (LMN) type sx" = excitation or increased activity in nervous system
{-} = "Negative (LMN) type sx" = deficit or decreased activity in nervous system

	Symmetry	Motor	Sensory	Pattern/Dist	Other
V. NMJ					
Myasthenia Gravis	Symmetric	{-} weakness/atrophy	0	**Descending?** Ocular sx: ptosis, diplopia, blurred (85%)	☐ Fatigable, improves w/ rest ☐ Resp sx (17%) → intubation? (use Rocuronium!) ☐ Tension test, Ice pack test ☐ Myasthenic vs Cholinergic crisis
Lambert-Eaton	Symmetric	{-} weakness/atrophy	0	**Proximal** muscle weakness (rise from chair, climb stairs, lift hands)	☐ Sx improve with use, IVIG? ☐ Paraneoplastic syndrome 2/2 malignancy?
Botulism	Symmetric	{-} weakness/atrophy	0	**Descending** flaccid paralysis (like GBS MF variant, MG) Bulbar/CN involved	☐ Pupils: fixed/dilated (vs MG) ☐ Anticholinergic sx ☐ Contaminated food source? Infected wound? ☐ Respiratory distress → intubate, Botulism Ig
Tick Paralysis	Symmetric	{-} weakness/atrophy	0	**Ascending** flaccid paralysis (like GBS)	☐ Pupils: fixed/dilated (vs MG) ☐ Anticholinergic sx ☐ REMOVE TICK!!!
VI. Muscle(Myopathy)					
Inflammatory (PM/DM)	Symmetric	{-} weakness/atrophy	0	**Proximal** muscle weakness Similar to LE (rise from chair, climb stairs, lift arms)	☐ Pain, tender muscles, Elevated CK ☐ Malar rash?
Metabolic	Symmetric	{-} weakness/atrophy	0	**Distal** Extremity weakness	☐ Electrolytes v periodic paralysis (K⁺)

92

VERTIGO

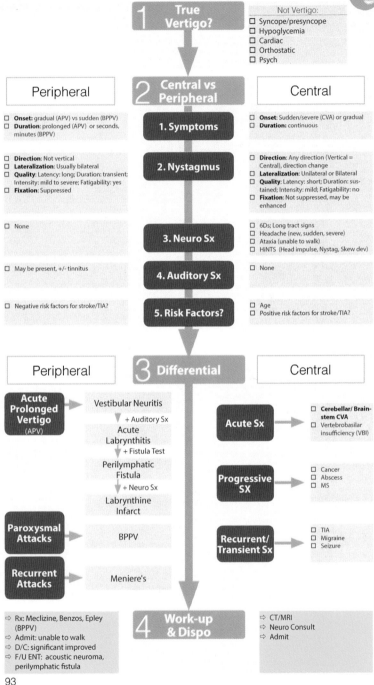

1. True Vertigo?

Not Vertigo:
- ☐ Syncope/presyncope
- ☐ Hypoglycemia
- ☐ Cardiac
- ☐ Orthostatic
- ☐ Psych

2. Central vs Peripheral

Peripheral

1. Symptoms
- ☐ **Onset:** gradual (APV) vs sudden (BPPV)
- ☐ **Duration:** prolonged (APV) or seconds, minutes (BPPV)

2. Nystagmus
- ☐ **Direction:** Not vertical
- ☐ **Lateralization:** Usually bilateral
- ☐ **Quality:** Latency: long; Duration: transient; Intensity: mild to severe; Fatigability: yes
- ☐ **Fixation:** Suppressed

3. Neuro Sx
- ☐ None

4. Auditory Sx
- ☐ May be present, +/- tinnitus

5. Risk Factors?
- ☐ Negative risk factors for stroke/TIA?

Central

1. Symptoms
- ☐ **Onset:** Sudden/severe (CVA) or gradual
- ☐ **Duration:** continuous

2. Nystagmus
- ☐ **Direction:** Any direction (Vertical = Central), direction change
- ☐ **Lateralization:** Unilateral or Bilateral
- ☐ **Quality:** Latency: short; Duration: sustained; Intensity: mild; Fatigability: no
- ☐ **Fixation:** Not suppressed, may be enhanced

3. Neuro Sx
- ☐ 6Ds; Long tract signs
- ☐ Headache (new, sudden, severe)
- ☐ Ataxia (unable to walk)
- ☐ HiNTS (Head impulse, Nystag, Skew dev)

4. Auditory Sx
- ☐ None

5. Risk Factors?
- ☐ Age
- ☐ Positive risk factors for stroke/TIA?

3. Differential

Peripheral

Acute Prolonged Vertigo (APV)
→ Vestibular Neuritis
  ↓ + Auditory Sx
  Acute Labrynthitis
  ↓ + Fistula Test
  Perilymphatic Fistula
  ↓ + Neuro Sx
  Labrynthine Infarct

Paroxysmal Attacks → BPPV

Recurrent Attacks → Meniere's

Central

Acute Sx →
- ☐ **Cerebellar/Brainstem CVA**
- ☐ Vertebrobasilar insufficiency (VBI)

Progressive SX →
- ☐ Cancer
- ☐ Abscess
- ☐ MS

Recurrent/ Transient Sx →
- ☐ TIA
- ☐ Migraine
- ☐ Seizure

4. Work-up & Dispo

Peripheral
- ⇨ Rx: Meclizine, Benzos, Epley (BPPV)
- ⇨ Admit: unable to walk
- ⇨ D/C: significant improved
- ⇨ F/U ENT: acoustic neuroma, perilymphatic fistula

Central
- ⇨ CT/MRI
- ⇨ Neuro Consult
- ⇨ Admit

VERTIGO

1. IS IT TRUE VERTIGO?
(Emerg Med Clin N Am 2012;30:681) (Essentials 2010-Swadron)

- The Approach (Questions)
  - ⇨ Is the dizziness true vertigo
  - ⇨ If so, is it central or peripheral vertigo
  - ⇨ Is the vertigo intermittent → likely benign
  - ⇨ Constant vertigo is either acute peripheral vestibulopathy (APV) or a posterior circulation/cerebellar CVA
- General Dizziness: 4 different etiologies
  - ⇨ Lightheadedness/Presyncope
  - ⇨ Vertigo
  - ⇨ Dysequilibrium (neuromuscular disorder)
  - ⇨ Psychiatric
- Definitions (Rosen's Emerg Med, 6th ed. Ch 13. 2006)
  - ⇨ True Vertigo: disorientation in space combined with a sense of motion
  - ⇨ Hallucination of movement of self (subjective vertigo) or of environment (objective vertigo)

2. CENTRAL VS PERIPHERAL?

General Approach
- Objective for vertigo is differentiating benign peripheral vertigo from life-threatening central vertigo, using the 5 criteria

Symptoms
- Cerebellar CVA: acute onset and continuous
  - ⇨ Other central vertigo is usually more gradual and continuous
- APV: gradual onset and continuous
- BPPV: Acute onset but intermittent

Nystagmus
- Central vertigo:
  - ⇨ Vertical
  - ⇨ Unilateral
  - ⇨ Non-fatigable
  - ⇨ Unsuppressed: not suppressed with fixation of gaze (nystagmus persistent when looking straight at your finger)
  - ⇨ Direction change: direction of nystagmus changes with eccentric gaze
- Vertical nystagmus ddx: central vertigo, PCP, EtOH, drugs

Neurologic symptoms
- Neuro exam: 6Ds of an abnormal neuro exam:
  - ⇨ Dizziness (vertigo)
  - ⇨ Diplopia (double vision)
  - ⇨ Dysphagia (difficulty swallowing)
  - ⇨ Dysarthria (difficulty speaking)
  - ⇨ Dysmetria (cerebellar ataxia)
  - ⇨ Dysdiadochokinesia (impaired ability to perform rapid, alternating movements)
- Long-tract signs
  - ⇨ Motor/sensory loss
- Ataxia
  - ⇨ Central vertigo/cerebellar pts usually unable to walk

6 Ds
☐ Dizziness
☐ Diplopia
☐ Dysphagia
☐ Dysarthria
☐ Dysmetria
☐ Dysdiadochokinesia

Auditory symptoms
- Auditory symptoms a sign of peripheral vertigo (acute labrynthitis)

HiNTS Test (Stroke 2009;40:3504-10)
- Head impulse test (Hi): (NEJM 2003;348:1027-32)
  - ⇨ Bedside test of horizontal VOR (vestibuloocular reflex)
  - ⇨ Start: Head turned to one side and eyes turned 10° from center to same side
  - ⇨ Motion: Apply brief high acceleration head turn so that eyes end looking at examiner's nose
  - ⇨ Test: Catch up saccades on one side, but not the other indicates **peripheral vestibular lesion** on that side
- Nystagmus (N)
  - ⇨ Nystagmus changes direction on eccentric gaze → central lesion
- Skew deviation (TS)
  - ⇨ Eyes are vertically misaligned because of imbalance of vestibular tone → central lesion
  - ⇨ Alternately cover each eye to test for realignment
- Positive test (central lesion-stroke)
  - ⇨ Normal horizontal head impulse test, direction-changing nystagmus in eccentric gaze, or skew deviation (vertical ocular misalignment)
  - ⇨ HINTS Test 100% sensitive, 96% specific for identifying stroke (Stroke 2009;40:3504-10)

Risk factor Assessment
- Isolated vertigo can be the only symptom in cerebellar stroke/TIA and posterior circulation hemorrhage
- Risk factors: Older age, male sex, and the presence of hypertension, coronary artery disease, diabetes mellitus, and atrial fibrillation

VERTIGO

3. PERIPHERAL VERTIGO

VESTIBULOPATHY (APV)
(NEJM 2003;348:1027-32)

Definition
- APV= Acute Peripheral Vestibulopathy or Acute Prolonged Vertigo
  - ⇨ Prolonged vertigo definition: continuous vertigo lasting more than a few hours
  - ⇨ Self limited, likely viral cause for symptoms → affecting peripheral vestibular portion of CN8
- Clinical
  - ⇨ Sx: gradual onset and continuous vertigo
  - ⇨ Neuro: Normal neuro exam and non-concerning type of nystagmus
  - ⇨ Head thrust test: positive, catch up saccades on one side

VESTIBULAR NEURITIS
- Clinical Presentation
  - ⇨ Develops over hours and resolves over days, usually post-viral
  - ⇨ May mimic infarct type symptoms
- Treatment
  - ⇨ General (Antihistamines, anticholinergics, anti-emetics, benzodiazepines)
  - ⇨ Directed treatment: Dexamethasone, valacyclovir

ACUTE LABYRINTHITIS
- Subtypes
  - ⇨ Toxic: usually medication induced, has auditory sx and tinnitus
  - ⇨ Serous: associated ENT infection, May have fever
  - ⇨ Suppurative: severe sx, febrile, toxic →Admit, IV Abx, ENT C/S

LABYRINTHINE INFARCT
- Abrupt onset, h/o vascular dz, associated with neuro signs (also considered central type vertigo)

PERILYMPHATIC FISTULA
- Associated with trauma, lifting, coughing, sneezing
- **Fistula test:** Vertigo and nystagmus induced by pressure in the external ear canal

BPPV

Etiology
- Free floating debris in posterior semicircular canal

Clinical
- Abrupt onset of vertigo seconds after change in head position, **lasting less than a minute**.

Diagnosis
- **Dix-Hallpike**
  - ⇨ Use: for diagnosis, presence of paroxysmal positional nystagmus is most reliable finding in patients with BPPV (Am J Otol 1995;16:806-10)
  - ⇨ Procedure:
    - ✓ Start: Seated with head turned 45° to side being tested
    - ✓ Motion: Quickly lower to supine position with head angled backward 45° off bed
    - ✓ Test positive: Nystagmus with affected side down, can continue to Epley from this position for treatment
    - ✓ Nystagmus is delayed in onset, fatiguable, and decreases with fixation

Treatment
- Canalith Repositioning Maneuvers
  - ⇨ **Epley and Semont** (Ann Emerg Med 2001;37:392-8)
    - ✓ See reference or **EMRAP.TV** Episode 9 for description of procedure
    - ✓ May not be better than standard medical therapy (J Emerg Med 2014;46(4):575)

MENIERE'S

Clinical
- Attacks of vertigo preceded/accompanied by **reduced hearing, tinnitus and pressure in ear**
- Attacks followed by residual hearing loss

Treatment
- Dietary restrictions (salt, caffeine, tobacco), Lasix, Betahistine, ENT referral

Other causes of Peripheral Vertigo
- Ear canal foreign body, trauma (labyrinth concussion), otitis media, cerumen impaction, medication (amino-glycosides)

VERTIGO

4. CENTRAL VERTIGO

CEREBELLAR STROKE
(Essentials 2011 "Stroke or Vertigo?" – Weingart)

Clinical Scenario
- Symptoms
  - ⇨ Sudden onset/continuous vertigo
  - ⇨ +/- Severe headache
- Nystagmus
  - ⇨ Vertical, unilateral, nonfatigable, unsupressed
  - ⇨ Skew deviation
- Neurologic symptoms
  - ⇨ 5Ds (Dizziness, Dysphagia, Dysphonia, Dysmetria, Diplopia)
  - ⇨ Long tract signs (motor/sensory)
  - ⇨ Ataxia (unable to ambulate)
- Isolated vertigo
  - ⇨ Definition: no other symptoms present except for vertigo
  - ⇨ May simulate sx of vestibular neuritis (VN)
  - ⇨ Cerebellar CVA vs VN (Neurology 2006;67:1178-83)
    - ✓ 10% isolated cerebellar infarct pts present with isolated vertigo symptoms (VN sx)
    - ✓ No patients with cerebellar infarct had a positive head thrust test

Caution!
10% isolated cerebellar infarct pts present with isolated vertigo

Diagnosis
- CT
  - ⇨ Can identify acute hemorrhage
  - ⇨ Not sensitive for acute stroke (especially of posterior fossa)
  - ⇨ Can identify large posterior CVA or mass effect (closed 4th ventricle)
- MRI
  - ⇨ Modality of choice to r/o infarctions
  - ⇨ Indication: (NEJM 1998;339:680-5)
    - ✓ **Neurologic** signs/symptoms
    - ✓ **Sudden onset** of vertigo in a patient with risk factors for stroke
    - ✓ **Headache**: new, severe headache accompanying the vertigo

MRI for Vertigo
☐ **Neurologic** symptoms
☐ **Sudden onset** of vertigo + stroke risk factors
☐ **Headache**: new and severe

HEADACHE

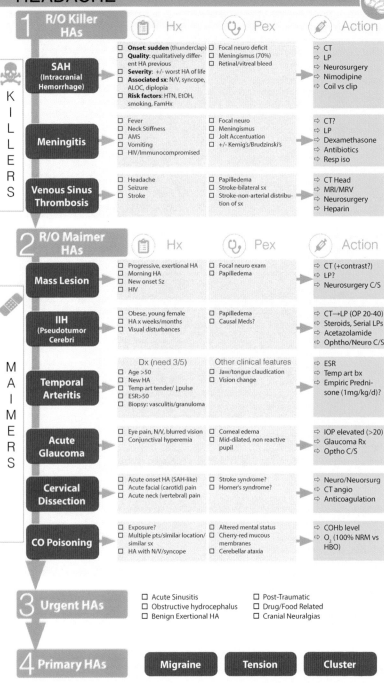

1 R/O Killer HAs

	Hx	Pex	Action

KILLERS

SAH (Intracranial Hemorrhage)
- ☐ **Onset: sudden** (thunderclap)
- ☐ **Quality**: qualitatively different HA previous
- ☐ **Severity**: +/- worst HA of life
- ☐ **Associated sx**: N/V, syncope, ALOC, diplopia
- ☐ **Risk factors**: HTN, EtOH, smoking, FamHx

Pex:
- ☐ Focal neuro deficit
- ☐ Meningismus (70%)
- ☐ Retinal/vitreal bleed

Action:
- ⇨ CT
- ⇨ LP
- ⇨ Neurosurgery
- ⇨ Nimodipine
- ⇨ Coil vs clip

Meningitis
- ☐ Fever
- ☐ Neck Stiffness
- ☐ AMS
- ☐ Vomiting
- ☐ HIV/Immunocompromised

Pex:
- ☐ Focal neuro
- ☐ Meningismus
- ☐ Jolt Accentuation
- ☐ +/- Kernig's/Brudzinski's

Action:
- ⇨ CT?
- ⇨ LP
- ⇨ Dexamethasone
- ⇨ Antibiotics
- ⇨ Resp iso

Venous Sinus Thrombosis
- ☐ Headache
- ☐ Seizure
- ☐ Stroke

Pex:
- ☐ Papilledema
- ☐ Stroke-bilateral sx
- ☐ Stroke-non-arterial distribution of sx

Action:
- ⇨ CT Head
- ⇨ MRI/MRV
- ⇨ Neurosurgery
- ⇨ Heparin

2 R/O Maimer HAs

	Hx	Pex	Action

MAIMERS

Mass Lesion
- ☐ Progressive, exertional HA
- ☐ Morning HA
- ☐ New onset Sz
- ☐ HIV

Pex:
- ☐ Focal neuro exam
- ☐ Papilledema

Action:
- ⇨ CT (+contrast?)
- ⇨ LP?
- ⇨ Neurosurgery C/S

IIH (Pseudotumor Cerebri)
- ☐ Obese, young female
- ☐ HA x weeks/months
- ☐ Visual disturbances

Pex:
- ☐ Papilledema
- ☐ Causal Meds?

Action:
- ⇨ CT→LP (OP 20-40)
- ⇨ Steroids, Serial LPs
- ⇨ Acetazolamide
- ⇨ Ophtho/Neuro C/S

Temporal Arteritis
Dx (need 3/5)
- ☐ Age >50
- ☐ New HA
- ☐ Temp art tender/ ↓pulse
- ☐ ESR>50
- ☐ Biopsy: vasculitis/granuloma

Other clinical features
- ☐ Jaw/tongue claudication
- ☐ Vision change

Action:
- ⇨ ESR
- ⇨ Temp art bx
- ⇨ Empiric Prednisone (1mg/kg/d)?

Acute Glaucoma
- ☐ Eye pain, N/V, blurred vision
- ☐ Conjunctival hyperemia

Pex:
- ☐ Corneal edema
- ☐ Mid-dilated, non reactive pupil

Action:
- ⇨ IOP elevated (>20)
- ⇨ Glaucoma Rx
- ⇨ Optho C/S

Cervical Dissection
- ☐ Acute onset HA (SAH-like)
- ☐ Acute facial (carotid) pain
- ☐ Acute neck (vertebral) pain

Pex:
- ☐ Stroke syndrome?
- ☐ Horner's syndrome?

Action:
- ⇨ Neuro/Neuorsurg
- ⇨ CT angio
- ⇨ Anticoagulation

CO Poisoning
- ☐ Exposure?
- ☐ Multiple pts/similar location/similar sx
- ☐ HA with N/V/syncope

Pex:
- ☐ Altered mental status
- ☐ Cherry-red mucous membranes
- ☐ Cerebellar ataxia

Action:
- ⇨ COHb level
- ⇨ O_2 (100% NRM vs HBO)

3 Urgent HAs
- ☐ Acute Sinusitis
- ☐ Obstructive hydrocephalus
- ☐ Benign Exertional HA
- ☐ Post-Traumatic
- ☐ Drug/Food Related
- ☐ Cranial Neuralgias

4 Primary HAs

Migraine **Tension** **Cluster**

HEADACHE

1. R/O KILLER HEADACHES

(Ann Emerg Med 2008;52:407-436)(Emerg Med Clin NA 2010;28:127-147)

General Approach:
- Emergency department evaluation relies on excluding life-threatening causes of HA (killers), specifically SAH and meningitis
- Then consider other serious causes of headache that can debilitate the patient (the maimers)
- When these have been excluded, we can then diagnose primary headache syndromes.

Testing
- Question 1: **Does this patient need a CT?** (ACEP Guidelines Ann Emerg Med 2008;52:407)
  - ⇨ Neuro exam-new abnormal findings (focal deficit, AMS) (ACEP Level B)
  - ⇨ New, sudden, severe HA
  - ⇨ HIV + with new HA
  - ⇨ Patients older than 50 with new type of HA (ACEP Level C)
- Question 2: **Does this patient need an LP?**
  - ⇨ R/O SAH: Sudden-onset, severe headache + CT Head (-) → LP to r/o SAH (ACEP Level B)
  - ⇨ Concern for Meningitis (Cell count, OP, gram stain)
  - ⇨ Concern for Idiopathic Intracranial Hypertension (Opening pressure)

SUBARACHNOID HEMORRHAGE

(J Emerg Med 2008;34:237-51) (Essentials 2011 "Bloody CSF" – Swadron)(EM:RAP 6/12-Swadron)

Clinical presentation
- **Onset: sudden (thunderclap)**
  - ⇨ Maximum severity is reached instantaneously in 50% and within 1-5 minutes in 19% of patients with SAH. (J Neurol Neurosurg Psychiatry 1998;65:791-3)
  - ⇨ Sudden severe HA: (Lancet 1994;344:590-3)
    - ✓ SAH in 25%
    - ✓ Benign thunderclap HA in 40%
    - ✓ Remaining will have another primary or secondary HA
  - ⇨ Therefore, all patients with sudden severe HA need to be worked-up for SAH

SAH HA Red Flags
☐ Sudden onset
☐ Maximal at onset
☐ Different from previous HAs

- Other qualities
  - ⇨ Quality: qualitatively different HA from previous
  - ⇨ Severity: +/- worst HA of life
  - ⇨ Associated sx: N/V, syncope, ALOC, diplopia
  - ⇨ Risk factors: HTN, EtOH, smoking, Fam Hx
- PEX:
  - ⇨ Focal neuro deficit
  - ⇨ Meningismus (70%)
  - ⇨ Retinal/vitreal bleed
- Clinical Presentation of SAH lies on a spectrum (Emerg Med Clin N Am 2003;21:73-87)
  - ⇨ The classic (middle of the spectrum) presentation is that of sudden onset and distinct HA, worst of their life associated with neck pain, N/V
  - ⇨ On the extreme end, they can present with focal neuro deficit and ALOC/AMS
  - ⇨ On the subtle end **1/3 present with only HA** without neuro deficits, and are likely to be misdiagnosed

Work-up
- **CT Head**
  - ⇨ CT sensitivity is extremely high early but rapidly diminishes with time
  - ⇨ Misses about 2% of SAH within 12 hours and 7% by 24 hours
  - ⇨ Therefore anyone with suspected SAH and normal CT requires an LP
  - ⇨ Journal Club (EM:RAP 3/14; 12/13)
    - ✓ CT within 6 hours (BMJ 2011;343:d4277)
      - i. Overall CT sensitivity is 93% (Sensitivity after 6h is 86%)
      - ii. CT **within 6 hours** of HA onset → Sensitivity 100%, Specificity 100%, NPV 100%
      - iii. Prospective cohort study
    - ✓ CT within 6 hours (Stroke 2012;43:2115)
      - i. CT within 6 hours of HA onset → Sensitivity 100% with 2 caveats
      - ii. Caveat 1: <6h rule only applies to pts with HA (not neck pain)
      - iii. Caveat 2: Experienced neuroradiologists needed to interpret CT
    - ✓ Editorial (Stroke 2012;43:2031)
      - i. "... we believe that practice should change. Neurologically intact patients who present with thunderclap headache and undergo **CT scan within 6 hours of symptom onset no longer need an LP** to exclude SAH if the CT scan is negative."

HEADACHE

- **Lumbar Puncture**
  - ⇨ Timing: Results depends on timing of HA (J Emerg Med 2002;23:67-74)
  - ⇨ <12h:
    - ✓ Xanthochromia may/may not be present; large RBCs should be present
    - ✓ Incompletely clearing RBCs?? (if suspected traumatic tap → repeat at different interspace)
  - ⇨ 12h-2weeks:
    - ✓ Xanthochromia highly suggestive of SAH; large RBC +/- present
  - ⇨ >2weeks: Both may be absent.

Treatment (See ICH Algorithm)
- ABC/Resus/Airway
  - ⇨ Treat like ICH patient
  - ⇨ Intubate if AMS, not protecting airway → document good neurologic exam prior
- Emergent Neurosurgical consultation
- Vasospasm prevention
  - ⇨ Nimodipine 60 mg po/NG q4h x 21d

MENINGITIS

(Emerg Med Clin N Am 2008;26:281-317) (Essentials "Meningitis: Bacterial vs Aseptic" 2011 – Williams)

Etiology
- Bacterial
  - ⇨ Meningococcus (Neisseria meningitidis)
  - ⇨ Streptococcus pneumoniae
  - ⇨ Haemophilus influenzae
  - ⇨ Listeria monocytogenes
- Viral
  - ⇨ Enteroviruses (≈ 85% of meningitis)
  - ⇨ Arboviruses (West Nile, etc...)
  - ⇨ Herpes viruses
  - ⇨ Others (Mumps, LCMV etc...)

Meningitis sx:	
Fever	85%
Stiff neck	70%
AMS	67%
HA	50%
Focal neuro	23%
Rash	22%

Clinical Presentation
- Classic triad
  - ⇨ All 3: fever, neck stiffness and AMS present in only 44%
    - ✓ Absence of all 3 virtually eliminates a diagnosis of meningitis
  - ⇨ 95% patients had 2 out of 4 of: (NEJM 2004;351:1849-59)
    - ✓ Headache
    - ✓ Fever
    - ✓ Neck stiffness
    - ✓ AMS
- Meningismus
  - ⇨ Jolt accentuation (JAMA 1999;282(2):175-81)
    - ✓ Procedure: Ask patient to turn head right/left, 2-3 rotations per second
    - ✓ Positive test: Worsening of headache
    - ✓ Absence of jolt accentuation has a sensitivity of 100% for ruling out meningitis
  - ⇨ Kernig's sign (inability to straighten the leg when the hip is flexed to 90 degrees)
  - ⇨ Brudzinski's sign (forced flexion of the neck elicits a reflex flexion of the hips)
    - ✓ Kernig/Brudzinski both have very low sensitivity ≈ 5%
- Other symptoms:
  - ⇨ Abnormal neurologic exam
  - ⇨ Leg pain, refusal to walk (Meningococcus)
  - ⇨ Photophobia, N/V, lethargy
  - ⇨ Petechial rash (Meningococcus)

Bottom Line
  - ⇨ **Triad**: Absence of all of the triad (fever, AMS, neck stiffness) → eliminates a diagnosis of meningitis
  - ⇨ **Meningismus**: Kernig/Brudzinski are not helpful in ruling out meningitis (low sensitivity)
    - ✓ If they are positive → can rule in meningitis (high specificity)
  - ⇨ **Jolt accentuation** negative essentially eliminates a diagnosis of meningitis

Work-up
- Lumbar puncture
  - ⇨ Tube 1&4: Cell count and diff
  - ⇨ Tube 2: glucose and protein
  - ⇨ Tube 3: Gram stain, culture, HSV PCR
- Do I need a **CT before LP**? (2 studies say not always) MAY omit if:
  - ⇨ Age<60, no immunocompromised/CNS disease/seizure within 1 week and has a non-focal neuro exam
    (NEJM 2001;345:1727-1733)
  - ⇨ Absence of AMS, focal neuro exam, papilledema and favorable clinical impression by doctor (Ann Int Med 1999;159:2681-2685)

HEADACHE

- CSF analysis (predictive of bacterial meningitis) (JAMA. 1989;262(19):2700)
  - ⇨ ↑WBC > 2000
    - ✓ Multiple studies show bacterial meningitis incidence of 5-19% in patients with CSF WBC < 100!
    - ✓ No single variable can r/o meningitis
  - ⇨ Neutrophil > 1180
  - ⇨ CSF glucose <34mg/dL
  - ⇨ CSF protein > 220 mg/dL
  - ⇨ Gram stain +

Treatment
- **Antibiotics**
  - ⇨ Timing
    - ✓ Administer as soon as possible-before LP
    - ✓ Multiple studies have shown an association between time of antibiotic administration and poor outcome (greater than 4-6 hours)
  - ⇨ Empiric antibiotics
    - ✓ Ceftriaxone 2gm IV or Cefotaxime 2gm IV immediately +
    - ✓ Vancomycin 1gm IV (15-20mg/kg) +
    - ✓ Ampicillin 2gm IV (adults > 50yo)
  - ⇨ Antimicrobial Choice: (CID 2004:39:1267-84) (see table)
- **Dexamethasone**
  - ⇨ Dose: 10mg IV q 6 hour x 4 days; start 15 minutes prior to, or with first dose of antibiotics
  - ⇨ Journal club (Cochrane Database 2010;9:CD00405)
    - ✓ No mortality benefit but helps prevent hearing loss and short-term neurologic sequelae
    - ✓ Benefits seen mostly in patients with *S. pneumoniae*
- **Acyclovir**
  - ⇨ Dose: 10mg/kg q 8h for HSV

Special Case: HA and HIV (CD4 < 200?)
- CT w/wo contrast:
  - ⇨ R/O mass lesion, toxo, lymphoma
- Serum
  - ⇨ If serum crypto Ag(-) → likely do not need LP (patient very unlikely to have crypto infection)
- Lumbar puncture
  - ⇨ Use: r/o cryptococcal meningitis
  - ⇨ India ink: round encapsulated yeast (75% patients)
  - ⇨ CSF crypto Ag: Sensitivity 93 to 100% and specificities 93 to 98%
  - ⇨ CSF culture: definitive diagnosis
- Treatment: Amphotericin + Fluconazole

CEREBRAL VENOUS THROMBOSIS
(EM:RAP 10-08) (Essentials 2009-D Williams)

General
- CVT = DVT of the brain = blood clots in brain (venous)
- CVT = Dural sinus thrombosis, (superior, sagittal, inferior) sinus thrombosis, cortical vein thrombosis

Risk factors
- Thrombophilia/Hypercoagulable state
- Pregnancy/Puerperium
- Medications (OCPs, Doxycycline)
- Cancer/Inflammatory/Hematologic disease

Clinical
- Presentation spectrum: HA → Seizure → Stroke
- Headache
  - ⇨ Headache type: No characteristic history, multiple types of HA symptoms
  - ⇨ PEX- Papilledema present in most cases (fundoscopic, pan-optic or US)
- Seizure
- Stroke
  - ⇨ Bilateral neuro deficit
  - ⇨ Non-arterial distribution

Diagnosis
- D-dimer-low sensitivity, not useful
- CT Head-normal in 30% of cases
  - ⇨ Highly suggestive:
    - ✓ Dense triangle sign (thrombosed sup sag sinus posteriorly)
    - ✓ Cord sign (thrombosed cortical vein)
    - ✓ Bilateral edema/ICH
  - ⇨ Diagnostic (CT w/ contrast-venogram): Empty delta sign (flow defect in sup sag sinus)
- MR Brain with venography (study of choice)

HEADACHE

Complications
- ICH → Coma → Death
- PE

Treatment
- Neurosurgical consultation
- Anticoagulation
  - ⇨ Heparin safe, even with hemorrhagic infarcts
- Journal Club-**Heparin anticoagulation**
  - ⇨ Cochrane Review of Heparin anticoagulation (Cochrane Database Syst Rev 2001;(4))
    - ✓ RR of death 0.33 (95% CI 0.08-1.21) → not statistically significant
    - ✓ Conclusion: CVT is a rare and fatal disease and no other treatment exists
  - ⇨ ISCVT-International Study on Cerebral vein and Dural Venous Thrombosis (Stroke 2004;35:664-70)
    - ✓ Prospective observational study 624 patients → 80% received anticoagulation
    - ✓ 6.8% mortality

2. R/O MAIMER HAs

BRAIN MASS LESION

Etiology
- Tumor, abscess, chronic SDH

Clinical Presentation
- Progressive, exertional HA, morning HA
- New onset seizure, nausea/vomiting
- H/O HIV (cryptococcus, toxoplasmosis, lymphoma, and tuberculosis)
- PEX: Focal neuro exam, papilledema, aphasia

Work-up
- CT Head w/wo contrast, MRI

Treatment
- Neurosurgical consultation, steroids, ventriculostomy

Vasogenic edema
- Etiology: tumor related disruption of BBB
- Treatment
  - ⇨ Glucocorticoids- indicated in all patients with peri-tumor edema
  - ⇨ Dexamethasone 10mg IV x 1 then 4mg IV q6h

HYDROCEPHALUS
- Cause: CNS infection, hemorrhage, tumor
- Types
  - ⇨ Communicating hydrocephalus
    - ✓ Symmetric dilation of all 4 ventricles
    - ✓ Extraventricular obstruction or impaired CSF absorption, usually in neonates/infants;
    - ✓ Adult causes: pseudotumor cerebri
  - ⇨ Non-communicating (Obstructive) hydrocephalus
    - ✓ Asymmetric dilation of ventricles
- Treatment
  - ⇨ Third Ventriculostomy-only effective for obstructive hydrocephalus
  - ⇨ Shunt (VP-Shunt)-can be used to treat either cause of hydrocephalus

SHUNT COMPLICATIONS
- **Shunt Infection (Ventriculitis)**
  - ⇨ 5 to 15 percent of procedures, most occurring in first 6 months
  - ⇨ Persistent fever → tap shunt
  - ⇨ Antibiotics, shunt may need removal
- **Shunt mechanical failure** (obstruction at the ventricular catheter)
  - ⇨ CT: Hydrocephalus
- **Overdrainage**
  - ⇨ Presentation: neurological symptoms → postural headache and nausea
  - ⇨ CT: Slit ventricle syndrome (small or slit-like ventricles)

HEADACHE

IIH

(EM:RAP 8/11 – Aubin)

General
- AKA Idiopathic Intracranial Hypertension, Pseudotumor cerebri

Presentation
- Obese, young female
- HA x weeks/months
- Visual disturbances
- Papilledema
  - ⇨ Not all patients with IIH have papilledema

Diagnosis
- Diagnostic criteria for IIH: (Neurology 2002;59:1492-95)
  1. S/Sx of elevated intracranial pressure
  2. Non focal neuro exam (except abducens nerve paresis)
  3. Normal neuroimaging study (CT w/ con or MRI/MRV)
  4. Increased CSF pressure (nonobese>200; obese>250 mm water)
  5. No other cause of increased intracranial pressure (CNS tumor, encephalitis, right heart failure)
- **Vision loss** secondary to papilledema is the only serious complication of IIH, is avoidable with appropriate treatment
- MRI/MRV to exclude CVT

Treatment
- Indications for treatment: Vision loss (emergent tx), headache (therapeutic)
- Weight loss
- Medications
  - ⇨ Acetazolamide (carbonic anhydrase inhibitor) reduces CSF pressure
  - ⇨ Topiramate (partial CAI) reduces CSF pressure
- Surgical
  - ⇨ VP Shunt (vision loss and HA refractory to treatment)
  - ⇨ Optic nerve sheath fenestration
  - ⇨ Venous stenting

TEMPORAL ARTERITIS

Clinical Presentation
- New HA
- Temp art tender/decr pulse
- Jaw/tongue claudication
- Vision change

Diagnosis (need 3/5)
- Age >50
- New HA
- Temp art tender/decr pulse
- ESR>50
- Biopsy: vasculitis/granuloma

Treatment
- No ischemic organ damage (eg, visual loss)→ begin empiric prednisone 40-60mg if medium or high suspicion until ESR or biopsy results return.
- Ischemic organ damage (AION)-Vision loss → Methylprednisolone 1000mg IV daily x 3 days

ACUTE GLAUCOMA

(See Acute Vision Loss Algorithm)

Clinical Presentation
- Eye pain, N/V, blurred vision
- Conjunctival hyperemia
- Corneal edema, mid-dilated, non reactive pupil
- Elevated IOP (>20)

Treatment
- Emergent Ophthalmology consultation
- Decrease IOP [See PDR for current recommendations and dosing]
  - ⇨ 0.5% timolol maleate (Timoptic)
  - ⇨ 1% apraclonidine (Iopidine)
  - ⇨ 2% pilocarpine (Isopto Carpine)
  - ⇨ Acetazolamide 500mg IV then 500mg po

HEADACHE

CERVICAL ARTERY DISSECTION
(EM:RAP 4-2011) (see Blunt Neck Trauma Algorithm)

General
- Cervical artery dissection = carotid artery dissection + vertebral artery dissection
- Common cause of pediatric strokes (1 in 5)
- Cause:
  ⇨ Major trauma: penetrating or blunt
  ⇨ Minor trauma: coughing, whiplash, cervical seatbelt signs, rotational routine neck movement, chiropractor manipulation

Presentation
- Stroke syndromes:
  ⇨ **Carotid artery dissection**: MCA, anterior circulation stroke syndromes (hemiplegia)
  ⇨ **Vertebral artery dissection**: posterior fossa symptoms (ataxia, vertigo, dysmetria)
  ⇨ **Wallenberg Syndrome**: ipsilateral facial numbness, contalateral body numbness
  ⇨ **Horner's Syndrome**: miosis, ptosis, anhydrosis (vertebral & carotid artery dissection)
- Facial (carotid), neck (vertebral) pain
- SAH like acute onset
- Cranial nerve abnormalities

Diagnosis
- Carotid duplex-poor sensitivity
- CT Angiography
- MRI/MRA
- Angiography

Treatment
- Neurological/Neurosurgery consultation
- Anticoagulation
  ⇨ Contraindicated if concomitant cerebral hemorrhage
  ⇨ Used to decrease risk of thrombus formation and embolization

CO POISONING

History and Physical
- Exposure?
- Multiple pts/similar location/similar sx
- HA with N/V/syncope
- Altered mental status
- Cherry-red mucous membranes
- Cerebellar ataxia

Action
- COHb level
- O_2 (100% NRM vs HBO)

3. URGENT HEADACHES
- Acute Sinusitis
- Obstructive hydrocephalus
- Benign Exertional HA
- Post-Traumatic
- Drug/Food Related
- Cranial Neuralgias

HEADACHE

4. PRIMARY HEADACHES

MIGRAINE HEADACHE

Presentation
- Common migraine
  - ⇨ Severe, throbbing, unilateral HA
  - ⇨ Photo/Phonophobia
  - ⇨ Hours to days
- Classic migraine
  - ⇨ Preceded by aura
  - ⇨ +/- GI distress
- POUNDing mnemonic
  - ⇨ Pulsating, duration 4-72 hOurs, Unilateral, Nausea, Disabling
  - ⇨ Highly predictive of migraine headache (JAMA 2006;296:1274-83)

Treatment
- IV Dopamine antagonist (Compazine, Reglan)
- IVF (Normal Saline)
- Opiates
- Triptans/NSAIDS
- Dexamethasone

CLUSTER HEADACHE

Presentation
- Middle aged men
- Sudden onset HA
- Unilateral blur vision/nasal congest/lacrimate/salivate/ sweat
- Lasts hours, recur same time of day
- Precipitated by exertion/stress

Treatment
- O_2
- Symptomatic relief
- Intranasal lidocaine
- Neurology referral

TENSION HEADACHE

Presentation
- Frontal/occipital/band-like
- No preceding event

Treatment
- Symptomatic relief (NSAIDS, Tylenol)

ACUTE CVA

1 Initial Eval

- ☐ ABCs
- ☐ IV/O₂/Monitor
- ☐ Airway compromise? Intubation?
- ☐ Asses neuro deficits
- ☐ Time of onset
- ☐ Severity? Stroke Scale (eg NIHSS)

2 True Stroke?

R/O Stroke Mimic
- ☐ Psychogenic
- ☐ Seizures
- ☐ Hypoglycemia
- ☐ Migraine with aura (complicated migraine)
- ☐ Hypertensive encephalopathy
- ☐ Other (Wernicke's, CNS tumor, Drugs, Bell's palsy, peripheral neuropathy)

3 Imaging (CT Head)

R/O ICH → See ICH Algorithm

ID Occlusive Vessel

ID Infarct

4 t-PA Candidate?

<3h onset

3-4.5h onset → See t-PA Algorithm

5 Other Stroke Treatments

Antiplatelet
- ⇨ ASA 325mg po within 24-48h
- ⇨ Plavix?

BP Control
- t-PA → Treat to goal BP < 180/105
- No t-PA → Consider treatment for BP>220/120

Neurology Consult

Endovascular?

Indications?
- ☐ Large vessel stroke
- ☐ Favorable penumbral pattern

6 Cause?

Acute thrombosis
Embolism-Cardiac
Embolism-Other
- ☐ Labs/Hypercoag
- ☐ EKG
- ☐ Echo TTE/TEE
- ☐ Carotid Duplex

ACUTE CVA

1. Initial Evaluation

(Review-Emergency Medicine Clinics of NA 2012:30) (CMEDownload: UCSF "Pitfalls in Stroke")
(AHA Guidelines-Stroke. 2013;44:870-947)

Initial Resuscitation

- Unstable?: If patient unstable, begin with ABCs and resuscitate as needed before a diagnosis is determined
- **Airway compromise?**
  - ⇨ Think: posterior circulation, brainstem ischemic stroke syndromes, massive anterior ischemic strokes, and hemorrhagic strokes
  - ⇨ **Intubation?:** May require airway protection/intubation because of altered level of consciousness (GCS<8, not protecting airway).
- Hypoxia: Common occurrence in acute stroke, treat with supplemental O_2

Asses neurologic deficit

- Timing of onset of symptoms (t_0)
  - ⇨ If patient **awoke with symptoms or unknown when symptoms started** → when was patient last awake and symptom-free or known to be normal?
  - ⇨ Neurological symptoms that completely **resolved, then recurred** → clock is reset and the time of symptom onset begins again
- Initial tests
  - ⇨ Blood glucose, CBC, CMP, cardiac markers, PT/PTT/INR
  - ⇨ Consider: Tox screen, Pregnancy, EKG, CXR
- Stroke severity measurement
  - ⇨ Use: quantify the degree of neurological deficits, facilitate communication, identify the location of vessel occlusion, provide early prognosis, help select patients for various interventions, and identify the potential for complications
  - ⇨ NIHSS (Stroke 1997; 28:307) go to www.mdcalc.com
- Cortical vs Lacunar stroke (Essentials 2011 "Cortical vs Lacunar")
  - ⇨ **Cortical** (as opposed to lacunar) has:
    - ✓ Altered sensorium
    - ✓ Motor AND Sensory deficit
    - ✓ Decreased higher executive function (language or neglect)
    - ✓ Poorer prognosis (large territory involved→ cerebral edema)

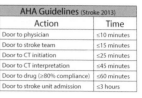

AHA Guidelines (Stroke 2013)	
Action	Time
Door to physician	≤10 minutes
Door to stroke team	≤15 minutes
Door to CT initiation	≤25 minutes
Door to CT interpretation	≤45 minutes
Door to drug (≥80% compliance)	≤60 minutes
Door to stroke unit admission	≤3 hours

2. R/O Stroke Mimic (3% patients)

(Stroke. 2009;40:1522–1525)(Emerg Med Clin N Am 2012;30:795–804)

Possible stroke mimics:

- **Psychogenic**-lack of objective cranial nerve findings, neurological findings in a nonvascular distribution, inconsistent examination
- **Seizures**-History of seizures, witnessed seizure activity, postictal period
- **Hypoglycemia**-History of diabetes, low serum glucose, decreased level of consciousness
- **Migraine with aura** (complicated migraine) -History of similar events, preceding aura, headache
- **Hypertensive encephalopathy**-Headache, delirium, significant hypertension, cortical blindness, cerebral edema, seizure
- **Wernicke's encephalopathy**-History of alcohol abuse, ataxia, ophthalmoplegia, confusion
- **CNS abscess**-History of drug abuse, endocarditis, medical device implant with fever
- **CNS tumor**-Gradual progression of symptoms, other primary malignancy, seizure at onset
- **Drug toxicity**-Lithium, phenytoin, carbamazepine

3. Imaging (R/O hemorrhage)

Goal

1. **Rule out hemorrhage (most important!)**
2. May identify the **occluded vessel**
3. May identify the **infarcted area** as well as the surrounding **ischemic penumbra** (depending on the imaging modality and elapsed time from the onset of symptoms)

CT Head

- **Noncontrast head CT scan is the initial imaging modality of choice**
- Perform within 25 minutes and interpret within 45 minutes of the patient's arrival (recommended in the 2010 AHA/ASA guidelines)
- Early infarct signs (cerebral ischemia)
  - ⇨ Loss of gray-white differentiation
    - ✓ Lenticular obscuration → loss of distinction among the nuclei of the basal ganglia
    - ✓ Insular ribbon sign → blending of the densities of the cortex and underlying white matter in the insula
    - ✓ Cortical ribbon sign → blending of the densities of the cortex and underlying white matter in the convexities
  - ⇨ Swelling of the gyri that produces sulcal effacement

ACUTE CVA

- MCA sign → increased density within the occluded artery, indicative of large-vessel occlusion
- MCA "dot" sign → clot within a branch of the MCA, smaller than the thrombus volume in the MCA and possibly a better target for intravenous t-PA

CT Angiography (CTA)
- Noninvasive gold standard imaging modality for locating occluded intracranial vessels.

MRI
- Excels at isolating even smaller areas of ischemia; higher sensitivity
- Diffusion-weighted MRI (DWI):
  - ⇨ Detects very early ischemic insults within the first few minutes
  - ⇨ Detects lesions in the posterior fossa (CT cannot)
- Full MRI sequence:
  - ⇨ DWI, perfusion-weighted, magnetic resonance angiography (MRA), gradient echo (GRE), and fluid-attenuated inversion recovery (FLAIR) sequences

4. T-PA CANDIDATE?

(Essentials 2012-"The Key is Consent")

Indication
- Intravenous fibrinolytic therapy is recommended in the setting of early ischemic changes (other than frank hypodensity) on CT, regardless of their extent (Class I; Level of Evidence A)

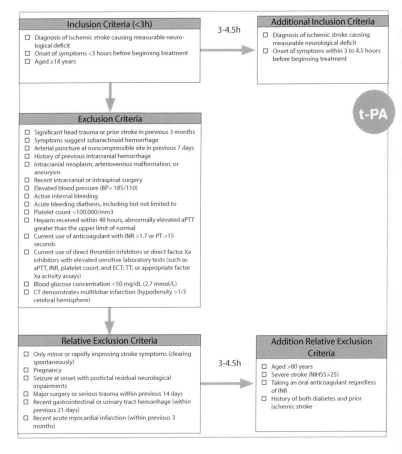

Inclusion Criteria (<3h)
- ☐ Diagnosis of ischemic stroke causing measurable neurological deficit
- ☐ Onset of symptoms <3 hours before beginning treatment
- ☐ Aged ≥18 years

3-4.5h →

Additional Inclusion Criteria
- ☐ Diagnosis of ischemic stroke causing measurable neurological deficit
- ☐ Onset of symptoms within 3 to 4.5 hours before beginning treatment

Exclusion Criteria
- ☐ Significant head trauma or prior stroke in previous 3 months
- ☐ Symptoms suggest subarachnoid hemorrhage
- ☐ Arterial puncture at noncompressible site in previous 7 days
- ☐ History of previous intracranial hemorrhage
- ☐ Intracranial neoplasm, arteriovenous malformation, or aneurysm
- ☐ Recent intracranial or intraspinal surgery
- ☐ Elevated blood pressure (BP> 185/110)
- ☐ Active internal bleeding
- ☐ Acute bleeding diathesis, including but not limited to
- ☐ Platelet count <100,000/mm3
- ☐ Heparin received within 48 hours, abnormally elevated aPTT greater than the upper limit of normal
- ☐ Current use of anticoagulant with INR >1.7 or PT >15 seconds
- ☐ Current use of direct thrombin inhibitors or direct factor Xa inhibitors with elevated sensitive laboratory tests (such as aPTT, INR, platelet count, and ECT; TT; or appropriate factor Xa activity assays)
- ☐ Blood glucose concentration <50 mg/dL (2.7 mmol/L)
- ☐ CT demonstrates multilobar infarction (hypodensity >1/3 cerebral hemisphere)

t-PA

Relative Exclusion Criteria
- ☐ Only minor or rapidly improving stroke symptoms (clearing spontaneously)
- ☐ Pregnancy
- ☐ Seizure at onset with postictal residual neurological impairments
- ☐ Major surgery or serious trauma within previous 14 days
- ☐ Recent gastrointestinal or urinary tract hemorrhage (within previous 21 days)
- ☐ Recent acute myocardial infarction (within previous 3 months)

3-4.5h →

Addition Relative Exclusion Criteria
- ☐ Aged >80 years
- ☐ Severe stroke (NIHSS>25)
- ☐ Taking an oral anticoagulant regardless of INR
- ☐ History of both diabetes and prior ischemic stroke

ACUTE CVA

Protocol (AHA)

- Dose: [See PDR for current dosing regimen]
- If the patient develops **severe headache, acute hypertension, nausea, or vomiting or has a worsening neurological examination**, discontinue the infusion and obtain emergent CT scan.
- BP and Neuro checks
  - ⇨ Every 15 minutes during and after IV tPA infusion for 2 hours → then every 30 minutes for 6 hours → then hourly until 24 hours after IV tPA treatment.
  - ⇨ Increase frequency of BP measurements if SBP is >180 mm Hg or DBP >105
  - ⇨ Antihypertensive medications to maintain blood pressure at or below these levels
- No concomitant heparin, warfarin, or aspirin during the first 24 hours after symptom onset
- Delay placement of nasogastric tubes, indwelling bladder catheters, or intra-arterial pressure catheters if the patient can be safely managed without them
- Obtain a follow-up CT or MRI scan at 24 hours after IV tPA before starting anticoagulants or antiplatelet agents
- Dispo: ICU or stroke unit for monitoring

tPA in Stroke (theNNT.com)
Benefits: **None** were helped (No stroke symptoms improved)
Harms: **5%** were harmed by a symptomatic intracranial hemorrhage

Contraindications

- See t-PA inclusion/exclusion algorithm
- For the most up to date indications/contraindications for t-PA in stroke please visit: http://www.stroke-site.org/guidelines/tpa_guidelines.html

Guidelines

- **AHA Guidelines** (Stroke 2013;44:870-947)
  - ⇨ Intravenous tPA (0.9 mg/kg, maximum dose 90 mg) is recommended for selected patients who may be **treated within 3 hours** of onset of ischemic stroke (Class I; Level of Evidence A)
  - ⇨ In patients eligible for intravenous tPA, benefit of therapy is time dependent, and treatment should be initiated as quickly as possible.
  - ⇨ The **door-to-needle time should be within 60 minutes** from hospital arrival (Class I; Level of Evidence A)
  - ⇨ Intravenous tPA (0.9 mg/kg, maximum dose 90 mg) is recommended for administration to eligible patients who can be treated in the time period of **3 to 4.5 hours** after stroke onset (Class I; Level of Evidence B)

Guidelines summary
t-PA in < 3hours
• AHA Level IA
• ACEP Level A
t-PA in 3-4.5hours
• AHA Level IB
• ACEP Level B

Journal Club: t-PA in Stroke
For a full breakdown of all 12 RCTs of tPA in stroke, go to www.theNNT.com

NINDS 1995 (N Engl J Med 1995;333:1581-7)
- **Benefit**: Treatment with intravenous rtPA was associated with an increase in the odds of a favorable outcome (OR, 1.9; 95% CI, 1.2–2.9)
  - ⇨ As compared with patients given placebo, patients treated with t-PA were at least 30 percent more likely to have minimal or no disability at three months on the assessment scales.
- **Harm**: Symptomatic intracerebral hemorrhage within 36 hours after the onset of stroke occurred in 6.4 percent of patients given t-PA but only 0.6 percent of patients given placebo (P<0.001).
- **Mortality**: mortality in the 2 treatment groups was similar at 3 months (17% versus 20%) and 1 year (24% versus 28%)

ECASS III (N Engl J Med 2008;359:131729)
- Goal: *We tested the efficacy and safety of alteplase administered between 3 and 4.5 hours after the onset of a stroke*
- **Favorable outcome**: alteplase > placebo (52.4% vs. 45.2%; odds ratio, 1.34; 95% CI=1.02 to 1.76; P=0.04).
- Global analysis: alteplase > placebo (odds ratio, 1.28; 95% CI, 1.00 to 1.65; P<0.05)
- **Intracranial hemorrhage**:
  - ⇨ Any intracranial hemorrhage: alteplase > placebo (27.0% vs. 17.6%; P=0.001)
  - ⇨ Symptomatic intracranial hemorrhage: alteplase > placebo (2.4% vs. 0.2%; P=0.008)
- **Mortality**: **No difference** between alteplase and placebo (7.7% and 8.4%, P=0.68)

IST-3 (Lancet 2012; 379: 2352–63) (EM:RAP 1/14)
- There is no evidence that tPA is better than placebo out to 6 hours.
- Although the authors claim improved functional benefit, the data does not support it

- Additional exclusion criteria:
  - ✓ Patients >80 years old
  - ✓ Oral anticoagulants regardless of INR
  - ✓ Baseline NIHSS score >25
  - ✓ Imaging evidence of ischemic injury involving more than one third of the MCA territory
  - ✓ History of both stroke and diabetes mellitus
- **ACEP Guidelines** (Ann Emerg Med. 2013;61:225-243)
  - **Level A recommendations**: IV tPA should be offered to acute ischemic stroke patients who meet National Institute of Neurological Disorders and Stroke (NINDS) inclusion/exclusion criteria and can be treated within **3 hours** after symptom onset.
  - **Level B recommendations:** IV tPA should be **considered** in acute ischemic stroke patients who meet European Cooperative Acute Stroke Study (ECASS) III inclusion/exclusion criteria and can be treated between **3 to 4.5 hours** after symptom onset

5. OTHER TREATMENT

Aspirin (Cochrane Database of Systematic Reviews 2008, Issue 3)
- Small but statistically significant **decline in mortality and unfavorable outcomes** with the administration of aspirin within 48 hours after stroke
- AHA recs:
  - Oral administration of aspirin (initial dose is 325 mg) within **24 to 48** hours after stroke onset is recommended for treatment of most patients (Class I; Level of Evidence A)
- **Do not give with tPA**: (Class III; Level of Evidence C)
- **Clopidogrel: Not well established** (Class IIb; Level of Evidence C)

Anticoagulation
- Several clinical trials demonstrate there is an increased risk of bleeding complications with early administration of either UFH or LMWH.
- Early administration of anticoagulants **does not lessen the risk of early neurological worsening**.

Endovascular treatments (EM:RAP 5/13; 11/13)
- Indications
  - Large Stroke (NIH stroke scale > 5-6) indicating large vessel occlusion
  - CT Angiography showing large vessel (carotid, basilar, MCA occlusion)
  - CT Perfusion showing favorable penumbral pattern

HTN
- General
  - Extreme hypertension: decreases perfusion to multiple organs, especially the ischemic brain, exacerbating ischemic injury, leads to encephalopathy, cardiac complications, and renal insufficiency
  - Moderate hypertension may be advantageous by improving cerebral perfusion of the ischemic tissue
- **BP management (no t-PA given)** (AHA Class I: Level C)
  - Treatment indications
    - ✓ Extreme HTN (BP> 220/120)
    - ✓ Other medical condition (MI, aortic dissection, and heart failure) necessitates lowering of BP
  - Treatment
    - ✓ If indicated → Lower SBP 15% and monitor for neurological deterioration related to the pressure lowering
    - ✓ If not indicated → start antihypertensives after 24h
  - Journal Club- **CATIS trial** (JAMA 2014;311:479) (EM:RAP 6/14)
    - ✓ Large RCT comparing BP reduction (10-25%) vs placebo in acute ischemic stroke
    - ✓ Results: Reduction of BP in acute ischemic stroke showed **no difference in death and disability**

ASA in Stroke (theNNT.com)

NNT=100 (death/dependency)

Benefits:
- 1 in 79 were helped (death, dependency avoided)
- 1 in 143 were helped (prevented repeat stroke)

Harms:
- 1 in 245 were harmed (major bleeding event)
- 1 in 574 were harmed (intracranial hemorrhage)

Journal Club: Endovascular treatments in Stroke

IMS 3 Trial (N Engl J Med 2013;368:893)
- Trial **stopped early due to futility** of endovascular therapy over t-PA alone
- No difference in clinical improvement (41% vs 39%) despite improvement of reperfusion rte by 40%

MR RESCUE (N Engl J Med 2013;368:914)
- Tried to select out patients who had an ischemic penumbra
- Conclusion: A favorable penumbral pattern on neuroimaging **did not** identify patients who would differentially benefit from endovascular therapy for ischemic stroke, nor was embolectomy shown to be superior to standard care.

SYNTHESIS trial (N Engl J Med 2013;368:904-13)
- Patients were randomized to **either** t-PA or endovascular treatment
- Conclusion: Endovascular therapy is **not** superior to standard treatment with intravenous t-PA.

Conclusion: 3 Randomized trials show neurointervention no better than standard therapy

ACUTE CVA

- **BP management (t-PA given)** (AHA Guidelines Class 1; Level B)
  - ⇨ Patient is **t-PA eligible** except that BP is >185/110 mm Hg:
    - ✓ **Labetalol** 10–20 mg IV over 1–2 minutes, may repeat 1 time; or
    - ✓ **Nicardipine** 5 mg/h IV, titrate up by 2.5 mg/h every 5–15 minutes, maximum 15 mg/h; when desired BP reached, adjust to maintain proper BP limits; or
    - ✓ Other agents (hydralazine, enalaprilat, etc) may be considered when appropriate
    - ✓ If BP is not maintained at or below 185/110 mm Hg, do not administer t-PA
  - ⇨ BP Management **during/after t-PA** → maintain BP at or below **180/105** mm Hg:
    - ✓ Monitor BP every 15 minutes for 2 hours from the start of t-PA therapy, then every 30 minutes for 6 hours, and then every hour for 16 hours
  - ⇨ If systolic BP >180–230 mm Hg or diastolic BP >105–120 mm Hg:
    - ✓ **Labetalol** 10 mg IV followed by continuous IV infusion 2–8 mg/min; or
    - ✓ **Nicardipine** 5 mg/h IV, titrate up to desired effect by 2.5 mg/h every 5–15 minutes, maximum 15 mg/h
  - ⇨ If BP not controlled or diastolic BP >140 mm Hg, consider IV sodium nitroprusside

Hyperthermia
- 1/3 of stroke patients will be hyperthermic in the first hours after stroke
- Associated with poor neurological outcome (increased metabolic demands, enhanced release of neurotransmitters, and increased free radical production)
- Cause
  - ⇨ Stroke itself: Acute stroke
  - ⇨ Cause of stroke: Infective endocarditis
  - ⇨ Complication of stroke: pneumonia, urinary tract infection (UTI), or sepsis
- Treatment
  - ⇨ Tylenol/NSAIDS modestly effective in treating hyperthermia

6. CAUSES

Thrombosis
- Large vessel vs small vessel
  - ⇨ Ddx: Atherosclerosis, arteritis, vasculitis, vasculopathy

Embolism
- Cardiac sources
  - ⇨ Atrial fibrillation, rheumatic valve disease, mechanical heart valves, recent MI (one month), SSS, dilated cardiomyopathy, cardiac thrombus, endocarditis
- Aortic source

Other Causes
- Endocarditis
- Dissection-Aortic or Vertebral
- Temporal Arteritis

ACUTE CVA

TIA

General (JAMA 2000;284:2901) (Essential 2010 "TIA"-Swadron)
- 90 day risk of stroke after TIA is 10.5%, half of which occur in the first 48 hours
- Short term risk of death, recurrent TIA and cardiovascular events is 25% in the first 90 days

> **TIA Definition**
>
> *A transient episode of neurological dysfunction caused by focal brain, spinal cord, or retinal ischemia, **without acute infarction***

Definition (Stroke 2009;40:2276–93)
- TIA: A transient episode of neurologic dysfunction caused by focal brain, spinal cord, or retina ischemia, without acute infarction
- Tissue based definition: 30% to 50% of patients with traditionally defined TIAs have evidence of infarction on MRI

Work-up
- MRI
  - ⇨ AHA/ASA currently recommends that all patients with TIA undergo emergent neuroimaging (MRI) within **24 hours** of symptom onset (class I, level B)
- Early Intervention (Lancet 2007; 370:1432)
  - ⇨ Early initiation of preventive treatments associated with decrease risk of recurrent TIA/stroke by 80%!
  - ⇨ Early work-up:
    - ✓ EKG
    - ✓ ECHO: TTE/TEE
    - ✓ Carotid US
  - ⇨ Early Preventive treatment:
    - ✓ ASA/Anti-platelet agent
    - ✓ Statin
    - ✓ BP control
    - ✓ Anticoagulation if indicated
    - ✓ Carotid endarterectomy for lesions >50%

ABCD2 Score	
A = Age >60 y	1
B = Blood pressure >140/90	1
C = Clinical features: unilateral weakness (**2**), speech difficulty without weakness (**1**)	2
D = Duration: >60 min (**2**), 10–59 min (**1**), <10 min (**0**)	2
D = Diabetes	1
Total	7

Stroke risk (Neurology 2011;77:1222–8)
- Risk increases with worsening clinical factors (ABCD2 score) and infarct on imaging
- TIA + **normal DWI** → 0.4% incidence of stroke at day 7 days
- TIA + normal DWI + **ABCD2 < 4** → 100% sensitivity in predicting the absence of stroke at 7 days

Score	@2 days	@ 7 days	@ 90 days
0-3 (Low risk)	1.0%	1.2%	3.1%
4-5 (mod risk)	4.1%	5.9%	9.8%
6-7 (high risk)	8.1%	11.7%	17.8%

Disposition(Controversial) (Emerg Med Clin N Am 2012;30:745)
- AHA and NICE incorporate the ABCD2 score and imaging findings into acute management and disposition recommendations
- AHA/ASA supports admission for patients with TIA with an ABCD2 score greater than 2, evidence of focal ischemia, or in any patient in whom rapid follow-up cannot be completed within 2 days as an outpatient

Dispo Algorithm
- **Strategy 1**: Admit ALL Patients
- **Strategy 2:** Risk stratify (ABCD2) and admit:
  - ⇨ ABCD2: ≥ 3 (Class IIa, Level C)
  - ⇨ ABCD2: 0 to 2 and uncertainty that outpatient workup can be completed within 2 days (Class IIa, C)
  - ⇨ ABCD2: 0 to 2 and other evidence that indicates the patient's event was caused by focal ischemia (Class IIa, C)
- **Strategy 3:** Risk stratify (ABCD2 + Imaging) (Neurology 2011;77:1222–8)
  - ⇨ MRI: No infarction + ABCD2 (0-3)
    - ✓ May d/c with Neurology follow up in 48h
    - ✓ If not possible → Admit
  - ⇨ MRI: No infarction + ABCD2 (≥4)
    - ✓ Admit, urgent neurologic consult and work-up
  - ⇨ MRI: + Infarction
    - ✓ If transient symptoms or symptoms resolved, patient with likely with TSI (Transient Symptoms with Infarction)

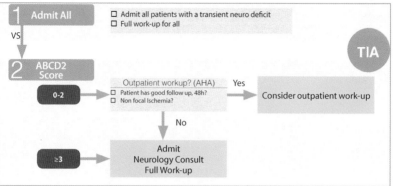

1 Admit All
- ☐ Admit all patients with a transient neuro deficit
- ☐ Full work-up for all

VS

2 ABCD2 Score

TIA

0-2

Outpatient workup? (AHA) → Yes → Consider outpatient work-up
- ☐ Patient has good follow up, 48h?
- ☐ Non focal Ischemia?

No

≥3 → Admit
Neurology Consult
Full Work-up

SEIZURE: STATUS EPILEPTICUS

1 Initial Tx

ABCs
⇨ ABCs, IV/O₂/Monitor; Intubation?
⇨ Maintain airway protection: oral/nasal airway

Rapidly Reversible Cause?
⇨ **Glucose:** give empirically or give if <80 (2-4ml/kg/dose)
⇨ **Opioid:** Naloxone 2mg (0.1mg/kg/dose)
⇨ **Alcoholic?:** Thiamine 100mg IV
⇨ **Pyridoxine:** Neonates/INH tox (50-100mg/dose)

Benzos
⇨ **Ativan:** (0.05-0.1mg/kg IV/IM) Adult:2mg/min (long duration of action)
⇨ **Valium:** (0.2-0.4mg/kg IV) Adult: 2mg/min or 0.5-1mg/kg PR (quicker onset, short duration)
⇨ **Versed:** 0.05-0.1mg/kg IV or 0.1-0.2 mg/kg IM (if no IV access)
• Benzos terminate 75-90% of seizures
• Versed IM and Valium IV→ same efficacy/time to sz cessation (Ind J Ped 2005;72:667)

2 AED

Phenytoin
⇨ **Phenytoin:** 10-20mg/kg IV (slower than 50mg/min)
⇨ **Fosphenytoin:** 10-20PE/kg (slower than 150mg/min)
• Onset: 10-30min, duration 24h
• No sedation/resp depression;
• +Hypotension with rapid administration of Phenytoin (propylene glycol)

Levetiracetam (Keppra)
⇨ **Levetiracetam:** 20 mg/kg IV (20-50mg/kg)
• Less resp depression and intubation risk
• (Pediatr Neurol 2009;41:37-39)

Valproate
⇨ **Valproic acid:** 15-20 mg/kg at 3-6 mg/kg/min
• Equal or greater efficacy vs Phenytoin as primary or secondary agent (Neurology 2006;67:340–342) (Seizure 2007;16:527)
• Consider before other agents that may require intubation (Emerg Med Clinic N Am 2011;29(1):51-64)

Phenobarbital
⇨ **Phenobarbital:** 20mg/kg IV over 5-10 min
• Divide doses into 260mg IV boluses
• +Sedation, resp depression (be ready to intubate), +hypotension
• Onset 15-30 min, duration 48h

Ketamine
⇨ **Ketamine:** 1.5-2 mg/kg
• Literature is sparse but is an option

INTUBATION?

3 Refractory Sz

NaHCO₃ Hypertonic Saline
⇨ **NaHCO₃:** 50ml of 7.5% solution
⇨ **3% Saline:** 100ml, repeat until seizure stops (for hyponatremia)
• Empiric treatment for **hyponatremic seizures, TCA overdose**

MgSO₄
⇨ **MgSO₄:** 4-6gm over 15 min, then 1-2gm/h gtt
• Consider in female → **eclampsia or EtOH withdrawal**
• Resp depression/hypotension at high doses (level >12)

Lidocaine
⇨ **Lidocaine:** 100mg (1mg/kg) IVP
• Used in neonates and some efficacy in adults (Epilepsia 1998;29:584)
• Beware if using after Phenytoin load as may induce arrhythmias

Pyridoxine
⇨ **Pyridoxine (B6)**
• Dose: 1gm Pyridoxine:1gm INH ingested (5gm if unknown)
• Empiric treatment for INH overdose

Refractory Status
⇨ **Propofol:** 3-5 mg/kg bolus then infuse at 1-15 mg/kg/h
⇨ Intubation/Ventilation
⇨ General Anesthesia/Coma (pentobarb, propofol, versed gtt)
⇨ Paralysis – no Succinylcholine due to possible rhabdo
⇨ Continuous EEG
⇨ Consults (Neuro/ICU/Anesthesia)
⇨ Hypotension: IVF, pressors

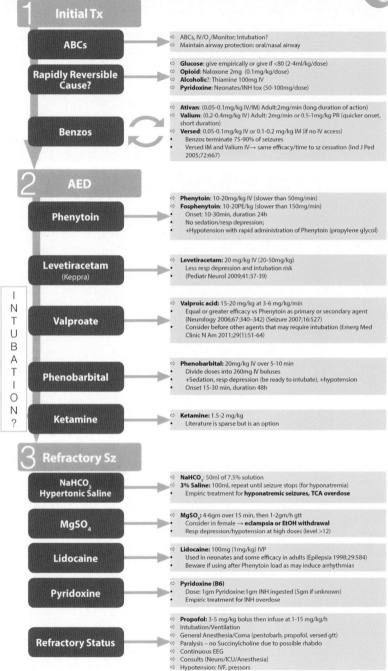

FEVER: < 29 DAYS OLD

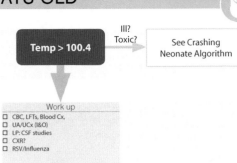

Temp > 100.4

Ill?
Toxic?

See Crashing
Neonate Algorithm

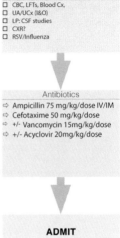

Work up
☐ CBC, LFTs, Blood Cx,
☐ UA/UCx (I&O)
☐ LP: CSF studies
☐ CXR?
☐ RSV/Influenza

Antibiotics
⇨ Ampicillin 75 mg/kg/dose IV/IM
⇨ Cefotaxime 50 mg/kg/dose
⇨ +/- Vancomycin 15mg/kg/dose
⇨ +/- Acyclovir 20mg/kg/dose

ADMIT

FEVER: < 29 DAYS OLD

GENERAL
(Emerg Med Clin N Am 2013:31;1073)

- 20% of febrile children have fever without an apparent source of infection (FWS) after history and physical exam
- A response to antipyretic medication does not change the likelihood of a child having a serious bacterial infection and should not be used for clinical decision-making (Level A ACEP recommendation Ann Emerg Med 2003;42:530-545).
- If parents report a fever at home but is afebrile in the ED, the child should still be considered as having had a fever

Work-up
- General
  - ⇨ **Full Sepsis work-up in all febrile infants < 29d**
  - ⇨ Infants between 1 and 28 days old with a fever should be presumed to have a serious bacterial infection (Level A ACEP recommendation Ann Emerg Med 2003;42:530-545)
  - ⇨ Using low risk criteria (Rochester) does not apply to the neonate (birth-29d) because too many serious bacterial infections can be missed → admission and further w/u is advised
- H&P
  - ⇨ Look for any obvious source of infection: cellulitis, abscess, omphalitis
- Labs
  - ⇨ CBC, LFTs, blood culture
  - ⇨ UA, urine culture
- CSF studies
  - ⇨ If the infant is critically ill, may postpone **LP** until stable.
  - ⇨ Positioning for LP may suppress respiratory drive → will need continuous pulse ox
  - ⇨ Sitting position may decrease risk of respiratory depression
- RSV +
  - ⇨ Will need admission to evaluate for apnea
- CXR
  - ⇨ Required only if resp sx present or toxic-appearing (tachypnea, retractions, grunting, abnormal lung exam or pulse ox)

CSF studies
☐ Tube 1: Culture/sensitivity
☐ Tube 2: Protein/glucose
☐ Tube 3: Cell count/diff
☐ Tube 4: HSV PCR

Disposition
- Admit all infants and await culture results

Antibiotics
- Ampicillin
  - ⇨ Dose: 200-300 mg/kg/d divided q 8h (<7d old infant) or q6h (>7d old)
- 3rd gen Cephalosporin
  - ⇨ Cefotaxime 150 mg/kg/day divided q6-8h
  - ⇨ Ceftriaxone contraindicated in neonates because can cause hyperbilirubinemia
- Vancomycin
  - ⇨ Dose: 15 mg/kg/dose
  - ⇨ Indication:
    - ✓ CSF gram stain → gram-positive cocci or ↑risk for Staph aureus infection
- Acyclovir
  - ⇨ Dose: 60 mg/kg/d IV divided every 8 hours
  - ⇨ Indications:
    - ✓ Ill-appearing, seizures, hepatitis(↑LFTs), mother with history of HSV, vesicular rash, pneumonitis (CXR)
    - ✓ CSF pleocytosis and a negative Gram stain until an alternative diagnosis is established or the HSV PCR becomes negative

HSV NEONATAL INFECTION

(Essentials 2012 "Who needs Acyclovir"-Claudius)

Spectrum of disease
- SEM (Skin-Eye-Mouth)
  - ⇨ Lowest mortality
  - ⇨ Presentation: vesicular skin lesions, keratitis, or chorioretinitis; affects face/scalp
  - ⇨ If untreated → can progress to disseminated and CNS disease
- CNS disease
  - ⇨ Irritable, focal neuro findings, bulging fontanelle, encephalitis, apnea, bradycardia
  - ⇨ Seizures and premature infant are risk factors for death
- Disseminated disease
  - ⇨ High mortality, multiple organs involved (liver/lungs)
  - ⇨ Sepsis with negative bacterial cultures, ↑AST/ALT

Consider acyclovir
☐ SEM-Skin-Eye-Mouth lesions
☐ Hypothermia
☐ Seizures
☐ <21 days old
☐ LFTs elevated
☐ Pneumonitis
☐ CSF pleocytosis
☐ ALL infants empirically?

Diagnosis
- HSV PCR- blood and CSF; negative result does not exclude HSV
- Viral culture, EEG
- CSF: Pleocytosis with gram stain negative suggestive
- ↑LFTs transaminitis (hepatitis)
- CXR (pneumonitis)

Treatment
- Acyclovir 60 mg/kg/d IV divided every 8 hours

FEVER: 4-8 WEEKS

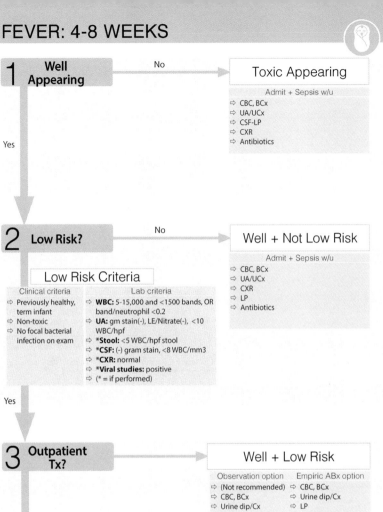

1 Well Appearing — No → **Toxic Appearing**

Admit + Sepsis w/u
⇨ CBC, BCx
⇨ UA/UCx
⇨ CSF-LP
⇨ CXR
⇨ Antibiotics

Yes ↓

2 Low Risk? — No → **Well + Not Low Risk**

Admit + Sepsis w/u
⇨ CBC, BCx
⇨ UA/UCx
⇨ CXR
⇨ LP
⇨ Antibiotics

Low Risk Criteria

Clinical criteria	Lab criteria
⇨ Previously healthy, term infant	⇨ **WBC:** 5-15,000 and <1500 bands, OR band/neutrophil <0.2
⇨ Non-toxic	⇨ **UA:** gm stain(-), LE/Nitrate(-), <10 WBC/hpf
⇨ No focal bacterial infection on exam	⇨ ***Stool:** <5 WBC/hpf stool
	⇨ ***CSF:** (-) gram stain, <8 WBC/mm3
	⇨ ***CXR:** normal
	⇨ ***Viral studies:** positive
	⇨ (* = if performed)

Yes ↓

3 Outpatient Tx? → **Well + Low Risk**

Observation option	Empiric ABx option
⇨ (Not recommended)	⇨ CBC, BCx
⇨ CBC, BCx	⇨ Urine dip/Cx
⇨ Urine dip/Cx	⇨ LP
⇨ Reevaluate in 24h	⇨ Ceftriaxone 50mg/kg IV/IM
	⇨ Re-evaluate in 24h

↓

4 Follow Up → **Outpatient Follow-Up**

Blood Cx (+)	Urine Cx (+)
⇨ Blood Cx positive: Admit for sepsis w/u and IV ABx	⇨ Persistent fever: Admit for sepsis w/u and IV ABx

FEVER: 4-8 WEEKS

(Emerg Med Clin N Am 2013;31:1073) (EM:RAP 6/13)

- Controversial: There are many approaches to the work-up of a febrile child...this is just one of them
- First, evaluate the infant and determine if they are toxic or ill appearing
- Then, use **low risk criteria** (Rochester, Boston, Philadelphia) to identify a cohort of infants that can safely be treated on an outpatient basis
- Separate those patients from those that have a higher risk of Serious Bacterial Illness (SBI) that includes UTI, occult bacteremia, bacterial enteritis and bacterial meningitis
- Risk of SBI in the three groups: (Pediatrics 1994;94:390-6)
  ⇨ Ill appearing **22.2%**
  ⇨ Well and not low risk **12.3%**
  ⇨ Well and low risk **1%**

1. ILL APPEARING

General
- 22.2% risk of serious bacterial illness (SBI)
- Use Pediatric assessment triangle (PAT) to help evaluate if infant is ill

Pediatric assessment triangle
- **Appearance**- Tone, interactiveness, consolability, look/gaze, speech/cry
- **Breathing**- Airway sounds, positioning, accessory muscle use
- **Circulatory status**- Pallor, cyanosis, delayed capillary refill, cool mottled skin

Full septic work-up
- CBC, LFTs, BCx
- UA/UCx
- CSF studies-LP
- CXR
- Antibiotics
  ⇨ Cefotaxime 50-100mg/kg
  ⇨ + Ampicillin 75mg/kg
  ⇨ + Vancomycin 15mg/kg
  ⇨ +/- Acyclovir 20mg/kg

Admit

2. LOW RISK?

Low Risk Work-up
- Using the **low risk criteria**, rate of SBI across multiple studies is **0.9%** (Ann Emerg Med 2000;36:602-614).
  ⇨ If the infant fails to meet low risk criteria, then they are at higher risk for SBI (**12.3%**) and should be admitted for sepsis w/u
  ⇨ Sensitivity of low risk criteria (Philadelphia) > 98% for identifying febrile children at low risk for SBI (NEJM 1993;329:1437-1441)
  ⇨ Other criteria show similar sensitivity: (Rochester criteria: Pediatrics1994;94:390) and (Boston criteria: J Pediatr 1992;120:22)-see table

Low risk criteria (Pediatrics 2001;108;311)
- Clinical criteria
  ⇨ Previously healthy
  ⇨ No focal bacterial infection on exam (except otitis media)
- Laboratory criteria
  ⇨ **WBC:** 5-15,000 and <1500 bands, OR band/neutrophil <0.2
  ⇨ **UA:** gm stain(-), LE/Nitrate(-), <10 WBC/hpf
  ⇨ *Stool: diarrhea if present: <5 WBC/hpf stool, no blood
  ⇨ *CSF: (-) gram stain, <8 WBC/mm³
  ⇨ *CXR: normal (if respiratory symptoms present)
  ⇨ *Positive viral testing: RSV, influenza, adenovirus, or enterovirus
     ✓   * = If performed

CSF studies
☐ Tube 1: Culture/sensitivity
☐ Tube 2: Protein/glucose
☐ Tube 3: Cell count/diff
☐ Tube 4: HSV PCR

- Lumbar Puncture
  ⇨ Lumbar Puncture is optional if the child is well appearing, has normal lab values and no other sources of infection found
  ⇨ Most experts **still recommend an LP in the 4-8wk old despite well appearance**
  ⇨ LP is indicated if discharging home on empiric antibiotics
  ⇨ LP is still indicated if another source of infection is found (i.e. UTI) because infants in this age group have difficulty containing infections to one organ system
- CXR
  ⇨ Obtain if temperature > 38°C and at least one clinical sign of pulmonary disease
  ⇨ Clinical signs: Tachypnea >50 breaths/min, cyanosis or O₂ saturation <95%, rales, rhonchi, retractions, wheezing, grunting, stridor, nasal flaring, or cough

FEVER: 4-8 WEEKS

Not Low Risk?
- If infant does not meet low risk criteria, they will require a full septic work-up, LP (if not already performed) and admission
- Treat as Ill appearing infant
- Begin empiric antibiotics (Ceftriaxone 50mg/kg IV)
- If CSF pleocytosis
  - ⇨ Ceftriaxone 100 mg/kg IV
  - ⇨ Acyclovir if < 42 days old
- Admit and await culture results
  - ⇨ Also consider admission if parents unreliable and not able to follow up in 24h

3. OUTPATIENT TREATMENT?

General
- Outpatient treatment reserved for only well appearing, low risk infants
- Must be able to follow up within 24h
- Must have reliable parents

Observation option
- Hold antibiotics until cultures become positive and re-evaluate in 24h
- No LP performed
- Most experts **do not recommend no LP/no antibiotics** option
- Re-evaluate patient and cultures in 24h

Empiric antibiotics option
- Treat empirically with antibiotics (Ceftriaxone)
- This option requires an **LP be done prior to Abx**
- Re-evaluate patient and cultures in 24h

4. FOLLOW UP

Blood culture +
- Blood Cx positive: Admit for sepsis w/u and IV ABx

Urine culture +
- Persistent fever: Admit for sepsis w/u and IV ABx

FEVER: >8 WEEKS OLD

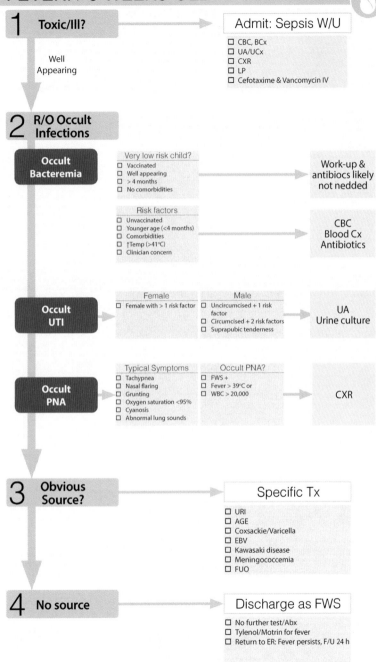

1 Toxic/Ill? ──────► Admit: Sepsis W/U
- □ CBC, BCx
- □ UA/UCx
- □ CXR
- □ LP
- □ Cefotaxime & Vancomycin IV

Well
Appearing

2 R/O Occult Infections

Occult Bacteremia

Very low risk child?
- □ Vaccinated
- □ Well appearing
- □ > 4 months
- □ No comorbidities

──────► Work-up & antibiocs likely not nedded

Risk factors
- □ Unvaccinated
- □ Younger age (<4 months)
- □ Comorbidities
- □ ↑Temp (>41°C)
- □ Clinician concern

──────► CBC
Blood Cx
Antibiotics

Occult UTI

Female
- □ Female with > 1 risk factor

Male
- □ Uncircumcised + 1 risk factor
- □ Circumcised + 2 risk factors
- □ Suprapubic tenderness

──────► UA
Urine culture

Occult PNA

Typical Symptoms
- □ Tachypnea
- □ Nasal flaring
- □ Grunting
- □ Oxygen saturation <95%
- □ Cyanosis
- □ Abnormal lung sounds

Occult PNA?
- □ FWS +
- □ Fever > 39°C or
- □ WBC > 20,000

──────► CXR

3 Obvious Source? ──────► Specific Tx
- □ URI
- □ AGE
- □ Coxsackie/Varicella
- □ EBV
- □ Kawasaki disease
- □ Meningococcemia
- □ FUO

4 No source ──────► Discharge as FWS
- □ No further test/Abx
- □ Tylenol/Motrin for fever
- □ Return to ER: Fever persists, F/U 24 h

FEVER: >8 WEEKS OLD

GENERAL APPROACH
(Emerg Med Clin N Am 2013;31:601)

- Controversial: There are many approaches to the work-up of a febrile child...this is just one of them
- Many febrile children in this age group will have a source of fever on history or physical (URI, gastroenteritis, Coxsackie, Varicella, etc.)
- Most will have a self-limiting viral illness
- Consider occult infections in this age group (bacteremia, UTI, pneumonia)
- If no source is found, then they are labeled Fever Without Source (FWS)

1. TOXIC/ILL APPEARING

Pediatric assessment triangle
- **Appearance**- Tone, interactiveness, consolability, look/gaze, speech/cry
- **Breathing**- Airway sounds, positioning, accessory muscle use
- **Circulatory status**- Pallor, cyanosis, delayed capillary refill, cool mottled skin

Full septic work-up
- CBC, LFTs, BCx
- UA/UCx
- CSF studies-LP
- CXR
- Antibiotics
  - ⇨ Cefotaxime 50-100mg/kg
  - ⇨ + Vancomycin 15mg/kg
  - ⇨ +/- Acyclovir 20mg/kg

Admit

2. R/O OCCULT INFECTIONS

PEDIATRIC UTI (AAP Practice Guidelines: Pediatrics 2011;128: 595–610)
- UTI risk factors-general
  - ⇨ See table
- Other source?
  - ⇨ Other potential source (gastroenteritis, otitis media, URI) does not r/o UTI
- Consider screening:(Pediatrics 2011;128: 595–610)
  - ⇨ Female <2yo
    - ✓ > 1 risk factor
  - ⇨ Male:
    - ✓ Uncircumcised + 1 risk factor
    - ✓ Circumcised + 2 risk factors
    - ✓ Suprapubic tenderness
- Urine collection
  - ⇨ I&O cath or suprapubic aspiration
  - ⇨ Bagged urine samples are likely to be contaminated and have an unacceptable false positive rate
- Diagnosis
  - ⇨ UA: >10 WBC/hpf or bacteriuria
  - ⇨ Urine culture: >50,000 cfu/ml
    - ✓ Obtain a urine culture in conjunction with other urine studies when UTI is suspected because a negative dipstick/UA does not always exclude UTI (**Level B** ACEP recommendation)

Girls UTI risk factors (AAP)
☐ White race
☐ Age less than 12 months
☐ Temp at least 39°C
☐ Duration of fever at least 2 days
☐ Absence of another source of infection

Boys UTI risk factors (AAP)
☐ Uncircumcised
☐ Race: non-black
☐ Temp at least 39°C
☐ Duration of fever > 24h
☐ Absence of another source of infection

Journal Club: Pediatric UTI
(Ann Emerg Med 2013;61:559)(BMJ 2010;340:c1594)

AAP position:
- UTI should be treated because can lead to renal scarring, renal failure and HTN

Does the Evidence Support Aggressively Pursuing the Diagnosis (Ann Emerg Med 2013;61:559)
- No evidence that renal scarring has long term sequelae
- Urosepsis rare in pediatric population
- Conclusion: May delay testing for UTI if other source of fever or fever present for < 4-5d

---

FEVER: >8 WEEKS OLD

- Treatment
  - ⇨ Antibiotics x 7-14 days
  - ⇨ Ceftriaxone, cefixime, cephalexin, or bactrim, depending on local antibiotic sensitivity patterns
- Admit
  - ⇨ Children < 2 months
  - ⇨ Unable to follow up within 48h
  - ⇨ Toxic/Ill/Urosepsis
  - ⇨ Not tolerating PO/medications
  - ⇨ Immunocompromised

PEDIATRIC PNEUMONIA

- Typical symptoms
  - ⇨ Tachypnea, nasal flaring, grunting, oxygen saturation <95%, cyanosis, abnormal lung sounds
  - ⇨ CXR indicated if any symptoms present
- Occult pneumonia
  - ⇨ 3% patients in this age group will have pneumonia without any of the above symptoms
- Consider screening CXR in FWS if:
  - ⇨ Fever > 39°C or
  - ⇨ WBC > 20,000

PEDIATRIC OCCULT BACTEREMIA (OB)

- No clear evidence for work-up of OB, controversial and based on clinician preference
- Low risk child?
  - ⇨ Definition
    - ✓ Vaccinated (2 Hib and 2 pneumococcal vaccines)
    - ✓ Well appearing
    - ✓ > 4 months
  - ⇨ Work-up likely not indicated (Academic Emerg Med 2009; 16:220)
    - ✓ Very low risk of occult bacteremia in this population(OB rate 0.25%)
- Risk factors?
  - ⇨ Definition
    - ✓ Unvaccinated
    - ✓ Younger age (<4 months)
    - ✓ Comorbidities
    - ✓ ↑Temp (41°C)
    - ✓ Clinician concern/other
  - ⇨ Consider further work up
    - ✓ CBC, blood culture, antibiotics
    - ✓ If child's only risk factor is being unvaccinated or younger age, may be able to send blood culture and have child follow up within 24 hours
- Pathogens
  - ⇨ Haemophilus influenzae Type b (Hib)
    - ✓ No longer a significant cause of bacteremia after introduction of Hib vaccine
  - ⇨ S. pneumo
    - ✓ Most common cause of bacteremia in this age group
  - ⇨ E. coli
    - ✓ Usually associated with concomitant UTI
  - ⇨ Salmonella
    - ✓ Most patients have concomitant diarrhea
  - ⇨ Neisseria meningitidis (see below)
    - ✓ Infrequent cause of bacteremia but high mortality (>10%)

FEVER: >8 WEEKS OLD

3. SOURCE OF INFECTION?

(EM:RAP 11/12 "Dangerous Pediatric Fevers"-Claudius)

Most have self-limiting viral illness
- URI
- AGE
- Coxsackie/Varicella

KAWASAKI DISEASE (KD)
- AKA: Mucocutaneous Lymph Node Syndrome
- Diagnosis
  - ⇨ Fever for 5 days or more and at least 4 of the 5 following clinical criteria:
    - ✓ Bilateral and nonexudative bulbar conjunctivitis
    - ✓ Oropharyngeal changes
    - ✓ Cervical lymphadenopathy
    - ✓ Rash: nonvesicular or bullous rash; nonspecific, diffuse maculopapular
    - ✓ Palms/soles: erythema or edema (in the acute phase)
  - ⇨ Incomplete KD
    - ✓ Definition: <5 days of fever or <4 symptoms
    - ✓ Screening test: CRP and ESR
- Treatment
  - ⇨ Admit
  - ⇨ IVIG 2g/kg over 12h
    - ✓ Helps decrease risk of cardiac complications (coronary artery aneurysm)
  - ⇨ Aspirin, high dose: 80-100 mg/kg in 4 divided doses until afebrile

MENINGOCOCCEMIA
- Syndromes: Disseminated Meningococcemia and Meningitis
- Presentation
  - ⇨ May have preceding URI or pharyngitis symptoms and diagnosed as viral illness
  - ⇨ Acute: sudden onset of fever, nausea, vomiting, headache, decreased ability to concentrate, and severe myalgias
  - ⇨ Poor perfusion → rapid progression to sepsis and shock/DIC in hours
  - ⇨ Rash
    - ✓ Usual progression: blanching maculopapular → petechiae → fulminant purpura
    - ✓ May start with non-blanching rash
- Risk factors
  - ⇨ Contact with patients with meningococcus, meningococcal disease outbreaks, and presence of fever and petechiae

FEVER UNKNOWN ORIGIN
- Definition: Fever with no obvious cause for > 3 weeks
- EBV (Epstein Barr virus)
  - ⇨ Most common cause of FUO
  - ⇨ Presentation: sore throat, cervical lymphadenopathy (LAD), splenomegaly, rash
  - ⇨ Dx: EBV titer
- Osteomyelitis- pain over bone?
- Cat scratch disease- pustule at inoculation site → LAD in 1-2 weeks
- Travel history?: Malaria, dengue fever, typhoid fever, rickettsial disease, Chikungunya
- Rheumatologic: JRA, Still's disease
- Oncologic: Leukemia

4. FEVER WITHOUT SOURCE
- No further testing or antibiotics
- Tylenol/Motrin for fever
- Return: fever persists, F/U 24 h

STRIDOR

1 Airway Emergency?

- ☐ ABC/IV/O₂/Monitor
- ☐ Racemic Epinephrine
- ☐ Nebulized steroids
- ☐ Steroids IV
- ☐ Emergent intubation?

2 Emergent Diagnosis

📋 H & P 🩺   ✏️ Action

Epiglottitis

- ☐ Age: 2-8yo
- ☐ Season: Winter
- ☐ Viral type prodrome
- ☐ **Toxic**, irritable
- ☐ Tripod position
- ☐ **Hyperextended neck**
- ☐ **Drooling**

- ☐ Dyspnea
- ☐ Dysphonia
- ☐ Dysphagia
- ☐ ↑Fever

- ⇨ Lateral Xray: **thumbprint sign**
- ⇨ Airway management in OR
- ⇨ Avoid anxiety
- ⇨ Gentle op exam
- ⇨ Antibiotics/Admit

RPA

- ☐ Age: 6m - 4y
- ☐ **Torticollis (stiff neck?)**
- ☐ Dysphagia
- ☐ Trismus
- ☐ Toxic
- ☐ Fever

- ☐ ↓neck extension
- ☐ ↓neck flexion
- ☐ **Neck mass**

- ⇨ Lateral Xray: soft tissue swelling
- ⇨ **CT neck**, U/S
- ⇨ ENT
- ⇨ Antibiotics
- ⇨ Airway management

Bacterial Tracheitis

- ☐ Age: 6m-8y
- ☐ Season: fall/winter
- ☐ Present similar to Epiglottitis/Croup
- ☐ Cough
- ☐ Toxic
- ☐ ↑Fever

- ☐ Resp distress
- ☐ No response to treatment

- ⇨ Frontal Xray: steeple sign?
- ⇨ Airway management in OR
- ⇨ Antibiotics
- ⇨ Admit

Foreign Body

- ☐ Age: Infants/toddlers
- ☐ Classic Triad (wheeze + cough + ↓BS)
- ☐ Triad present in only 1/3

Symptoms
- ☐ 3 Stages
- ☐ Violent cough
- ☐ Asymptomatic interval
- ☐ Complications

- ⇨ **Xrays** (nl in 2/3)
- ⇨ Bilateral decubitus
- ⇨ Insp/Exp
- ⇨ Position of comfort
- ⇨ ENT

3 Croup?

📋 H & P 🩺   ✏️ Action

Croup

- ☐ Age: 6m-4y
- ☐ Season: fall-winter
- ☐ Viral prodrome
- ☐ **Barky cough (seal)**
- ☐ Hoarse
- ☐ ↑fever/toxicity →rare
- ☐ Croup score?

- ⇨ Frontal Xray: steeple sign
- ⇨ Cool mist?
- ⇨ Decadron
- ⇨ Racemic Epi

4 Congenital Cause?

Stridor present since birth?
- ☐ Laryngomalacia
- ☐ Subglottic stenosis
- ☐ Vocal cord paralysis
- ☐ Vascular ring
- ☐ Webs
- ☐ Papillomas

STRIDOR

Empiric treatment
- Racemic Epi
- Nebulized steroids
- Steroids IV
- Emergent intubation?

Types of stridor:
- Inspiratory → subglottic
- Expiratory → supraglottic
- Biphasic → subglottic, glottic
- Sonorous → nasal

2. R/O EMERGENT DIAGNOSIS

EPIGLOTTITIS

General
- Acute inflammation of epiglottis and surrounding structure → serious, life threatening, airway emergency

Clinical
- Age: 2-8yo; Season: Winter
- Viral type prodrome
- Toxic, irritable, fever
- Tripod position, hyperextended neck
- The D's: Drooling, Dyspnea, Dysphonia, Dysphagia

Diagnosis
- Lateral neck Xray → "thumb print sign"
  - ⇨ Can be negative in up to 20% of cases (Prim care 1990;17(2):335-45)
- Diagnosis made on visualization of inflamed epiglottis

Treatment
- Avoid agitation of child as this can worsen the airway (no IV, oral examination)
- If emergent airway needed → use tube size 0.5-1 smaller than age
- Ideal airway should be obtained in the OR, controlled conditions
- Antibiotics (3rd gen Cephalosporin)

RETROPHARYNGEAL ABSCESS

General
- Clinical Presentation similar to meningitis but usually has normal mental status
- Pathology: Deep neck space infection (URI vs penetrating trauma to oropharynx), can spread through neck → danger space → cause mediastinitis

Clinical: (Pediatrics 2003;111:1394-8)
- Torticollis (stiff neck?)(36.5%)
- ↓Neck extension (45%), ↓Neck flexion (12.5%)
- Dysphagia
- Trismus, toxic, fever
- Stridor rare (3%)
- Age:
  - ⇨ 50% of cases occur between 6-12mos, 96% occur before 6 years of age (Arch Dis Child 1991;66:1227-30)
  - ⇨ Lymph nodes of Rouviere that drain the retropharyngeal space atrophy after 6 years
- Appearance: Child with neck in neutral, difficulty extending neck and uses eyes to look up
- **Often confused with meningitis:**
  - ⇨ ↓Neck flexion in meningitis vs ↓neck extension in RPA (Pediatrics 2003;111:1394-8)

> Fever, Stiff Neck, AMS??
>
> Consider RPA along
> with meningitis!!!
> (Similar presentations)

Work-up
- Xray, lateral neck
  - ⇨ Low yield, not widely used
- CT neck
  - ⇨ Helps localize where problem is
  - ⇨ Difficult to differentiate between pus and cellulitis
- US neck
  - ⇨ May help distinguish between purulence vs adenitis vs abscess

STRIDOR

Treatment
- ENT Consultation
- Antibiotics (alone treat 37%):
  - ⇨ Clindamycin
- OR if not improve

Complications
- Airway compromise
- **Descending necrotizing mediastinitis**
  - ⇨ Spread from RP space → retrovisceral space → pierce alar fascia → Danger space
  - ⇨ Rare in children
- Internal jugular vein thrombosis
- Mycotic aneurysms

BACTERIAL TRACHEITIS

General
- Croup-like illness + toxic + not respond to therapy
- Pathology: laryngeotracheobronchitis, subglottic edema and membranous secretions

Clinical
- BT vs epiglottitis (J Otolaryngol 1989;18(3):101-4)
  - ⇨ Tracheitis children have a cough, comfortable lying down, no drool
- Age: 6m-8y; Season: fall/winter
- Present similar to Epiglottitis/Croup
- Cough, toxic, ↑fever, resp distress
- No response to treatment

Diagnosis
- Frontal neck X-ray → Steeple sign (non-specific finding)
- Endoscopic visualization of normal supraglottic structures and subglottic inflammation, pus in airway, ulcers, secretions

Treatment
- Emergent airway → use tube size smaller than what is appropriate for their age
- Ideally intubated , diagnosed, cultured in the OR under optimal conditions
- Antibiotics: anti-Staph (Nafcillin/Oxacillin + 3rd gen Ceph)

FOREIGN BODY ASPIRATION

Clinical
- Age: Infants/toddlers
- Classic Triad (wheeze + cough + ↓BS) present in only 1/3
- Symptoms (3 stages)
  - ⇨ Violent cough
  - ⇨ Asymptomatic interval
  - ⇨ Complications

Diagnosis
- History
  - ⇨ Only 50% diagnosed in first 24h
  - ⇨ **Usually asymptomatic in ED**
  - ⇨ Witnessed foreign body aspiration?
  - ⇨ Elicit a choking/coughing episode in the history (sudden onset dyspnea/choking/cyanosis)
- Xrays (normal in 2/3)
  - ⇨ Sensitiivty 68%, specificity 68% (Pediatr Radiol 1989;19:520)
  - ⇨ Bilateral decubitus (not helpful)
  - ⇨ Insp/Exp
- CT

Treatment
- Position of comfort
- ENT
- Referral for bronchoscopy

Complications:
- Obstruction, infection, fever, cough

STRIDOR

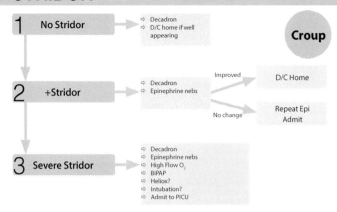

1 No Stridor → ⇨ Decadron
⇨ D/C home if well appearing

Croup

2 +Stridor → ⇨ Decadron
⇨ Epinephrine nebs

Improved → D/C Home

No change → Repeat Epi
Admit

3 Severe Stridor → ⇨ Decadron
⇨ Epinephrine nebs
⇨ High Flow O₂
⇨ BiPAP
⇨ Heliox?
⇨ Intubation?
⇨ Admit to PICU

3. CROUP TREATMENT

CROUP
(EM:RAP 2/13 "Notes from the Community: Croup 2013 Style" – Sloas)

General
• Peak incidence in 1-2yo
• Organisms: Parainfluenza I (most common-80%), II and III, M. pneumoniae, RSV, Influenza (severe form), adenovirus

Clinical
• Age: 6m-4y; Season: fall-winter
• Viral prodrome
• Barky cough, hoarse (subglottic airway narrowing)
• Fever: common in croup, but usually not toxic
• Lateral Neck Xray: Steeple sign (non-specific finding)
• Croup score? (See table)
• Sx peak over 2 days and resolve over 1 week
• Croup score: mild (0-4), mild/mod (5-6), moderate (7-8), severe (9-14), terminal (15)

Croup Score:	0	1	2	3
Color:	Normal	Dusky	Cyanotic	Cyanotic on O2
Air mvmt:	Normal	Mild↓	Mod↓	Marked↓
Retractions:	None	Mild	Mod	Severe
Mentation:	Normal	Restless	Lethargic	Obtunded
Stridor:	None	Mild	Mod	Severe

Treatment
• **Cool mist**
  ⇨ Sooths inflamed mucosa
  ⇨ Multiple studies show minimal efficacy in treating croup (JAMA 2006;295(11):274)
  ⇨ Generally not helpful
• **Steroids**
  ⇨ Indication: all croup in the ED?
  ⇨ Decreased mortality for croup from 1/200 to 1/30,000
  ⇨ Multiple studies show efficacy, associated with a decrease in ED stay and ED bounce backs (Ann Emerg Med 2002;30(3):353)
  ⇨ Efficacious for even **mild** croup, less likely to return for croup related care (NEJM 2004;351(13):1306)
  ⇨ Dose:
    ✓ 0.15mg/kg vs 0.3mg/kg vs 0.6mg/kg?? (Max 10 mg)
    ✓ All equally efficacious PO or IM or inhaled (Acad Emerg Med 2003;10:16)
    ✓ IV formulation can be given po

STRIDOR

- **Racemic epinephrine**
  - ⇨ Indication: mod/severe croup; stridor at rest → can help reduce need for emergent intubation
  - ⇨ Dose: 0.25-0.5ml of 2.25% solution with saline to total of 3ml
  - ⇨ Racemic Epi vs Epinephrine?
    - ✓ Equivalent: substitute with epinephrine 0.5ml /kg of 1:1000, 5ml max with equal efficacy (Pediatrics 1992;89(2):302) (Cochrane Database Syst Rev. 2011 Feb 16)
  - ⇨ Rebound phenomenon?
    - ✓ No need for admission for observation, if significantly improved → can be safely discharged after 3 hours (Ann Emerg Med 1995;25:331-7)
  - ⇨ Repeat Epinephrine
    - ✓ Usually 2 doses of epi = Admit
    - ✓ But, if they respond to the 2nd epinephrine, well-appearing and observed 2-4 hours without decompensation → can possibly d/c home
- **Summary: may give cool mist, steroids for all kids in ED, epinephrine only if they have stridor**

Disposition

- Discharge: well-appearing, normal color, no stridor at rest, no ALOC
- Admit: Moderate croup score, toxic appearing, respiratory distress, received more than 2 doses of nebulized epinephrine

D/C Criteria:
☐ Good PO intake
☐ RR < 40
☐ Sat > 94%
☐ Well appearing

4. CONSIDER CONGENITAL CAUSE

Stridor present since birth?

- Laryngomalacia
- Subglottic stenosis
- Vocal cord paralysis
- Vascular ring
- Webs
- Papillomas

CRASHING NEONATE

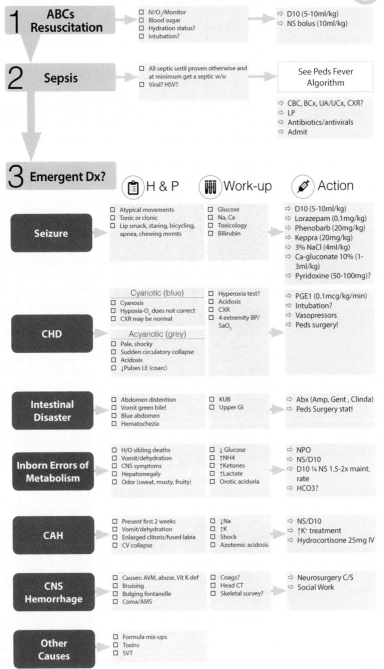

1 ABCs Resuscitation
- ☐ IV/O₂/Monitor
- ☐ Blood sugar
- ☐ Hydration status?
- ☐ Intubation?

⇨ D10 (5-10ml/kg)
⇨ NS bolus (10ml/kg)

2 Sepsis
- ☐ All septic until proven otherwise and at minimum get a septic w/u
- ☐ Viral? HSV?

See Peds Fever Algorithm

⇨ CBC, BCx, UA/UCx, CXR?
⇨ LP
⇨ Antibiotics/antivirals
⇨ Admit

3 Emergent Dx?

📋 H & P   🏥 Work-up   💉 Action

Seizure
- ☐ Atypical movements
- ☐ Tonic or clonic
- ☐ Lip smack, staring, bicycling, apnea, chewing mvmts

- ☐ Glucose
- ☐ Na, Ca
- ☐ Toxicology
- ☐ Bilirubin

⇨ D10 (5-10ml/kg)
⇨ Lorazepam (0.1mg/kg)
⇨ Phenobarb (20mg/kg)
⇨ Keppra (20mg/kg)
⇨ 3% NaCl (4ml/kg)
⇨ Ca-gluconate 10% (1-3ml/kg)
⇨ Pyridoxine (50-100mg)?

CHD
Cyanotic (blue)
- ☐ Cyanosis
- ☐ Hypoxia-O₂ does not correct
- ☐ CXR may be normal

Acyanotic (grey)
- ☐ Pale, shocky
- ☐ Sudden circulatory collapse
- ☐ Acidosis
- ☐ ↓Pulses LE (coarc)

- ☐ Hyperoxia test?
- ☐ Acidosis
- ☐ CXR
- ☐ 4 extremity BP/SaO₂

⇨ PGE1 (0.1mcg/kg/min)
⇨ Intubation?
⇨ Vasopressors
⇨ Peds surgery!

Intestinal Disaster
- ☐ Abdomen distention
- ☐ Vomit green bile!
- ☐ Blue abdomen
- ☐ Hematochezia

- ☐ KUB
- ☐ Upper GI

⇨ Abx (Amp, Gent , Clinda)
⇨ Peds Surgery stat!

Inborn Errors of Metabolism
- ☐ H/O sibling deaths
- ☐ Vomit/dehydration
- ☐ CNS symptoms
- ☐ Hepatomegaly
- ☐ Odor (sweat, musty, fruity)

- ☐ ↓ Glucose
- ☐ ↑NH4
- ☐ ↑Ketones
- ☐ ↑Lactate
- ☐ Orotic aciduria

⇨ NPO
⇨ NS/D10
⇨ D10 ¼ NS 1.5-2x maint, rate
⇨ HCO3?

CAH
- ☐ Present first 2 weeks
- ☐ Vomit/dehydration
- ☐ Enlarged clitoris/fused labia
- ☐ CV collapse

- ☐ ↓Na
- ☐ ↑K
- ☐ Shock
- ☐ Azotemic acidosis

⇨ NS/D10
⇨ ↑K⁺ treatment
⇨ Hydrocortisone 25mg IV

CNS Hemorrhage
- ☐ Causes: AVM, abuse, Vit K def
- ☐ Bruising
- ☐ Bulging fontanelle
- ☐ Coma/AMS

- ☐ Coags?
- ☐ Head CT
- ☐ Skeletal survey?

⇨ Neurosurgery C/S
⇨ Social Work

Other Causes
- ☐ Formula mix-ups
- ☐ Toxins
- ☐ SVT

130

CRASHING NEONATE

General Approach

(Essentials 2011"Peds Resuscitation Course")(CMEDownload "Resuscitation Conference 2013" - Cantor)
(Pediatr Clin N Am 2006;53:69-84)

- Definition: Full-term newborn, born well and d/c home by pediatrician → returns in first month looking sick, hypotensive and dehydrated
- Always begin with ABCs and decide whether or not to emergently intubate.
- Begin fluid resuscitation if not in overt CHF and check/correct hypoglycemia
- Consider and rule-out emergent causes starting with focused H&P, labs and possibly imaging
- At minimum, these neonates will get a septic work-up including labs, antibiotics and possibly LP, then admission

1. ABCs & Resuscitation

Resuscitation
- Early IV access
  ⇨ Scalp vein, IO line, umbilical line
- Vital signs:
  ⇨ 4 extremity BP; Pre and post ductal O_2 saturation
  ⇨ Minimally acceptable SBP = 60
- Initial labs
  ⇨ Full sepsis work-up (Accucheck, CBC/CMP/BCx/Lactate/NH_4/UA/UCx)

Ddx: THE MISFITS
☐ **T**rauma
☐ **H**eart disease/Hypovolemia
☐ **E**ndocrine (CAH)
☐ **M**etabolic (electrolytes)
☐ **I**nborn errors metabolism
☐ **S**eizures
☐ **F**ormula mishaps
☐ **I**ntestinal disaster
☐ **T**oxins
☐ **S**epsis

Treat reversible causes
- Hypoglycemia always present→treat early with D10 (5-10ml/kg IV)
- Begin fluid resuscitation → NS boluses (10ml/kg IV)

2. Begin Sepsis W/U

Neonatal Sepsis

(See "Fever <29 days" Algorithm)

Full septic work-up
- All ill appearing neonates are septic until proven otherwise
- CBC, LFTs, BCx
- UA/UCx
- CSF studies-LP
- CXR
- Antibiotics
  ⇨ Cefotaxime 50-100mg/kg
  ⇨ + Ampicillin 75mg/kg
  ⇨ + Vancomycin 15mg/kg
  ⇨ +/- Acyclovir 20mg/kg
- Admit

3. Emergent Differential

Seizure

Presentation
- Atypical seizure
  ⇨ Presents with atypical movements → usually not tonic-clonic
  ⇨ Usually staring spell, lip smacking, bicycling, tonic, migratory clonic

Diagnosis
- Differential diagnosis is large: (Emerg Med Clinics North Am 2002;20:27-48)
  ⇨ Hypoxic-Ischemic encephalopathy → most common cause(50-65%)
  ⇨ Intracranial hemorrhage: IVH/SDH/SAH (15%)
  ⇨ Electrolyte abnormalities: ↑Ca, ↑↓Na, ↑Phosphate, ↑↓ glucose
  ⇨ Other: Infection, IEM, metabolic, drug withdrawal, toxins, trauma, hypertension, formula mix-up (↓Na)
- Work-up
  ⇨ Labs
    ✓ Check labs even if seizures have stopped
    ✓ Check glucose immediately
    ✓ Check and correct Na, glucose, Ca
  ⇨ CT Head
  ⇨ Sepsis work-up

CRASHING NEONATE

- Treatment
  - ⇨ Correct hypoglycemia: D10: (5 to 10 ml/kg)
  - ⇨ Benzo: Lorazepam 0.1mg/kg initial drug of choice
  - ⇨ Anticonvulsant
    - ✓ Phenobarbital 20mg/kg IV
    - ✓ Levetiracetam (Keppra) 20mg/kg IV
    - ✓ Fosphenytoin 15-20 mg/kg IV
  - ⇨ Treat hypocalcemia (≤7mg/dl): Ca gluconate 10% (100–300 mg/kg IV)
  - ⇨ Treat hyponatremia (<125 mg/dl): 3% saline (4 ml/kg)
  - ⇨ Pyridoxine (50-100mg)
    - ✓ Consider if refractory seizures
  - ⇨ Sepsis
    - ✓ Begin sepsis work-up and broad antibiotics (see peds fever algorithm)
    - ✓ Treat for HSV (LP and begin acyclovir)

CONGENITAL HEART DISEASE

(EM:RAP 9/13 "Neonatal Cardiology" & 10/11 - C3 Project)(Essentials 2011 "CHD" -Rose)

General

- Neonate with congenital heart disease may rely on a patent ductus arterious (PDA) to shunt blood for pulmonary blood flow or systemic blood flow
- PDA usually closes within 2 weeks → ductus arteriosus no longer able to shunt blood past CHD lesion → rapid clinical deterioration depending on site of lesion
- May have ductal dependent pulmonary blood flow (Cyanotic CHD) or ductal dependent systemic blood flow (Acyanotic CHD)

	Acyanotic	Cyanotic
Color	Grey ($\downarrow$PBF)	Blue
Path	Ductal dependent systemic blood flow	Ductal dependent pulmonary blood flow R→L shunt
Examples	Coarctation, AS, Hypoplastic LV	$\downarrow$PBF: TOF, Tricus atresia, $\uparrow$PBF: TA, TAPVR, TGA
Present	1-2 weeks, sudden	1-2 weeks, sudden
Sx	Sudden circulatory collapse, hypotension, acidosis	Cyanotic, hypoxia not responsive to O_2
PEX	Shock, CHF, $\downarrow$LE pulses	Cyanotic
CXR	Normal	Boot shaped heart (TOF) Egg on a string (Transposition) Snowman (TAPVR)
PDA	Need PDA for systemic blood flow	Need PDA for pulm blood flow
Tx	PGE1	PGE1

Cyanotic CHD

- General
  - ⇨ Ductal dependent **pulmonary** blood flow
  - ⇨ When duct closes → $\downarrow$ pulmonary blood flow → $\downarrow O_2$ to body → infant becomes cyanotic/blue
  - ⇨ Cardiovascular consult immediately → OR?
- Diagnosis
  - ⇨ PEX: Cyanosis (blue baby)
  - ⇨ Hypoxia
    - ✓ $\downarrow O_2$ saturation → likely ductal dependent lesion
    - ✓ Hyperoxia test:
      - i. 10-15 min of 100% FiO_2
      - ii. If ABG PaO_2 <150 → indicative of cyanotic CHD
  - ⇨ CXR
    - ✓ Rule out other causes for hypoxia
- Treatment
  - ⇨ O_2
  - ⇨ PGE1
  - ⇨ IV fluids if hypotensive
  - ⇨ Vasopressors: Dopamine/Dobutamine if needed

Acyanotic CHD

- General
  - ⇨ Ductal dependent **systemic** blood flow
  - ⇨ When duct closes → $\downarrow$blood flow to body → **shock**
  - ⇨ Likely lesion: critical coarctation, aortic stenosis, hypoplastic LV

CRASHING NEONATE

- Diagnosis
  - ⇨ Shock?
    - ✓ Poor perfusion, tachycardia, hypotension
  - ⇨ 4 extremity BP and SaO$_2$
    - ✓ Look for gradient between extremities
- Treatment
  - ⇨ PGE1
  - ⇨ IVF if not in CHF
  - ⇨ Vasopressors: Dopamine, Dobutamine, Milrinone

Treatments
- PGE1
  - ⇨ Dose
    - ✓ 0.1 mcg/kg/min
  - ⇨ Side effects
    - ✓ Hypotension
    - ✓ Apnea
      - i. Dose-dependent and occurs early
      - ii. May need to intubate before transfer (do not stop PGE1)
  - ⇨ Check for clinical improvement → Perfusion, pH, BP, SaO$_2$, Urine output
- Vasopressors
  - ⇨ Cyanotic CHD:
    - ✓ Dopamine/Dobutamine
  - ⇨ Acyanotic CHD:
    - ✓ Dopamine/Dobutamine (5-10 mcg/kg/min), Milrinone
    - ✓ Do not use Levophed or Epinephrine → may worsen coarctation
- Other
  - ⇨ IV fluids
  - ⇨ Acidosis? → Consider HCO$_3$ for pH < 7.0
  - ⇨ Anemia? → Consider transfusion

INTESTINAL EMERGENCIES

VOLVULUS
- Presentation
  - ⇨ Congenital malrotation
  - ⇨ Irritable, vomiting: gastroenteritis symptoms
  - ⇨ Unexplained Bilious Vomiting in young infant = malrotation and midgut volvulus until proven otherwise
- Work-up
  - ⇨ KUB: usually normal but can have "double-bubble" sign with severe duodenal obstruction
  - ⇨ UGI: corkscrewing of intestine
- Treatment
  - ⇨ Antibiotics
  - ⇨ Surgical emergency!
  - ⇨ Complete volvulus can lead to bowel necrosis in 1-2 hours! (Emerg Med Clinics North Am 2002;20:139-153)

Vomit Pearl
Bilious vomit = Volvulus

NECROTIZING ENTEROCOLITIS
- Usually in premies but can be in full term infants
- Presentation: similar to volvulus → feeding difficulties, irritability, abdominal distention, and hematochezia
- KUB
  - ⇨ Low sensitivity-usually normal
  - ⇨ Late: pneumatosis intestinalis (gas in bowel wall) or portal free air
- Tx: Bowel rest, antibiotics, surgical consultation

Other Intestinal emergencies
- Incarcerated hernia
- Diaphragmatic hernia
- Toxic Megacolon
- Duodenal atresia
- Pyloric stenosis

Treatment for all
- ABCs and resuscitation: Saline and Dextrose as above
- NPO
- Antibiotics
- Upper GI contrast study
- Surgical Consult

CRASHING NEONATE

INBORN ERRORS OF METABOLISM (IEM)

Pathophysiology
- Biochemical defect that causes accumulation of toxic metabolite (NH_4, ketones, lactic acid)

Presentation
- AMS, vomiting, lethargy, coma, dehydration
- H/O sibling deaths
- CNS symptoms
- Hepatomegaly
- Odor (sweat, musty, fruity, like urine)
- Family history of siblings with same presentation?

Work-up and treatment
- Labs
  - ⇨ ↓ Glucose
  - ⇨ ↑NH_4
  - ⇨ ↑Ketones
  - ⇨ ↑Lactate
- NPO
- Hypoglycemia: D10 (5-10ml/kg IV)
- Rehydrate
  - ⇨ Bolus: 10cc/kg NS boluses
  - ⇨ Maintenance: D10 ¼ NS 1.5-2x maint rate after fluid boluses
- HCO_3? (if pH<7.1 for organic acidemia)

Acidosis → yes → ↑NH_4 → yes → Organic acidemia / Urea cycle defect; no → Amino acid defect

CAH (CONGENITAL ADRENAL HYPERPLASIA)

Pathophysiology
- 21-hydroxylase deficiency (90%)
  - ⇨ Deficiency in cortisol and aldosterone → hyponatremia, hyperkalemia
  - ⇨ Accumulation of androgens → changes in female genitalia

Presentation
- Vomiting, dehydration, lethargy, decreased po intake
- Shock in the first 2 weeks of life
- Hyponatremia, hyperkalemia and hypoglycemia

Treatment
- Hypoglycemia treatment → D10 (5 to 10 ml/kg)
- Resuscitate: 10cc/kg NS boluses
- Treat hyperkalemia
  - ⇨ Ca-gluconate for hyperK and EKG changes
  - ⇨ (See bradycardia algorithm-remember to adjust dosages for peds)
- Steroids: Hydrocortisone 25mg IV/IM/IO

NON-ACCIDENTAL TRAUMA

Presentation
- May have no external signs of trauma
- Scalp hematoma → associated with ↑risk of intracranial hemorrhage
- Retinal hemorrhages

Work-up
- CT head
- Admit
- Social work/child services

OTHER CAUSES

- NAT (Non accidental Trauma)
- Arrhythmias
- Formula-mix ups
- Omphalitis
- AVM (Arteriovenous Malformation)
- Bronchiolitis

1 Unstable?

Resuscitation →

Ruptured Ectopic?
⇨ ABCs
⇨ IV/O₂/Monitor/Hb
⇨ IVF resuscitate
⇨ T&C→Transfusion?
⇨ FAST US: Free fluid? Mass?
⇨ Emergent GYN consult for OR

Stable

2 R/O Ectopic

US

ß-HCG

+ Ectopic

⇨ US: Free Fluid?
⇨ GYN C/S
⇨ MTX vs Surgery vs Expectant mgmt

Unstable

OR

Indeterminate

HCG < DZ

Non-Diagnostic

⇨ GYN C/S
⇨ Serial ß-HCG (48h)

HCG > DZ

Abnormal Pregnancy

⇨ GYN C/S
⇨ Expectant mgmt vs MTX vs Surgery

+ IUP

☐ No Ectopic
☐ Heterotopic? (Infertility drugs?...)
☐ Eval for SAB (below)

3 Eval for SAB

OS

POC

Tx

Threatened

☐ Os closed
☐ No POC

⇨ Expectant mgmt
⇨ D/C Home
⇨ GYN F/U

Inevitable

☐ Os open
☐ No POC

⇨ GYN C/S
⇨ Surgical vs medical management

Incomplete

☐ Os open
☐ + POC

⇨ Remove POC
⇨ GYN C/S
⇨ Surgical vs medical management

Complete

☐ Os closed
☐ POC expelled

⇨ Expectant mgmt
⇨ D/C Home
⇨ GYN F/U

4 Rh Status →

RhoGAM if Rh(-)

5 Other Dx

☐ Exclude Vaginal/Cervical/Uterine Pathology
☐ Molar pregnancy
☐ Physiologic/Implantation Bleeding (Dx of exclusion)
☐ Abruption

VAGINAL BLEEDING: PREGNANT

1. GENERAL APPROACH AND RESUSCITATION

ACEP Guidelines (Ann Emerg Med. 2012;60:381-390.) (EM:RAP 10/13)

- General
  - ⇨ Start with initial resuscitation and ABCs depending on stability of the patient
  - ⇨ Then rule-out ectopic pregnancy using pelvic ultrasound and HCG level
  - ⇨ If ultrasound shows IUP and no concern for ectopic, then evaluate for SAB based on os and POC on exam
  - ⇨ Final steps are to consider RhoGAM and other benign causes for vaginal bleeding
- Unstable patient
  - ⇨ Treat as ruptured ectopic
  - ⇨ Clinical: Severe abdominal pain, peritonitis, hypotension/shock
  - ⇨ FAST US: Intraperitoneal free fluid, complex adnexal mass
  - ⇨ Type and Cross vs transfusion
  - ⇨ Emergent Gyn consult for OR

2. R/O ECTOPIC PREGNANCY

Work-up

- Based on results of U/S → 3 possibilities:
  - ⇨ If U/S shows **ectopic**, Gyn consult for operative vs conservative management
  - ⇨ If U/S shows **IUP** and no concern for heterotopic, eval for SAB
  - ⇨ If U/S **indeterminate**, classify into non-diagnostic or abnormal pregnancy based on ß-HCG level

Gestational Age	Transabdominal Landmarks	Transvaginal Landmarks	β-HCG Level
4-5 weeks	+/- Gestational sac	Gestational sac	1000
5 weeks	Gestational sac +/- yolk sac	Gestational sac, yolk sac +/-fetal pole	1000-2000
6 weeks	Yolk sac and fetal pole	Yolk sac, fetal pole with cardiac activity	10,000-20,000

A. INTRAUTERINE PREGNANCY (IUP)

U/S criteria for IUP
- See table for normal US appearance in pregnancy
- Gestational sac + "double decidual sac" sign is earliest sign of pregnancy, although most believe it is the yolk sac

Pitfall: Pseudosacs
- Pseudosacs are false sacs that can be confused with gestational sacs
- Pseudosacs can occur in 10-20% of ectopic pregnancies
- Centrally located → compared to eccentric location of true gestational sacs

Management
- Ectopic?
  - ⇨ IUP in uterus essentially rules-out ectopic pregnancy unless concerned about heterotopic pregnancy
- **Heterotopic** (ectopic + IUP) incidence:
  - ⇨ General population: 1:4,000-30,000
  - ⇨ Incidence in assisted reproduction: 1 in 100, therefore cannot exclude ectopic and further work-up needed in this population
- Miscarriage
  - ⇨ See Eval for Spontaneous Abortion section → patient is, at minimum having a threatened miscarriage

B. INDETERMINATE: NON DIAGNOSTIC

(β-HCG < DZ)

Discriminatory Zone (DZ):
- Definition: β-HCG level at which it is assumed that all viable intrauterine pregnancies can be visualized by ultrasound
- Level varies by institution and by experience of ultrasonographer
- DZ level
  - ⇨ Discriminatory zone for ß-HCG for transvaginal U/S is classically 1500-3000 (depending on institution)
  - ⇨ New evidence shows discriminatory zone may actually be higher, even greater than 3500 in one study (Obstet Gynecol 2013;121:65–70)(N Engl J Med 2013;369:1443)
  - ⇨ Caution in using a strict β-HCG cutoff to rule out a viable gestation

Indeterminate U/S below Discriminatory Zone (DZ):
- Ddx: early viable IUP vs nonviable IUP vs ectopic
- If pt stable:
  - ⇨ Gyn consult
  - ⇨ Serial ß-HCG
  - ⇨ U/S repeat when ß-HCG above DZ
  - ⇨ OK to d/c home if patient stable and reliable
- **Pitfall**: Low ß-HCG
  - ⇨ U/S should still be obtained if ß-HCG is below discriminatory zone because may still be able to diagnose both IUP and ectopic (Level C ACEP Recommendation)

VAGINAL BLEEDING: PREGNANT

C. INDETERMINATE: ABNORMAL PREGNANCY
(β-HCG > DZ)

General
- Definition: Indeterminate U/S + β-HCG above the discriminatory zone
- Ddx: Recent spontaneous AB, multiple gestation, molar pregnancy, ectopic pregnancy, viable or non-viable pregnancy
- Indeterminate U/S + ß-HCG > DZ: Diagnostic of ectopic pregnancy? (Fertil Steril 1998;70:972-981)

Follow up
- Follow-up needed in abnormal pregnancy because of **increased likelihood of ectopic** (Level B ACEP Recommendation Ann Emerg Med 2003;41:123)
- Serial β-HCG
  - ⇨ Standard approach for serial ß-HCG is a rise of 66% at 48hours (considered normal) although:
  - ⇨ A normal rise may be seen in up to 15% of ectopics and an abnormal rise (<66%) may be seen in 15% of IUPs (Obstet Gynecol 1981;58:162-6)
  - ⇨ Serial ß-HCG values at 48h: (Level B ACEP Recommendation Ann Emerg Med 2003;41:123)
    - ✓ **66% increase:** IUP, Ectopic (15%)
    - ✓ **Plateau:** nonviable IUP, Ectopic Pregnancy (EP)
    - ✓ **<66% increase:** Ectopic, non-viable IUP, nl IUP(15%)
    - ✓ **Decreasing:** SAB, resolving ectopic
- Ectopic pregnancy can resolve spontaneously by tubal abortion or regression, but >90% of women with ectopic and ß-HCG>2,000 will require surgery (CMAJ 2005;173(8);905-912)

ECTOPIC PREGNANCY

Diagnosis
- U/S signs suggestive of ectopic pregnancy (Ma OJ, First Trimester Pregnancy. In: Emergency Ultrasound, McGraw Hill. 2003, pp. 239)
  - ⇨ Definite: Extra-uterine embryo with cardiac activity (seen in 15-20% of ectopic pregnancies)
  - ⇨ Suggestive: Free pelvic or Intra-peritoneal fluid, tubal ring, complex adnexal mass
- Incidence of **heterotopic** (ectopic + IUP) in
  - ⇨ General population: 1:4,000-30,000
  - ⇨ Incidence in assisted reproduction: 1 in 100, therefore cannot exclude ectopic and further work-up needed in this population

Treatment
- Unstable
  - ⇨ Treat as ruptured ectopic
  - ⇨ Clinical: Severe abdominal pain, peritonitis, hypotension/shock
  - ⇨ FAST US: Intraperitoneal free fluid, complex adnexal mass
  - ⇨ Type and Cross vs transfusion
  - ⇨ Emergent GYN consult for OR
- Stable
  - ⇨ Expectant management
    - ✓ Indication: unknown location pregnancy or suspected ectopic with low/declining β-HCG
    - ✓ Contraindications: Risk factors for rupture (increasing abdominal pain), not able to follow-up, and lack of timely access to medical care
  - ⇨ Methotrexate
    - ✓ See table for indications
  - ⇨ Surgery
    - ✓ Indications: Hemodynamic instability, contraindications to methotrexate, suspicion or risk factors for rupture, or failed medical therapy

Indications for Medical Therapy for Ectopic Pregnancy

- ☐ Hemodynamically stable
- ☐ Patient desires future fertility
- ☐ Ability to return for follow-up
- ☐ No contraindications to MTX
- ☐ Unruptured mass <3.5cm
- ☐ No fetal cardiac activity
- ☐ Quantitative ß-hCG < 6,000-15,000

VAGINAL BLEEDING: PREGNANT

3. Eval for Spontaneous Abortion

SPONTANEOUS ABORTION

General
- Evaluate for spontaneous abortion in the patient with an IUP and vaginal bleeding
- Classify into type of SAB based on cervical OS and POC (Products of Conception)

Classification
- Threatened miscarriage
  - ⇨ Os closed and no POC
- Inevitable
  - ⇨ Os open and no POC
- Incomplete
  - ⇨ Os open and POC on exam in os
- Complete
  - ⇨ Os closed and POC expelled

Incidence of miscarriage: (BMJ 1997;315:32-4)
- 21% of pregnant patients bleed before 20th wk
  - ⇨ 57% of those will miscarry
    - ✓ 80% of those will miscarry before 12 weeks
- After detection of fetal cardiac activity, <5% of pregnancies with normal sonographic appearance will abort(Ann Emerg Med 2003;41:123,)

4. RhoGAM?

Indication
- RhoGAM 50 mcg for Rh(-) women at time of first trimester pregnancy loss (Level B ACEP Recommendation Ann Emerg Med 2003;41:123,)
- No recommendations for after first trimester, but standard dose is 300 mcg IM

5. Non Emergent Causes of Vaginal Bleeding

MOLAR PREGNANCY
- Diagnosis by U/S showing "snowstorm" pattern or cystic structures
- Treatment is surgical evacuation with close monitoring of ß-HCG levels

IMPLANTATION BLEEDING
- Definition: spotting from implantation of embryo around the time of expected menses

ANEMBRYONIC PREGNANCY
- Development of a gestational sac without embryonic structures
- They may present with vaginal bleeding and abdominal pain
- The diagnosis is confirmed with ultrasound. Treatment is misoprostol and/or uterine aspiration

ROUND LIGAMENT SYNDROME
- Usually presents with abdominal or low back pain, not vaginal bleeding
- Normal occurrence due to growth of the uterus
- The majority have pain on the right side as the uterus tilts to that side

ACUTE PELVIC PAIN

1 Resuscitation
- ☐ ABCs
- ☐ IV/O₂/Fluids
- ☐ β-HCG

2 R/O GYN Causes

📋 H & P	🔊 U/S	✏️ Action

Ovarian Torsion

H & P
- ☐ Risk Factors: Reproductive age, pregnant, infertility tx, vigorous activity, h/o ov cyst
- ☐ Acute severe unilateral pelvic pain
- ☐ Radiation back, flank, groin
- ☐ N/V

U/S
- ☐ Cystic/Solid mass (>70%)
- ☐ Free Fluid (>50%)
- ☐ Doppler (Art/venous flow, whirlpool sign)

Action
- ⇨ Pain control
- ⇨ GYN consult
- ⇨ OR

TOA

H & P
- ☐ Abd/Pelvic pain
- ☐ Vaginal d/c
- ☐ PID sx
- ☐ CMT/adnexal pain
- ☐ Palpable mass
- ☐ Fever
- ☐ ↑WBC

U/S
- ☐ Cystic/Solid mass (>70%)
- ☐ Free Fluid (>50%)
- ☐ Doppler (Art/venous flow, whirlpool sign)

Action
- ⇨ Antibiotics
- ⇨ GYN consult
- ⇨ CT?
- ⇨ IR guided drainage
- ⇨ OR

PID

H & P
- ☐ Abd/Pelvic pain
- ☐ Vaginal d/c
- ☐ Fever
- ☐ STD risk factors
- ☐ CMT/Adnexal tenderness
- ☐ Febrile
- ☐ ↑WBC/ESR

U/S
- ☐ Can use to r/o TOA

Action
- ⇨ Cultures
- ⇨ Antibiotics
- ⇨ GYN consult

3 R/O Non-GYN Causes

GI Causes
- ☐ Appendicitis
- ☐ Diverticulitis
- ☐ Hernia, Obstruction, other
- ☐ (See Abdominal Pain Algorithm)

Action
- ⇨ Labs
- ⇨ CT A/P?
- ⇨ Surgery C/S

GU Causes
- ☐ UTI/Pyelonephritis
- ☐ Kidney stone/ Renal Colic

Action
- ⇨ UA
- ⇨ U/S
- ⇨ CT Stone protocol

4 Other GYN Causes
- ☐ Ruptured ovarian cyst (can be emergent if hemoperitoneum present)
- ☐ Mittleschmerz
- ☐ Endometriosis
- ☐ Leiomyoma

ACUTE PELVIC PAIN

1. GENERAL APPROACH AND RESUSCITATION

- The approach to the woman with pelvic pain is to start with the initial resuscitation and β-HCG
- Then the focus should be on emergent gynecologic disease, such as ovarian torsion and PID/TOA
- Then expand the differential to think about non-gynecologic causes from GU or GI origin, most commonly appendicitis
- If that work-up is negative, consider treating empirically for PID, and think about other causes of pelvic pain

2. EMERGENT GYN CAUSE?

OVARIAN TORSION

General
- Definitive diagnosis of ovarian torsion is based on surgical findings
- Difficult diagnosis → correct pre-operative diagnosis made in only 38% of cases (J Reprod Med 2000;45:831)

Clinical Presentation
- Risk Factors: Reproductive age, pregnant, infertility tx, vigorous activity
- Acute severe unilateral pelvic pain
- Radiation to back, flank, groin
- N/V

U/S
- **Cyst/Mass** (Clin Exp Obstet Gynecol 2004;31:34)
    ⇨ Found in >94% of torsion cases
    ⇨ Most commonly, mass is greater than 5cm
    ⇨ Normal ovaries (absence of cyst/mass) does not completely rule-out torsion
    ⇨ Normal ovaries found in 6% of adult cases and over 50% of children under age 15 (Arch Pediatr Adolesc Med 2005;159:532-535)
- **Doppler blood flow** (J Clin Ultrasound. 2009;37(8):436)
    ⇨ Predictive of non-viability of the ovary
    ⇨ Blood flow preserved in early/incomplete torsion or torsion/detorsion
- **Whirlpool sign** (J Ultrasound Med 2004;23:1643–1649)
    ⇨ Sonographic appearance of twisted vascular pedicle
    ⇨ Earliest and most definitive sign for torsion
- Caution
    ⇨ Ovaries have dual blood supply, therefore, the presence of normal flow does not exclude torsion
    ⇨ If high clinical suspicion (persistent pain) → may need laparoscopy despite negative ultrasound

Treatment:
- Pain control
- Gyn consult for surgical evaluation

TOA
(EM:RAP 1/11 "Imaging in TOA"-Swadron)

General: Tuboovarian Abscess
- Definition: Inflammatory mass in fallopian tube/ovary/pelvic organs, found most commonly in reproductive age women and typically results from upper genital tract infection
- Etiology: PID (most common), pelvic surgery, intra-abdominal process
- Microbiology: same as PID, polymicrobial, anaerobes

Clinical Presentation
- Abd/Pelvic pain
- PID symptoms, Vaginal d/c
- CMT/adnexal pain
- Palpable mass
- Fever, ↑WBC

Diagnosis
- Consider in any woman suspected of PID
- U/S:
    ⇨ Homogeneous, cystic mass with air/fluid levels and septations
    ⇨ Utility (Journal Emerg Med 2011;40:170)
        ✓ Newer studies show **sensitivities that range from 56% to 93%**, with a specificity of **86% to 98%**
        ✓ Low sensitivity of US → cannot rule out TOA, especially in the high risk patient
        ✓ If US negative → may need CT to continue evaluation for TOA
    ⇨ Helps differentiate TOA vs TOC (tubo-ovarian complex)→ perfused inflammatory living tissue without abscess wall, amenable to medical therapy

Treatment
* Medical: Trial of medical therapy (antibiotics) vs
* IR guided drainage vs
* Surgery: operative drainage

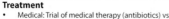

PID

General
* Represents a spectrum of disease from endometritis to fatal intra-abdominal sepsis

Clinical Presentation
* Abd/Pelvic pain
* Vaginal d/c
* Fever
* STD risk factors
* CMT/adnexal tenderness
* ↑WBC/ESR

Diagnosis
* US
  * ⇨ Rule-out TOA
  * ⇨ May be diagnostic of PID
* CDC has issued a **minimum set of criteria for treatment of PID** for women with **abdominal pain** and at least **one** of the criteria (See Table) (MMWR Recomm Rep 2010;59:1-110)

Criteria for Treatment: (MMWR Recomm Rep 2010;59:1-110)

☐ CMT or uterine/adnexal tenderness	☐ Vaginal secretions with WBC on saline microscopy
☐ Oral Temp>101F	☐ Elevated ESR
☐ Leukocytosis/left shift	☐ Elevated CRP
☐ Abnormal cervical/vaginal discharge	

Treatment (EM:RAP 7/13)
* Outpatient treatment
  * ⇨ If stable, well appearing, tolerating po, pain controlled → can be discharged on po antibiotics
  * ⇨ Antibiotics (see most recent CDC guidelines)
* Inpatient treatment
  * ⇨ If patient meets criteria for hospitalization → start IV antibiotics, admit

Criteria for Hospitalization: (MMWR Recomm Rep 2010;59:1-110)

☐ Surgical emergencies (e.g., appendicitis) cannot be excluded	☐ Unable to follow or tolerate an outpatient oral regimen;
☐ Pregnant	☐ Severe illness, nausea and vomiting, or high fever; and
☐ Does not respond clinically to oral antimicrobial therapy	☐ Tubo-ovarian abscess

3. R/O NON-GYN CAUSES
* See Abdominal Pain algorithms for more detailed explanation of GI and GU causes of abdominal pain
* Consider Appendicitis vs Diverticulitis (possible CT AP)
* Consider UTI (Check UA)
* Consider renal colic (UA, US, CT Stone?)

4. OTHER GYN CAUSES

OVARIAN CYST RUPTURE
* Sudden onset, unilateral abdominal pain, +/-vaginal bleeding, +/- peritoneal signs (blood irritating peritoneum)
* Uncomplicated (follicular or corpus luteum cyst) → follow expectantly for enlarging hemoperitoneum
* Complicated: may need surgical management, blood transfusion

MITTELSCHMERZ
* Mid-cycle pain from rupturing of follicle during ovulation

TRAUMA: PRIMARY SURVEY

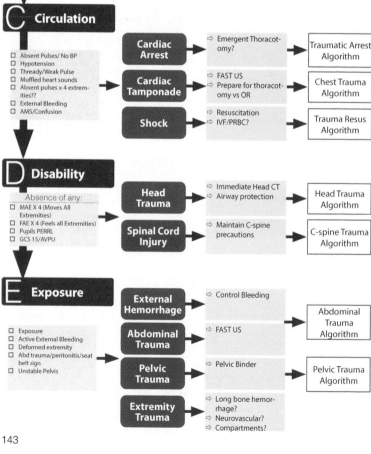

A Airway

Critical Dx

Critical Action

Absence of any:
- ☐ Patent
- ☐ Protected
- ☐ Phonating

→ **Airway Obstruction**

→
- ⇨ Clear obstruction
- ⇨ OP/NP airway
- ⇨ Open airway
- ⇨ Prepare for intubation
- ⇨ Cont Primary Survey

→ Airway Algorithm

B Breathing

- ☐ No breath sounds/not ventilating
- ☐ Unequal Breath sounds / chest excursion
- ☐ Crepitus
- ☐ Tracheal deviation
- ☐ JVD
- ☐ Flail Chest

→ **Respiratory Arrest**

→
- ⇨ Airway control and intubation
- ⇨ BVM until ready for intubation

→ Airway Algorithm

→ **Tension PTX**

→
- ⇨ Needle Thoracostomy
- ⇨ Set up for Chest Tube
- ⇨ Continue Primary Survey

→ Chest Trauma Algorithm

C Circulation

- ☐ Absent Pulses/ No BP
- ☐ Hypotension
- ☐ Thready/Weak Pulse
- ☐ Muffled heart sounds
- ☐ Absent pulses x 4 extremities??
- ☐ External Bleeding
- ☐ AMS/Confusion

→ **Cardiac Arrest**

→
- ⇨ Emergent Thoracotomy?

→ Traumatic Arrest Algorithm

→ **Cardiac Tamponade**

→
- ⇨ FAST US
- ⇨ Prepare for thoracotomy vs OR

→ Chest Trauma Algorithm

→ **Shock**

→
- ⇨ Resuscitation
- ⇨ IVF/PRBC?

→ Trauma Resus Algorithm

D Disability

Absence of any:
- ☐ MAE X 4 (Moves All Extremities)
- ☐ FAE X 4 (Feels all Extremities)
- ☐ Pupils PERRL
- ☐ GCS 15/AVPU

→ **Head Trauma**

→
- ⇨ Immediate Head CT
- ⇨ Airway protection

→ Head Trauma Algorithm

→ **Spinal Cord Injury**

→
- ⇨ Maintain C-spine precautions

→ C-spine Trauma Algorithm

E Exposure

- ☐ Exposure
- ☐ Active External Bleeding
- ☐ Deformed extremity
- ☐ Abd trauma/peritonitis/seat belt sign
- ☐ Unstable Pelvis

→ **External Hemorrhage**

→
- ⇨ Control Bleeding

→ Abdominal Trauma Algorithm

→ **Abdominal Trauma**

→
- ⇨ FAST US

→ **Pelvic Trauma**

→
- ⇨ Pelvic Binder

→ Pelvic Trauma Algorithm

→ **Extremity Trauma**

→
- ⇨ Long bone hemorrhage?
- ⇨ Neurovascular?
- ⇨ Compartments?

TRAUMA: PRIMARY SURVEY

GENERAL

- In severe trauma, assessment and resuscitation should be done simultaneously
- Always continue with the primary survey, even while doing procedures
- The purpose of the Primary Survey is to address and manage life threatening emergencies as early as possible in the evaluation of the trauma patient

A: AIRWAY

(**Essentials** 2010 "ABCs"-Arora) (EM:RAP 4/13)

Airway obstruction?:
☐ Patent?
☐ Protected/Gag reflex present?
☐ Phonating, patient able to speak?
  ✓ **Eval for airway obstruction**
    1. Open airway: Lift angle of jaw or chin to open airway while maintaining strict **C-spine precautions**
    2. Clear obstruction: Suction, McGills forceps
    3. OP/NP airway
    4. Able to Clear?
  ✓ **Persistent obstruction → Prepare to intubate**
    1. Prepare for intubation
    2. Continue Primary Survey while setting up
    3. Go to Airway Algorithm

B: BREATHING

Respiratory arrest?:
☐ Breath sounds/ventilating
  ✓ **No: Respiratory arrest?**
    1. Immediate intubation/airway control
    2. BVM until ready for intubation
    3. Go to airway algorithm

Tension Pneumothorax?:
☐ Unequal breath sounds/chest excursion
☐ Crepitus
☐ Tracheal deviation
☐ JVD
☐ Flail Chest
  ✓ **Does pt have a __Tension__ pneumothorax?** (Pneumothorax + Hypotension/Hypoxia/Tracheal Deviation)
    ✓ **If Yes: Immediate Needle Thoracostomy**
      1. Set up for immediate Chest Tube
      2. Go to Chest Trauma Algorithm
    ✓ **If No: Pt with stable Pneumothorax?** → Further evaluation needed
      1. US, CXR
      2. Set up for chest tube
      3. Continue Primary Survey
      4. Other pulmonary disease: Flail chest, sucking chest wound?

C: CIRCULATION

Cardiac Arrest?:
☐ Absent pulses, No BP
  ✓ **Yes: Resuscitate, thoracotomy?**
    1. Prepare for emergent thoracotomy
    2. FAST for cardiac tamponade
    3. Go to Traumatic Cardiac Arrest Algorithm

Cardiac Tamponade?:
☐ Hypotension
☐ Thready, weak pulses
☐ Muffled Heart tones
☐ ↓Pulses x 4 extremities
☐ Altered Mental Status/Confusion
  ✓ **If Yes: FAST US → positive for pericardial effusion?**
    ✓ **If Yes: OR vs thoracotomy**
      1. Prepare for thoracotomy if patient decompensates
      2. Prepare patient for OR immediately
      3. Go to Chest Trauma Algorithm

144

TRAUMA: PRIMARY SURVEY

Shock?
☐ ↓BP, HR, Shock index>0.9, cool clammy skin, AMS, ↑lactate
- ✓ **If Yes: Resuscitation**
  1. Begin Resuscitation-large bore IVs/Central line, Crystalloids,PRBC
  2. Identify cause of shock
  3. Stop active bleeding
  4. Go to Trauma Resuscitation Algorithm

D: DISABILITY

Head Trauma/Injury?
☐ Move all extremities (MAE) X 4
☐ Feel all extremities (FAE) X 4
☐ Pupils PERRL
☐ GCS 15, AVPU (Alert, Voice, Pain, Unresponsive)
- ✓ If concern for Head Trauma:
  1. Stabilize airway (consider intubation for GCS<8)
  2. Immediate Head CT
  3. Go to Head Trauma Algorithm

Is there concern for Spinal Cord injury?
- ✓ **Yes: Spinal immobilization**
  1. Maintain C-spine precautions
  2. Rectal and neuro exam before intubation
  3. Go to C-spine trauma algorithm

E: EXPOSURE

Active External Bleeding?:
- ✓ Yes: Control bleeding

Deformed extremity?:
1. Evaluate for internal long bone hemorrhage (femur)
2. Evaluate for Neurovascular status
3. Evaluate for compartment syndrome
4. Immobilize/splint early (↓pain, ↓bleeding, ↓ risk of fat embolism, ↓neurovascular damage)

Abdominal Trauma/Peritonitis/Seat Belt sign?
1. FAST to evaluate for internal hemorrhage
2. Peritonitis →prepare for OR
3. Go to Abdominal trauma algorithm

Pelvic Trauma
1. Unstable Pelvis
2. Pelvic Binder
3. Go to abdominal Trauma algorithm

F: 5 Fs

Finger:
• Rectal exam for rectal tone

FAST
• US

Foley
• Contraindications: blood at meatus and high riding prostate

Fentanyl
• Pain control

Family

TRAUMA: PRIMARY SURVEY

HISTORY: AMPLEF

A: Allergies

M: Meds

P: PMH

L: Last Meal, LMP

E: Events of Trauma

F: Family, friends, field information

SECONDARY SURVEY AND WORK-UP

Head to toe Exam

Imaging
- CXR
- Pelvis
- C-spine
- Other injuries?
- Labs
  - ⇨ POC: Accucheck, Hgb (serial)
  - ⇨ CBC, Chem, LFTs, Coag, lactate, Tox/EtOH, troponin, T&C
  - ⇨ Urine: U preg, UA, U Tox
  - ⇨ ABG

TRAUMA: RESUSCITATION

1. ABCs

Continue primary and secondary survey as per usual
See Trauma Primary Survey Algorithm

2. CAUSE OF SHOCK?

- See Shock Algorithm
- Obstructive shock
  - ⇨ Cardiac tamponade
  - ⇨ Tension pneumothorax
- Cardiogenic shock
  - ⇨ Blunt cardiac injury (BCI)
  - ⇨ ACS
- Neurogenic shock
  - ⇨ Spinal cord injury
- Hypovolemic shock
  - ⇨ Hemorrhage

3. RESUSCITATION STRATEGIES

(Essentials 2011-Inaba)

OR ASAP?
- Do not delay OR if indicated
- Indication: hypotensive penetrating abdominal/chest trauma
- Presume vascular injury as the cause

Permissive Hypotension option
- Use: Penetrating trauma to chest/abdomen
- Contraindication: Intracranial injury (hypotension reduces cerebral perfusion)
- Mechanism:
  - ⇨ **Limit fluid resuscitation** (at least until hemorrhage is controlled by natural hemostasis, external pressure, angiography or surgery)
  - ⇨ Aggressive fluid administration might, via increasing BP → cause dilution of clotting factors and hypothermia → disrupt thrombus formation and enhance bleeding
- Goal: **Target fluid resuscitation to SBP of 70mm Hg**
- **Conclusion: Consider "permissive hypotension" in patients with suspected active bleeding, SBP of about 90mmHg and good mentation** (Demetriades-"The Red Book")

> #### Journal Club: Permissive Hypotension in Trauma
>
> **NEJM 1994** (NEJM 1994;331:1105)
> - Delayed fluid resuscitation associated with increased survival (70% vs 62%)
> - **No difference in morbidity**
>
> **Dutton et al** (J Trauma. 2002;52:1141)
> - Series of blunt and penetrating trauma patients compared target SBP 70mmHg vs 100mmHg
> - **No difference in mortality** in the two groups
>
> **Morrison et al** (J Trauma. 2011;70: 652– 663)
> - Patients stratified into Low goal MAP (LMAP) group of 50mmHg vs High goal MAP (HMAP) of 65mmHg
> - LMAP group had lower postoperative mortality (6 versus 10 deaths), received fewer blood products, and did not develop coagulopathy or multiple organ failure
> - **No significant difference in overall mortality** at 30 days.

Massive Transfusion (MT) protocol (LAC+USC specific)
- Definition: Patient requiring >10 Units blood in 12-24h
- General: Coagulopathy is present on arrival in 25% of patients because of loss of factors and platelets
- Indication: Severe hemorrhage/blood loss resulting in severe hypotension/shock
- Protocol (Goal of 1:1:1 Ratio in MT patient)
  - ⇨ Begin with 1-2L NS or LR
  - ⇨ PRBC Transfusion:
    - ✓ Whole blood (autotransfused) vs uncrossed vs type specific vs cross matched
  - ⇨ Plasma (FFP)
    - ✓ Indication: >6 Units PRBC, elevated INR, Coumadin use
    - ✓ Ratio: 1:1 with PRBC, beginning on the 6th Unit (Begin on first unit if Warfarin use)
  - ⇨ Platelets
    - ✓ Indication: >6 Units PRBC
    - ✓ Ratio: Apheresis platelets in 1:6 ratio with PRBC
    - ✓ Note: 1 Unit apheresis platelets = 6-8 units random pooled donor platelets

- Adverse effects
  - ⇨ Use of plasma had no effect on outcome if massive transfusion was not achieved, irrespective of ratio
  - ⇨ Increased complications with plasma if MT not achieved: (J Am Coll Surg 2010;210:957)
    - ✓ Pneumonia (2x), Sepsis (2x),
    - ✓ Multi-system organ failure (MSOF 6x)
    - ✓ ARDS (12x)
  - ⇨ End point?
    - ✓ Damage control infusion of FFP and PLT should be rapidly terminated when it becomes clear that a massive transfusion will not be required. (J Trauma. 2011;71: S329–S336)

> ### Journal Club: Massive Transfusion in Trauma
> (EM:RAP 7/13)
>
> **Teixeira 2009** (J Trauma. 2009;66:693)
> - A high FFP:RBC is an independent predictor of survival in MT
>
> **Inaba 2010** (J Am Coll Surg 2010;211: 573)
> - Increasing platelet transfusion, in ratios approaching 1:6 was associated with a stepwise improvement in survival at 12 and 24 hours and in overall survival to discharge
>
> **PROMMTT** (JAMA Surg. 2013;148(2):127)
> - Increased ratios of plasma:RBCs and platelets:RBCs were independently associated with decreased 6-hour mortality
> - The survival was strongest in the first 6 hours and there was no association by 30 days.
> - If the ratio of FFP:PRBC < 1:2 → 3-4 fold increase in death when compared to a 1:1 ratio

---

ADJUNCTIVE THERAPIES

Tranexamic acid (TXA) (EM:RAP 12/12) (Essentials 2013 "Tranexamic acid"-Mallon)
- CRASH-2 Trial (Lancet 2010; 376: 23–32)
  - ⇨ **All cause mortality decreased with TXA** (16% vs 14.5%)
  - ⇨ Risk of death due to bleeding reduced (5.7% to 4.9%)
  - ⇨ Many criticisms with trial (probably underestimated benefit of TXA)
  - ⇨ No safety issues with TXA
- CRASH-2 secondary analysis (Lancet 2011;377:1096)
  - ⇨ Early treatment (**<1h) decreased death** due to bleeding from 7.7% (TXA) to 5.3% (placebo)
  - ⇨ Treatment between **1 and 3 h also reduced the risk of death** due to bleeding 4.8% (TXA) to 6.1% (placebo)
  - ⇨ Treatment **after 3h increased death** due to bleeding 4.4% (TXA) to 3.1% (placebo)
- MATTERS Trial (Arch Surg. 2012;147(2):113)
  - ⇨ TXA group had **lower mortality** despite being more severely injured (17.4% vs 23.9%)
  - ⇨ More mortality benefit if patient received massive transfusion (14.4% vs 23.9%)
  - ⇨ TXA survival OR = 7.23
  - ⇨ Independent predictor of survival in patients receiving MT (OR = 7.2)
- TXA Use [See PDR for current dosing regimen]
  - ⇨ 1 gram over 10 min, may repeat (then1 gram over 8 hours)
  - ⇨ Give early (3 hour window for improved benefit)

Hypertonic Saline
- 8 RCTs show **no survival benefit**
- Traumatic Brain Injury- TBI (JAMA. 2004;291:1350-1357)
  - ⇨ Hypertonic saline showed **no difference in survival or neurologic outcome**
- ROC Trial (JAMA. 2010;304(13):1455-1464)(Ann Surg. 2011; 253(3):431)
  - ⇨ Stopped early for **futility**
  - ⇨ Hypertonic saline had no difference in survival, neurologic outcome or MSOF
- Hypertonic saline use (Inaba)
  - ⇨ Non-shock fluid resuscitation → No
  - ⇨ Shock, fluid challenge → No
  - ⇨ TBI requiring fluid → No
  - ⇨ **TBI + Increased ICP → MAYBE**

1 Initial Resuscitation

A: Airway
- IV/O₂/Monitor
- Intubation

B: Breathing
- Lung US vs
- Bilateral Chest tubes

C: Circulation
- Central line
- IV Fluid
- Blood transfusion?

2 Thoracotomy vs US

No SOL?

Signs of Life (SOL)?
- Pulse
- Pupils
- Movement
- Breathing
- PEA
- Cardiac motion (US)

SOL + → See Trauma Resus Algorithm

No SOL

Prolonged CPR?

Prolonged Resus?
- Blunt trauma, CPR >10min
- Penetrating trauma torso, CPR > 15min
- Penetrating trauma neck/ extremity, CPR >5 min

Yes → DEAD

No

ED Thoracotomy vs ECHO

Cardiac activity?
or
Cardiac tamponade?

No → DEAD

Yes

Release pericardial tamponade
Repair cardiac injury

TRAUMA: CARDIAC ARREST

1. INITIAL RESUSCITATION

(**Essentials** 2012-Weingart)(EM:RAP 5/2012)
(J Am Coll Surg 2003;196:106-112) (J Trauma Acute Care Surg 2012;73:1359)

A: Airway
- Oxygen/BVM
- Intubation

B: Breathing
- Tension pneumothorax/hemothorax?
- Tx: US chest(diagnosis) vs bilateral chest tubes (empiric treatment)

C: Circulation
- IV Fluids/Blood transfusion
- Cardiac tamponade: Thoracotomy (see below)

2. THORACOTOMY VS ECHO

(Western Trauma Association Guidelines: westerntrauma.org)

Signs of Life?
- Signs of life:
  - ⇨ Pulse
  - ⇨ Pupils
  - ⇨ Movement
  - ⇨ Breathing
  - ⇨ PEA
  - ⇨ Cardiac motion (US)
- If SOL (+) → follow further ATLS guidelines and resuscitate patient
  - ⇨ See Trauma Resuscitation algorithm
- Profound refractory shock?
  - ⇨ CPR with SOL or SBP < 60
  - ⇨ Indication for resuscitative thoracotomy

No Signs of Life (SOL):
☐ No pulse
☐ No pupils
☐ No movement
☐ No breaths
☐ No PEA
☐ No cardiac motion (US)

Prolonged downtime?
- Time limits:
  - ⇨ Blunt trauma, CPR > 10min
  - ⇨ Penetrating trauma, CPR > 15min
  - ⇨ Penetrating trauma to neck/extremity > 5 min
- If prolonged downtime → further efforts futile
- If within time-frame → continue to ED thoracotomy
  - ⇨ Can do ED US/ECHO as substitute for thoracotomy

ED Thoracotomy Indications:
Trauma + CPR + no SOL +:
☐ Blunt trauma, CPR < 10min
☐ Penetrating trauma, CPR < 15min
☐ Penetrating trauma to neck/ extremity < 5 min

ED Thoracotomy/ECHO
- Goal:
  - ⇨ Look for **cardiac activity**
  - ⇨ Look for **pericardial effusion/tamponade**
  - ⇨ **If no cardiac activity and no effusion/tamponade → DEAD**
- Procedure: ED Thoracotomy (Essentials 2013-"Crack to Cure")
  - ⇨ **Release pericardial tamponade**
  - ⇨ Advance ET tube to right mainstem
  - ⇨ Address hemorrhage inside chest
  - ⇨ Cross clamp aorta → diverts blood away from intra-abdominal hemorrhage
  - ⇨ Open cardiac resuscitation
  - ⇨ Chest tube on right: if + blood → clamshell
- ED Thoracotomy Survival rates:
  - ⇨ Overall survival rate 7.4%, dictated by location & mechanism of injury (J Am Coll Surg 2000;190:288-98)
    - ✓ Thoracic injury 10.7% (Cardiac-19.4%), **abdominal injury 4.5%**
    - ✓ Penetrating injury 8.8% (stab wounds 17%, GSW 4.3%) **blunt trauma 1.4%**

TRAUMA: BLUNT HEAD

1 CT Decision Rules

Nexus II

If ALL criteria present:
- ☐ No evidence of cranial trauma (skull fx, scalp hematoma)
- ☐ Normal neurologic exam (no AMS, no abnormal behavior, non-focal)
- ☐ Age < 65
- ☐ No persistent vomiting
- ☐ No coagulopathy

→ **No CT**

ACEP Policy

LOC or amnesia plus:
- ☐ Headache
- ☐ Vomiting
- ☐ Age > 60 years
- ☐ Drug or
- ☐ Alcohol intoxication
- ☐ Deficits in short-term memory
- ☐ Trauma above the clavicle
- ☐ Post traumatic seizure
- ☐ GCS <15
- ☐ Focal neurologic deficit
- ☐ Coagulopathy

→ **CT**

2 CT Minor Decision Rules

Canadian Rules

High Risk
- ☐ GCS<15 at 2h post injury
- ☐ Suspected open or depressed skull fx
- ☐ Age >65
- ☐ Vomiting >2x
- ☐ Any sign of basal skull fx

Medium Risk
- ☐ Amnesia before impact >30mins
- ☐ Dangerous Mechanism (auto v ped, fall from height >3ft, ejected)

→ **CT**

New Orleans Criteria

- ☐ Headache
- ☐ Drug/ETOH Intoxication
- ☐ Age >60
- ☐ Vomiting
- ☐ Persistent anterograde amnesia
- ☐ Soft tissue/bony injury above the clavicles
- ☐ Seizure

→ **CT**

3 Delayed Bleed Risk?

Coumadin
Plavix
Other Anticoagulant

→ Observation

VS

D/C Home with Return Precautions

4 Special Population

Coagulopathy
Anticoagulants
Elderly
Pediatrics

TRAUMA: BLUNT HEAD

1. HEAD CT RULES

Nexus II (J Trauma 2005;59:954–959)
- Criteria highly associated with intra-cranial injury:
  - ⇨ Evidence of significant skull fracture
  - ⇨ Scalp hematoma
  - ⇨ Neurologic deficit
  - ⇨ Altered level of alertness
  - ⇨ Abnormal behavior
  - ⇨ Coagulopathy
  - ⇨ Persistent vomiting
  - ⇨ Age 65 years or more.
- Evidence:
  - ⇨ Clinically significant injuries: Sens 98.3; NPV 99.1%; Specificity-13.7%
  - ⇨ Expected miss rate: approximately 1.7% of cases with "clinically important" intracranial injuries
- Use: Identify patients that are low risk that don't need further imaging, not useful in deciding who does need imaging

ACEP Clinical Policy (Ann Emerg Med. 2008;52:714-748)
- A head CT is indicated in head trauma patients with **loss of consciousness or posttraumatic amnesia** only if one or more of the following is present **(Level A Recommendation)**:
  - ⇨ Headache
  - ⇨ Vomiting
  - ⇨ Age greater than 60 years
  - ⇨ Drug or alcohol intoxication
  - ⇨ Deficits in short-term memory
  - ⇨ Physical evidence of trauma above the clavicle
  - ⇨ Posttraumatic seizure
  - ⇨ GCS score less than 15
  - ⇨ Focal neurologic deficit
  - ⇨ Coagulopathy
- A head CT should be considered in head trauma patients with **no LOC or posttraumatic amnesia** if there is **(Level B Recommendation)**:
  - ⇨ Focal neurologic deficit
  - ⇨ Vomiting, severe headache
  - ⇨ Age 65 years or greater
  - ⇨ Physical signs of a basilar skull fracture
  - ⇨ GCS score less than 15
  - ⇨ Coagulopathy
  - ⇨ Dangerous mechanism of injury*
    - ✓ * Dangerous mechanism of injury includes ejection from a motor vehicle, a pedestrian struck, and a fall from a height of more than 3 feet or 5 stairs.

2. OTHER HEAD CT RULES (FOR YOUR CONSIDERATION)

Canadian (Lancet. 2001;357:1391-6)
- Clinically important brain injury Sens 98%, Specificity 50%
- Neurosurgical intervention Sens 100%, Specificity 68%
- Complicated algorithm, extensive inclusion criteria for study, difficult to use in practice
- Inclusion Criteria:
  - ⇨ LOC, amnesia, disorientation
  - ⇨ GCS >13
  - ⇨ Age >16
  - ⇨ No penetrating skull injury
  - ⇨ Not pregnant
  - ⇨ No focal deficit
  - ⇨ No coagulopathy
  - ⇨ No seizure
  - ⇨ No unstable vital signs

Glasgow Comas Scale (GCS)		
(E) Best Eye Response	Spontaneous-open with blinking	4
	Opens to verbal command, speech, shout	3
	Opens to pain	2
	None	1
(V) Best Verbal Response	Oriented	5
	Confused conversation, able to answer questions	4
	Inappropriate response	3
	Incomprehensible speech	2
	None	1
(M) Best Motor Response	Obeys commands for movement	6
	Purposeful movement to painful stimulus	5
	Withdraws from pain	4
	Abnormal (spastic) flexion, decorticate posture	3
	Extensor (rigid) response, decerebrate posture	2
	None	1

New Orleans (NEJM 2000;343(2):100)
- Too sensitive and non-specific (Sens 100%, Spec 24%)
- Limitations: limited applicability, wide confidence intervals, has not been validated, used any injury as outcome measure
- Imaging obtained for any patient with trauma above clavicles → decreases specificity
- Inclusion criteria
  - ⇨ Age >3yo
  - ⇨ +LOC
  - ⇨ Normal neuro exam
  - ⇨ GCS 15

TRAUMA: BLUNT HEAD

3. DELAYED BLEED RISK?

Delayed bleed Evidence (BHT + Anticoagulation) (EM:RAP 1/14-Arora/Menchine) (Essentials 2013 #67)
- **Immediate intracranial hemorrhage** (BHT + Anticoagulation)
  - ⇨ ICH is a real entity with occurrence of 10-15%
  - ⇨ Any patient with head trauma on warfarin or clopidogrel should get an initial Head CT scan
- **Delayed intracranial hemorrhage** (BHT + Anticoagulation + CT neg)
  - ⇨ Delayed ICH is also a real entity
  - ⇨ **Increased risk in elderly and ↑INR >3**
  - ⇨ **Observation option**: admit for 24 h observation and repeat CT?
  - ⇨ **D/C option:** Low risk, reliable, family present and able to return for any subtle changes

INR Reversal (CHEST 2012;141(2)(Suppl):e152S)(EM:RAP 12/13- Arora)
- FFP
  - ⇨ 15cc/kg begins working immediately
  - ⇨ Use if PCC not readily available
- Vitamin K
  - ⇨ INR > 10 → Vit K 2.5-5mg po
  - ⇨ Serious/Life threat bleed → 10mg IV over 30 min (prevents anaphylactoid rxn)
  - ⇨ Begins working at 4 hours, full effect at 24h
- Prothrombin Complex Concentrate (PCC, KCentra)
  - ⇨ Concentrated clotting factors affected by warfarin (factors II, VII, IX and X)
  - ⇨ Use: Any serious or life threatening bleed
  - ⇨ VS FFP: PCC has a smaller volume, higher concentration of factors, complete reversal, only one dose in 24h, no need for thawing
  - ⇨ PCC in the ER (Circulation. 2013;128:360)
    - ✓ ↓Adverse event: **FFP:19.5%** patients and PCC: 9.7%
    - ✓ PCC: faster time to reversal (5.7 to 11.8 hours) and about half as much blood transfused vs FFP
    - ✓ No increase in blood clots/DVT/PE

Elevated INR (Chest 2012)

INR	Bleeding	Action
INR < 4.5	No significant bleeding	☐ Lower/omit next warfarin dose
INR > 4.5 <10	No significant bleeding	☐ Omit next 1-2 warfarin doses ☐ Vitamin K not routinely recommended
INR > 10	No significant bleeding	☐ Hold warfarin until therapeutic ☐ **Vitamin K** 2.5-5mg po, even if not bleeding
Any INR	**Serious/life threatening bleeding**	☐ Hold warfarin ☐ **Vitamin K** 5-10 mg IV ☐ **PCC** 25-50 U/kg ☐ Repeat INR 30min post infusion ☐ FFP if PCC not available

Kcentra (4-factor PCC) dosing (FDA)

Pre-treatment INR:	2-4	4-6	>6
Dose of 4-PCC (U/kg)	25	35	50
Max dose:	2500	3500	5000

Journal Club: Delayed Bleed Risk in BHT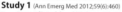

Study 1 (Ann Emerg Med 2012;59(6):460)
- **Immediate bleed** higher with Clopidogrel:
  - ⇨ Clopidogrel **12.0%**; vs Warfarin **5.1%**; (relative risk 2.3)
- **Delayed bleed** only seen in Warfarin:
  - ⇨ Warfarin: **0.6%** (4 of 687 pts) vs Clopidogrel: **0%** (0 of 243pts)
  - ⇨ Patients with delayed bleeds on warfarin, all had a GCS of 15 and 50% died

Study 2 (Ann Emerg Med 2012;59:451)
- Prospective case series of patients with BHT on warfarin with normal initial CT
- 6% (5 pts) delayed bleed risk on repeat CT, only 1 had neuro changes
- 2% returned with bleeds even after the 24 hour observation period and two negative head CTs.
- The relative risk of delayed hemorrhage with an initial INR > 3.0 was 14 (RR = 14)

4. SPECIAL POPULATIONS

Loss of Consciousness
- Increased prevalence of injury but not present as an independent predictor when control for other variables
- Do not use as indicator for CT imaging

Seizure
- Not associated with increased prevalence of injury
- Infrequently seen, difficult to assess if truly had a seizure vs syncope

Intoxication
- Decreased prevalence of injury → likely because of over-imaging intoxicated patients
- Need to improve risk stratification

Elderly
- High prevalence of occult head injury and delayed bleeds
- Does not require high mechanism of injury (usually GLF) and increased use of anticoagulants
- Have low threshold for CT, admission, correction of coagulopathy and re-imaging

Normal CT
- AMS on presentation → concern for Diffuse Axonal Injury (DAI)
- Coagulopathy → Observation for delayed intracranial hemorrhage vs D/C home with strict return precautions

CONCUSSION

(Br J Sports Med 2013;47:250–258) (EM:RAP 10/13-Spangler/Baird)

Diagnosis
- Symptoms: somatic (e.g. headache), cognitive (e.g. feeling like in a fog) and/or emotional symptoms (e.g. lability)
- Physical signs (e.g. loss of consciousness (LOC), amnesia)
- Behavioral changes (e.g. irritability)
- Cognitive impairment (e.g. slowed reaction times)
- Sleep disturbance (e.g. insomnia)

On-field evaluation
- Concussion assessment using SCAT3, SAC or other assessment tool
- Serial monitoring and **NO Return To Play (RTP) on same day**

Treatment
- Physical and cognitive rest until the acute symptoms resolve and then a graded program of exertion prior to medical clearance and RTP
- Graduated RTP (Return To Play) protocol
  - ⇨ 6 step program, each step lasting 24h → RTP in 7 days
  - ⇨ Must be symptoms free 24h to go to next step
- Second impact syndrome.
  - ⇨ Diffuse cerebral edema if the patient experiences a second concussion while still symptomatic from the first concussion → increased ICP → coma/death.
  - ⇨ Rare: 1.5 deaths/yr
- Post-concussion syndrome: persistence of symptoms >3mos

Gradual RTP Steps
1. No activity
2. Light aerobic exercise
3. Sport-specific exercise
4. Non-contact training drills
5. Full-contact practice
6. Return to play

Pediatric Head Trauma

General(Emerg Med Clin N Am 2013;31:653–675)

- Must weigh risks and benefits in child when deciding whether or not to obtain CT
  ⇨ Radiation risk: The lifetime risk of fatal cancer from a single head CT has been estimated to be 1 in 1500 for a 1-year-old and 1 in 5000 for a 10-year-old (Am J Roentgenol 2001;176(2):289–96)(N Engl J Med 2007;357(22):2277–84)
- Skull films as screening?
  ⇨ For ICI?: 1/2 of children with intracranial injury do not have skull fracture (not good enough)
  ⇨ For skull fracture?: Plain films miss 2.9% of skull fractures (not recommended as sole modality)

PECARN(Lancet 2009;374:1160-70)(Essentials 2012 "Head trauma in kids"-Claudius)

- General: Large (n=42,412), prospective multicenter trial, <18 yo assessed for clinically important traumatic brain injury (ciTBI)
- Goal: identify which head-injured children were at very low risk of clinically important traumatic brain injuries and therefore did **not** require head CT scans
- **Children >2 yo:** sensitivity of 96.8% for ciTBI and a **NPV 99.95%** if none of the predictors were present
- **Children <2yo:** Sensitivity 100%; **NPV 100%** if none of the criteria were present
- **Severe mechanism of injury** and no other predictors:
  ⇨ Lower risk of ciTBI than children with more than one predictor (RR 0.07 for children <2 years and 0.11 for children >2 years) (Arch Pediatr Adolesc Med 2012;166(4):356)
  ⇨ Define "Severe Mechanism": MVA w/ejection, death, or rollover; unhelmeted peds vs. auto; fall >5ft or 3 ft (<2y)
- Scalp hematoma (SH)
  ⇨ Most important predictor variable: scalp hematoma present in 14/15 (93%)
  ⇨ 6-30% of infants with SH will have skull fracture (SF).
  ⇨ 15-30% of infants with skull fracture will have intracranial injury
  ⇨ 1/2 of infants with intracranial injury will have SF

Pediatric Glasgow Comas Scale (GCS)

(E) Best Eye Response	Spontaneous-open with blinking	4
	Opens to verbal command, speech, shout	3
	Opens to pain	2
	None	1
(V) Best Verbal Response	Smiles, coos, babbles, interacts, oriented to sounds	5
	Cries but consolable	4
	Cries to pain	3
	Moans to pain	2
	None	1
(M) Best Motor Response	Normal spontaneous movement	6
	Withdraws to touch	5
	Withdraws from pain	4
	Abnormal (spastic) flexion, decorticate posture	3
	Extensor (rigid) response, decorticate posture	2
	None	1

PECARN RULE (Lancet 2009)

<2 yo	> 2yo
☐ GCS ≤14	☐ GCS ≤ 14
☐ Palpable skull fx	☐ Basilar skull fx
☐ AMS	☐ AMS
☐ Scalp hematoma, non-frontal	☐ LOC
☐ LOC ≥ 5s	☐ Vomiting
☐ Not acting normal	☐ Severe HA
☐ Severe mechanism	☐ Severe mechanism

NEXUS II pediatrics (Pediatrics 2006;117;e238)

- Good sensitivity and NPV but poor specificity
- Performed as well in children as in adult population
- Sensitivity 98.6% and NPV 99.1%

Discharge precautions

- Indications to return to the ED include:
  ⇨ Persistent vomiting, worsening headache, or worsening neurologic symptoms
- In the absence of neurologic decline, repeat CT imaging is not indicated for patients with an initial negative scan
- Children should be instructed not to return to gym class or sports until all of their symptoms have resolved and they have been reevaluated by a physician

Nexus II (Pediatrics 2006)

☐ Significant skull fracture (diastatic, depressed, open, or basilar)
☐ Altered level of alertness
☐ Neurologic deficit
☐ Persistent vomiting
☐ Scalp hematoma
☐ Abnormal behavior
☐ Coagulopathy

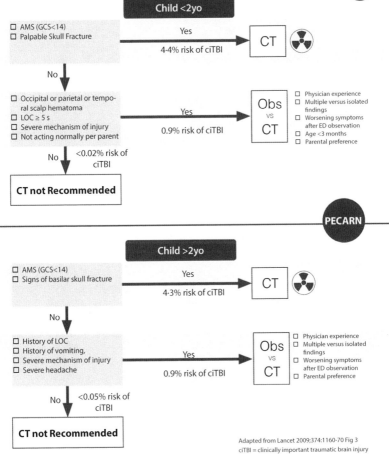

Child <2yo

☐ AMS (GCS<14)
☐ Palpable Skull Fracture

Yes — 4·4% risk of ciTBI → CT

No ↓

☐ Occipital or parietal or temporal scalp hematoma
☐ LOC ≥ 5 s
☐ Severe mechanism of injury
☐ Not acting normally per parent

Yes — 0.9% risk of ciTBI → Obs vs CT

☐ Physician experience
☐ Multiple versus isolated findings
☐ Worsening symptoms after ED observation
☐ Age <3 months
☐ Parental preference

No ↓ <0.02% risk of ciTBI

CT not Recommended

PECARN

Child >2yo

☐ AMS (GCS<14)
☐ Signs of basilar skull fracture

Yes — 4·3% risk of ciTBI → CT

No ↓

☐ History of LOC
☐ History of vomiting,
☐ Severe mechanism of injury
☐ Severe headache

Yes — 0.9% risk of ciTBI → Obs vs CT

☐ Physician experience
☐ Multiple versus isolated findings
☐ Worsening symptoms after ED observation
☐ Parental preference

No ↓ <0.05% risk of ciTBI

CT not Recommended

Adapted from Lancet 2009;374:1160-70 Fig 3
ciTBI = clinically important traumatic brain injury

156

TRAUMA: C-SPINE CLEARANCE

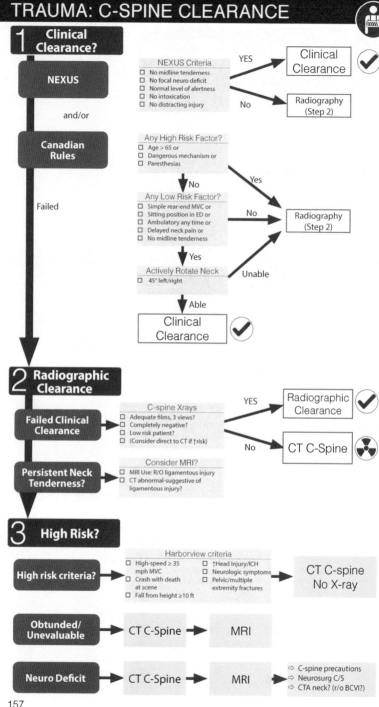

1 Clinical Clearance?

NEXUS

and/or

Canadian Rules

Failed

NEXUS Criteria
- ☐ No midline tenderness
- ☐ No focal neuro deficit
- ☐ Normal level of alertness
- ☐ No intoxication
- ☐ No distracting injury

YES → Clinical Clearance ✓

No → Radiography (Step 2)

Any High Risk Factor?
- ☐ Age > 65 or
- ☐ Dangerous mechanism or
- ☐ Paresthesias

↓ No

Any Low Risk Factor?
- ☐ Simple rear-end MVC or
- ☐ Sitting position in ED or
- ☐ Ambulatory any time or
- ☐ Delayed neck pain or
- ☐ No midline tenderness

Yes → Radiography (Step 2)

No → Radiography (Step 2)

Yes ↓

Actively Rotate Neck
- ☐ 45° left/right

Unable → Radiography (Step 2)

Able ↓

Clinical Clearance ✓

2 Radiographic Clearance

Failed Clinical Clearance

C-spine Xrays
- ☐ Adequate films, 3 views?
- ☐ Completely negative?
- ☐ Low risk patient?
- ☐ (Consider direct to CT if ↑risk)

YES → Radiographic Clearance ✓

No → CT C-Spine ☢

Persistent Neck Tenderness?

Consider MRI?
- ☐ MRI Use: R/O ligamentous injury
- ☐ CT abnormal-suggestive of ligamentous injury?

3 High Risk?

High risk criteria?

Harborview criteria
- ☐ High-speed ≥ 35 mph MVC
- ☐ Crash with death at scene
- ☐ Fall from height ≥10 ft
- ☐ ↑Head Injury/ICH
- ☐ Neurologic symptoms
- ☐ Pelvic/multiple extremity fractures

→ CT C-spine No X-ray

Obtunded/ Unevaluable → CT C-Spine → MRI

Neuro Deficit → CT C-Spine → MRI

⇨ C-spine precautions
⇨ Neurosurg C/S
⇨ CTA neck? (r/o BCVI?)

TRAUMA: C-SPINE CLEARANCE

1. CLINICAL CLEARANCE-LOW RISK PATIENT

NEXUS

Definitions
- **Midline posterior bony cervical-spine tenderness** is present if the patient reports:
  ⇨ Pain on palpation of the posterior midline neck from the nuchal ridge to the prominence of the first thoracic verte-bra, or if the patient evinces pain with direct palpation of any cervical spinous process

C-Spine Clearance
☐ Asymptomatic/↓Risk: → NEXUS +/-CCR
☐ Failed NEXUS/CCR → C-spine xrays
☐ High risk mechanism: → CT C-spine
☐ Unevaluable patient: → CT C-spine
☐ Neuro deficit → CT & MRI

- **Intoxication**: Patients should be considered intoxicated if they have either of the following:
  ⇨ A recent history provided by the patient or an observer of intoxication or intoxicating ingestion
  ⇨ Evidence of intoxication on physical examination such as an odor of alcohol, slurred speech, ataxia, dysmetria, or other cerebellar findings
  ⇨ Any behavior consistent with intoxication
  ⇨ Patients may also be considered intoxicated if tests of bodily secretions are positive for alcohol or drugs that affect the level of alertness
- **An altered level of alertness** can include any of the following:
  ⇨ Glasgow Coma Scale score of 14 or less
  ⇨ Disorientation to person, place, time, or events
  ⇨ Inability to remember three objects at five minutes
  ⇨ Delayed or inappropriate response to external stimuli or other findings
- A **focal neurologic deficit** is any focal neurologic finding on motor or sensory examination
- **Distracting injury:** No precise definition of a painful distracting injury is possible
  ⇨ This category includes any condition thought by the clinician to be producing pain sufficient to distract the patient from a second (neck) injury
  ⇨ Such injuries may include, but are not limited to, any long-bone fracture; a visceral injury requiring surgical consultation; a large laceration, degloving injury, or crush injury; large burns; or any other injury causing acute functional impairment
  ⇨ Physicians may also classify any injury as distracting if it is thought to have the potential to impair the patient's ability to appreciate other injuries

---

Journal Club: NEXUS C-Spine Rules

NEXUS validation study (NEJM 2000;343:94-9)
- Nexus identified all but **8/818** patients with any C-Spine Injury (CSI) and all but **2/578** patients with clinically significant injury (CSI)
- Cervical Spine injury (Sens 99%, NPV 99.8%)
- Clinically significant injury (Sens 99.6%, NPV 99.9%)

CCR vs Nexus study (NEJM 2003;349:2510-8)
- Retrospective study done by developers of Canadian rule
- **Sensitivity 90.7% for NEXUS vs 99.4% for CCR**
- CCR identified 161 of 162 CSI in patients in whom the range of motion was evaluated
- Nexus missed 1/10 injuries

Do we need each of the 5 criteria? (Ann Emerg Med 2001;38:22-25)
- A substantial number of patients (29%) with clinically significant CSI met only **one** of the criteria
- **Posterior mid-line tenderness** was the only criteria present in 61% of these patients
- **Distracting injury** was sole criterion present in **45/578** of patients with clinically significant CSI

NEXUS vs CT (J Trauma 2007;62:1405)
- Clinical exam (NEXUS) had a sensitivity of only 58% (7/17 injuries missed) when compared to CT C-spine results (gold standard)

158

CANADIAN C-SPINE RULES (CCR)

- Definitions
  - ⇨ For patients with trauma who are alert (GCS = 15), stable and cervical spine injury is a concern, the determination of risk factors guides the use of cervical spine radiography.
  - ⇨ A dangerous mechanism is considered to be:
    - ✓ Fall from an elevation ≥3 ft or 5 stairs
    - ✓ Axial load to the head (e.g., diving)
    - ✓ Motor vehicle collision at high speed (>100 km/hr) or with rollover or ejection
    - ✓ Collision involving a motorized recreational vehicle
    - ✓ Bicycle collision
  - ⇨ A simple rear-end motor vehicle collision excludes being pushed into oncoming traffic, being hit by a bus or a large truck, a rollover, and being hit by a high-speed vehicle.

Journal Club: Canadian C-Spine Rules

CCR validation study (JAMA 2001;286:1841-1848)
- Sensitivity 100%

CCR better than physician judgment? (Ann Emerg Med 2003;42:395)
- **Physician judgment had 92% sensitivity** for predicting a probability of clinically important fracture
- **CCR had 100%** sensitivity for predicting a probability of clinically important fracture

CCR vs Nexus study (NEJM 2003;349:2510-8)
- Retrospective study done by developers of Canadian rule
- **Sensitivity 90.7% for NEXUS vs 99.4% for CCR**
- CCR identified 161 of 162 CSI in patients in whom the range of motion was evaluated
- Nexus missed 1/10 injuries

2. RADIOGRAPHIC CLEARANCE

Plain X rays
- Use: Low risk patients that fail clinical c-spine clearance
- Negative criteria
  - ⇨ Xrays must be **3 views, adequate, and no abnormality detected** to be considered negative
  - ⇨ If not all criteria met → CT
- Journal Club
  - ⇨ Mixed results on utility of plain Xrays
  - ⇨ Flexion/Extension views are not useful/inadequate to evaluate for ligamentous injury (J Orthop Trauma 2011;25:51)

Journal Club: Plain films for C-spine Clearance

NEXUS breakdown (Ann Emerg Med 2001;38:1-7)
- Total misses: Of 818 pts with CSI, Xrays identified 498 patients **(Missed 320/818; 39.1%)**
- Normal & Adequate: 47 CSI patients xrays were interpreted as normal and adequate **(miss rate 47/818; 5.7%)**
- Conclusion: "... *in many patients with blunt trauma, plain films are not adequate, and adjunctive studies are required before cervical spine injury can be excluded.*"

Diaz et al. (J Trauma. 2005;59:897)
- Plain Xray failed to identify 299 of 416 cervical spine injuries (72%)

Meta-analysis (J Trauma. 2005;58:902)
- The pooled sensitivity for cervical spine plain radiography was 52%

EAST Trauma Guidelines (J Trauma 2009;67:651)
- Plain radiographs contribute no additional information and should not be obtained

CT C-spine
- Multiple studies show high sensitivity (100%) if done with lateral reconstructions (to eval alignment)
- Straight to CT? (i.e. no plain films?)
  - ⇨ High risk patient (>1 Nexus criteria, bad mechanism of injury)
  - ⇨ Low likelihood of adequate films: DJD, obese, ALOC
- **Harborview Criteria** (AJR 2000;174:713)
  - ⇨ Study identified high risk criteria → Patient should go directly to CT (no plain films)
  - ⇨ Pts with > 5% risk of CSI

TRAUMA: C-SPINE CLEARANCE

MRI
- Indications:
  - ⇨ Neurologic deficit
  - ⇨ Abnormal CT
  - ⇨ Persistent cervical pain/tenderness
  - ⇨ Obtunded patient, unable to clear C-spine
- R/O Ligamentous injury (Ann Emerg Med 2011;58:521)
  - ⇨ MRI obtained for: CT negative + persistent midline tenderness
  - ⇨ 78/178 patients (44%) had acute cervical injury detected on MRI
  - ⇨ 2.8% of these were managed surgically
  - ⇨ Consider MRI for patient that has persistent midline cervical tenderness, even after negative CT

3. HIGH RISK PATIENT

High risk criteria
- **Harborview Criteria** (AJR 2000;174:713)
  - ⇨ Study identified high risk criteria → Patient should go direct-ly to CT (no plain films)
  - ⇨ Pts with > 5% risk of CSI
- Work-up
  - ⇨ Straight to CT
  - ⇨ Plain Xrays not indicated

AMS
- Plain Xrays not indicated
- CT C-spine to r/o bony injury
- Consider MRI to r/o ligamentous and cord injury

Neurologic deficit
- Strict C-spine precautions
- Plain Xrays not indicated
- CT C-spine to evaluate for bony injury
- MRI C-spine to evaluate for ligamentous and spinal cord injury
- Neurosurgery consult
- CTA neck?
  - ⇨ R/O blunt cerebrovascular injury (BCVI)? (See Neck trauma algorithm)

> **High risk criteria: Harborview**
> - ☐ High-speed ≥ 35 mph MVC
> - ☐ Crash with death at scene of motor vehicle accident
> - ☐ Fall from height (≥10 ft)
> - ☐ Significant closed head injury (or intracranial hemorrhage seen on CT
> - ☐ Neurologic symptoms or signs referred to the cervical spine
> - ☐ Pelvic or multiple extremity fractures

C-SPINE ALGORITHM AT LAC+USC

- Awake/alert/not intoxicated: NEXUS and/or Canadian C-spine Rules
- Neck tenderness w/low mechanism: plain radiographs/C-spine xrays
- Neck tenderness w/high mechanism: CT C-spine
- Unevaluable patient: CT C-spine
- Evaluable patient w/neurological deficit & normal CT: MRI

NEUROGENIC SHOCK
(Resuscitation 2008;76:57-62)

Incidence
- Cervical injury (19%), Thoracic injury (7%)

Definition
- High cord lesion causing decreased sympathetic outflow resulting in **hypotension** and **bradycardia**
- Depressed spinal reflexes caudal to spinal cord injury
- Phase 1 (0-1days)
  - ⇨ Areflexia/hyporeflexia
  - ⇨ DPR (delayed plantar response) is first reflex to appear and may be present in the ED
- Phase 2 (1-3 days)
  - ⇨ Initial reflex return
  - ⇨ Return of reflexes: cutaneous return first (Cremaster, BC, anal wink) before DTRs
- Phase 3 (4 days-1month)
  - ⇨ Early hyperreflexia
  - ⇨ DTRs re-appear early in this phase (AJ → KJ) and DPR will be lost
- Phase 3 (1-12 months)
  - ⇨ Spasticity/hyperreflexia

Treatment
- R/O Hemorrhage
- Fluid resuscitation (NS or LR)
- Vasopressors (DA vs NE vs Phenylephrine) to target MAP (unknown)

TRAUMA: PENETRATING NECK

1 Airway Control

- ☐ ABCs
- ☐ Cardiac arrest? Thoracotomy indicated?
- ☐ Emergent airway? Procedure of choice → RSI
- ☐ Back-up plan?: LMA, nasotracheal, fiberoptic, cric, direct tracheal, awake intubation
- ☐ C-collar → ?remove for airway eval if neuro intact

2 Bleeding Control

- ☐ Direct pressure
- ☐ No clamps, no ties (except EJ)
- ☐ Platysma violated?
- ☐ Resuscitation: IVF, blood transfusion
- ☐ Unstable → OR

3 Evaluate Injury

	Hard Signs 🏴	Soft Signs	☢ Selective W/U
Airway	☐ **Respiratory distress** ☐ **Air bubbling** through wound ☐ **Major hemoptysis**	☐ SQ emphysema ☐ Hoarseness ☐ Minor hemoptysis ☐ Trachea deviated	⇨ CXR/ soft tissue neck ⇨ CT neck ⇨ Bronchoscopy
Vascular	☐ **Severe active bleeding** ☐ **Expanding hematoma** ☐ **Peripheral pulse absent/** diminished (ABIs) ☐ **Bruit/Thrill** ☐ Unexplained **hypotension/ shock** ☐ **Pulsatile Bleeding** ☐ **CNS Ischemia** (hemiplegia)	☐ Small/moderate hematoma ☐ Minor bleeding ☐ Proximity wound ☐ Peripheral ischemia	⇨ Color flow Doppler ⇨ CT angio (4 vessel) ⇨ Angiography
Digestive Tract	None	☐ Odynophagia ☐ SQ emphysema ☐ Hematemesis	⇨ Gastrografin swallow ⇨ Flexible endoscopy ⇨ Rigid endoscopy
Neuro	None	☐ Spinal cord deficit ☐ Cranial nerve deficit ☐ Horner's syndrome ☐ Brachial plexus injury	⇨ C-spine series ⇨ CT C-spine/Head ⇨ Vascular eval

4 Work-up

Hard Signs → **OR** 🖊

Soft Signs → **CTA** ☢
- + Injury → OR
- Indeterminate CT? Trajectory? → Directed Evaluation
- No injury Normal Trajectory → D/C vs Obs

Asymptomatic → **Observation** 👁

TRAUMA: PENETRATING NECK

1. AIRWAY MANAGEMENT

(Essentials 2010-Inaba)

Cardiac arrest
- ED thoracotomy
  - ⇨ Indication: Penetrating neck trauma + No signs of life + CPR < 5min
  - ⇨ Cross clamp aorta and treat for air embolism?
  - ⇨ Trendelenburg and attempt to aspirate air from right ventricle

Initial Evaluation
- Platysma violation?
  - ⇨ If no platysma violation → likely no need for further w/u
- Anterior vs Posterior triangle of neck
  - ⇨ Most critical structures are anterior to sternocleidomastoid muscle (anterior triangle)
- What Zone of neck? (See table)

Airway control
- Airway best controlled in OR
  - ⇨ Unnecessary intubation may further damage airway
  - ⇨ May intubate directly through neck laceration
- Indications for emergent airway:
  - ⇨ Hypoxia
  - ⇨ Unable to protect airway (loss of gag, ↑secretions…)
  - ⇨ Altered Mental Status
  - ⇨ Shock
  - ⇨ Consider early intubation for expanding hematoma, other signs of airway distortion
- Emergent airway in neck trauma (Ann Emerg Med 2000;35:221-5)
  - ⇨ 11% needed emergent airway management
  - ⇨ 100% successful with RSI if clinician deemed airway to be RSI capable

Zones of Neck		
Zone I	Sternal notch→ inferior cricoid	Trachea, esophagus, great vessels, thoracic duct, upper mediastinum, lung apices
Zone II	Cricoid cartilage→ angle of mandible	Carotid and vertebral arteries, jugular veins, pharynx, larynx, esophagus, trachea
Zone III	Angle of mandible→ base of skull	Distal carotids and vertebral arteries, jugular veins

2. CONTROL BLEEDING

Bleeding
- Persistent bleeding from Zone I injury → possible subclavian artery injury
  - ⇨ Direct pressure with one finger to visualized bleed
  - ⇨ May temporarily tamponade bleed by inserting foley into entrance wound
  - ⇨ Impaled objects → do not remove, to be removed in OR

3. INJURY EVALUATION

Airway injury
- Hard signs
  - ⇨ **Respiratory distress**
  - ⇨ **Air bubbling** through wound
  - ⇨ **Major hemoptysis**
- Soft signs
  - ⇨ Hoarseness → likely laryngeal fracture/injury or recurrent laryngeal nerve injury
  - ⇨ Minor Hemoptysis → ask patient to cough to evaluate for hemoptysis
  - ⇨ SQ emphysema
  - ⇨ Trachea deviated
- Work-up
  - ⇨ Plain films (CXR, AP/lat neck) → may show cervicofacial emphysema, mediastinal emphysema
  - ⇨ CT → extrapulmonary air, tracheal disruption
  - ⇨ Bronchoscopy → gold standard

Vascular Injury
- Hard signs
  - ⇨ **Severe active bleeding**
  - ⇨ **Expanding hematoma**
  - ⇨ **Peripheral pulse absent**/ diminished (ABIs)
    - ✓ Zone I injury: check **ABI** of each arm → if <0.9, assume vascular injury
  - ⇨ **Bruit/Thrill**
    - ✓ 50% of carotid injuries have bruits, pathognomonic of AV fistula that needs repair
  - ⇨ Unexplained **hypotension/ shock**
  - ⇨ **Pulsatile Bleeding**
  - ⇨ **CNS Ischemia** (hemiplegia)

- Soft signs
  - ⇨ Small/moderate hematoma
  - ⇨ Minor bleeding
  - ⇨ Proximity wound
  - ⇨ Peripheral ischemia
- Physical exam (J Trauma 2000;48:208-13)
  - ⇨ Normal PEX and CXR showed NPV 100% for vascular injury in one series
- Work-up
  - ⇨ CT angio → sensitivity 90-100%
  - ⇨ If suspect venous injury → place patient in Trendelenburg to prevent air embolism

Digestive tract
- Hard signs: None
- Soft signs
  - ⇨ Odynophagia
  - ⇨ SQ emphysema
    - ✓ Can be esophageal or tracheal injury
  - ⇨ Hematemesis
- Work-up (Am J Surg 1987;54:619-22) (EAST Guidelines J Trauma 2008;64:1392)
  - ⇨ Esophageal injury is most commonly missed injury → early diagnosis and treatment is critical
  - ⇨ CT Neck
    - ✓ Not sensitive enough to detect all esophageal injuries
    - ✓ If ↑suspicion → need further work-up
  - ⇨ Combination rigid endoscope + barium swallow → 100% sensitivity for esophageal injuries
  - ⇨ No blind NG tube

Nerve injury
- Hard signs: None
- Soft signs
  - ⇨ Spinal cord deficit
  - ⇨ Cranial nerve deficit
  - ⇨ Horner's syndrome
  - ⇨ Brachial plexus injury
- Physical Exam
  - ⇨ Lower cranial nerves
    - ✓ **CN 9** (Glossopharyngeal nerve) → say aaahhhhh, is palate rising, midline
    - ✓ **CN 10** (Vagus, recurrent laryngeal nerve) → hoarseness
    - ✓ **CN 11** (Accessory nerve) → shrug shoulders
    - ✓ **CN 12** (hypoglossal nerve) → tongue midline
  - ⇨ **Spinal Cord injury**
    - ✓ Moving all extremities, sensation in all extremities, rectal tone, priapism
    - ✓ C-spine clearance (ok to clear clinically?)
      - i. Stab wounds → no reports of unstable fractures
      - ii. GSW → all unstable c-spine fx patients also presented with neurological signs (Spine 2005;30:2274-9)
  - ⇨ **Horner's syndrome** → Carotid injury
    - ✓ Ptosis, miosis, anhidrosis
  - ⇨ Brachial Plexus injury
    - ✓ Increased in Zone I injuries
    - Median n. → fist
    - Radial n. → wrist extension
    - Ulnar n. → finger abduction/adduction
    - Musculocutaneous n. →flex forearm
    - Axillary n. → abduction of arm
- Work-up
  - ⇨ Plain films for C-spine fracture? (vs CT?)
  - ⇨ CT angio to evaluate carotids
  - ⇨ No role for steroids in penetrating spinal cord injury (Neurosurgery 1997;41:576-83)

4. WORK-UP

(EM:RAP 3/13 "Penetrating Neck Injury-CT Scan" Inaba)

Hard Signs
- Patient with hard signs → 89.7% have clinically significant injury
- Absolute indications for OR (Hard signs):
  - ⇨ Shock
  - ⇨ Uncontrolled bleeding
  - ⇨ Absent radial pulse
  - ⇨ Respiratory distress

Soft Signs
- Traditional work up
  - ⇨ Neck injuries no longer evaluated by zones → workup dictated by physical exam
  - ⇨ Traditional work up replaced by CTA
- CT angiography (J Trauma Acute Care Surg 2012;72:576)
  - ⇨ Initial modality of choice
  - ⇨ Directed evaluation based on symptoms and zone of injury
    - ✓ Physical and CTA combined are **sensitive (100%) and specific (97.5%)** for clinically significant injury
    - ✓ Consider CTA as first test, with more specific tests base on physical exam and imaging findings.
  - ⇨ Results:
    - ✓ Positive CTA → likely to OR
    - ✓ Negative CTA → D/C vs observation
    - ✓ Indeterminate CT/concerning trajectory?
      - i. May need further directed/traditional workup
      - ii. Bronchoscopy, DL, esophagoscopy, contrast swallow etc...

Traditional work up	
Zone I	• Four vessel angiogram • Bronchoscopy • Barium swallow • EGD
Zone II	• Surgical exploration
Zone III	• Four vessel angiogram • Bronchoscopy • Barium swallow • EGD

C-Spine: Work-up
☐ Hard signs → OR
☐ Soft signs → CTA
☐ No signs → Obs

Asymptomatic patients (World J Surg 1997;21:41-48)
- Observation
- Absence of signs/symptoms suggestive of vascular or aerodigestive injury excluded significant injury (NPV 100% for both)

TRAUMA: BLUNT NECK

BLUNT CEREBROVASCULAR INJURY (BCVI)

(westerntrauma.org)

Definition
- BCVI = Blunt carotid injury (BCI) + blunt vertebral injury

Mechanism of injury:
- Trauma → intimal tear can lead to:
  - ⇨ Thrombosis → embolism → stroke
  - ⇨ Dissection → vessel occlusion
  - ⇨ Pseudoaneurysm → occlusion or rupture → hemorrhage or AV fistula

Signs/symptoms of BCVI
- Arterial hemorrhage from neck, nose, or mouth
- Expanding cervical hematoma
- Cervical bruit in patient < 50 years old
- Focal neurologic defect (neuro deficit inconsistent with CT/MRI findings)

Risk factors for BCVI
- Any high energy mechanism:
  - ⇨ Displaced mid-face fracture (LeForte II or III)
  - ⇨ Basilar skull fracture with carotid canal involvement
  - ⇨ Closed head injury consistent with diffuse axonal injury and GCS < 6
  - ⇨ Cervical vertebral body or transverse foramen fracture, subluxation, or ligamentous injury at any level
  - ⇨ Any fracture at C1-C2
  - ⇨ Near hanging with anoxia
  - ⇨ Clothesline type injury or seat belt abrasion with significant swelling, pain, or altered mental status

Work up
- CT angiography (initial study of choice)
- Angiography

Treatment
- Antithrombotic treatment (Heparin)
- Endovascular treatment

BLUNT CAROTID INJURY (BCI)

Seatbelt sign
- The seatbelt sign is usually not an isolated finding
- If no hard findings → not need work-up? Based on clinical suspicion (see above) (J Trauma 2002;52:618-23)

Other symptoms (see above)
- Horner's syndrome
- Expanding hematoma
- Bruit/ thrill (particularly in those <50 years old)
- Stroke findings with negative CT head

Treatment
- Heparin and Coumadin

Journal Club
- Mayberry et al (Arch Surg 2004;139:609)
  - ⇨ Rare diagnosis: 10 yrs & 35,000 blunt trauma patients → only 17 had BCI
  - ⇨ Most patients with BCI develop stroke symptoms within a few hours of presentation

VERTEBRAL ARTERY INJURY

- Can embolize to ipsilateral or contralateral side
- Clinical
  - ⇨ HA + neck pain +/- Brainstem sx (vertigo, ataxia, CN findings)
  - ⇨ 5Ds (Dizziness, Diplopia, Dysphagia, Dysarthria, Dysmetria, Dysdiadochokinesia)

STRANGULATION

Injuries:
- Larynx, hyoid, trachea, rare cervical spine injury (only in judicial hangings, ↑height)

Pitfall
- Well appearing on arrival → hypoxic lung injury and florid pulmonary edema after 4-6 hours
  - ⇨ Inspiration against a closed airway causes negative pressure → pulmonary edema
  - ⇨ Check for petechiae to face and neck
  - ⇨ CXR prior to discharge for pulmonary edema

Work-up
- CT neck (especially if hoarse, crepitus)

CLOTHESLINE INJURY

- Can cause transection of trachea
- Consider fiberoptic or awake intubation
  - ⇨ RSI causes loss of muscle tone and ↑risk of soft tissue intubation
- Work-up → CT scan

TRAUMA: PENETRATING CHEST

A | Arresting

ED Thoracotomy? → See Traumatic Cardiac Arrest Algorithm

U | Unstable

| (US) W/U (cart) | | (pen) Treatment |

Begin Resuscitation

Resus to SBP>90
- ☐ IV Fluids/Blood/FFP
- ☐ R/O Other areas of blood loss (abdomen, pelvis, extremities, external...)
- ☐ Stop blood loss

→ See Trauma Resuscitation Algorithm

R/O Tamponade — US

⇒ US: Pericardial effusion
⇒ US: Tamponade phenomenon, collapse of RV

OR Immediately
⇒ Pericardiocentesis if OR delay?
⇒ ED Thoracotomy (if decompensates/arrest)

R/O Tension PTX — US / CXR

⇒ US: anterior air, no sliding lung
⇒ CXR: PTX, deep sulcus sign, SQ air
⇒ Chest Tube-empiric?

Chest Tube
⇒ Needle Thoracostomy
⇒ Tube Thoracostomy

R/O Hemothorax/ Hemorrhage — US / CXR

⇒ US: Blood in pleural cavity
⇒ CXR: haziness in lung fields
⇒ Chest Tube-empiric?

Resusc/Chest Tube
⇒ Tube Thoracostomy
⇒ PRBC Transfusion
⇒ CT (source of bleeding?)
⇒ OR?

S | Stable

R/O Cardiac Injury → US
- effusion → CTA
+ effusion → OR

R/O PTX/HTX → US / CXR
No → Serial CXR
Yes → Chest Tube?

R/O Trans-mediastinal injury → CTA
− → Done
+ → Directed Tx

R/O L Diaphragm Injury
⇒ Obs 12 hours
⇒ R/O GI injury
⇒ Laparoscopy

A: ARRESTING PATIENT

(CMEDownload-Resus 2012-Penetrating Chest Trauma) (Essentials 2010-Inaba) (westerntrauma.org)

ED Thoracotomy indications:
- Trauma patient, CPR, no signs of life (SOL) +:
  - ⇨ Blunt trauma with CPR <10min
  - ⇨ Penetrating trauma with CPR <15min
  - ⇨ Penetrating trauma to neck/extremity < 5 min

ED Thoracotomy Indications:
Trauma + CPR + no SOL +:
☐ Blunt trauma, CPR < 10min
☐ Penetrating trauma, CPR<15min
☐ Penetrating trauma to neck/ extremity < 5 min

Procedure:
- Resuscitative Thoracotomy (Open the left chest)
  - ⇨ Release tamponade and open resuscitation of heart
  - ⇨ Control bleeding
  - ⇨ Cross-clamp aorta → Shunt blood up
- Right Chest Tube
  - ⇨ Blood? → Clamshell thoracotomy to control bleeding

Survival rates:
- Overall survival rate 7.4%, dictated by location & mechanism of injury (J Am Coll Surg 2000;190:288-98)
  - ⇨ **Thoracic injury 10.7% (Cardiac-19.4%)**, abdominal injury 4.5%
  - ⇨ **Penetrating injury 8.8% (stab wounds 17%, GSW 4.3%)** blunt trauma 1.4%

No Signs of Life (SOL):
☐ No pulse
☐ No pupils
☐ No movement
☐ No breaths
☐ No PEA
☐ No cardiac motion (US)

U: UNSTABLE PATIENT

Resuscitation (See Trauma Resuscitation Algorithm)
- Critical Actions
  - ⇨ Crystalloid resuscitation
  - ⇨ Initiate cross-matching
  - ⇨ See Trauma Resuscitation Algorithm
- Remains Unstable?
  - ⇨ Continue resuscitation
    - ✓ Blood transfusion → uncross-matched or type specific
    - ✓ Thaw FFP
    - ✓ Target endpoint → SBP 90, talking

Localize bleeding (See Blunt Chest Trauma Algorithm)
- Cardiac U/S
  - ⇨ Pericardial effusion
  - ⇨ Tamponade phenomenon, collapse of RV
- Lung US
  - ⇨ PTX: Anterior air-no sliding lung
  - ⇨ HTX: Blood in pleural cavity
- CXR
  - ⇨ PTX: deep sulcus sign, SQ air
  - ⇨ Hemothorax: haziness in lung fields
- Chest tube, Clinically directed
  - ⇨ Indications
    - ✓ Hemothorax/Pneumothorax
    - ✓ Clinical exam/diagnostic
  - ⇨ OR
    - ✓ Output>1-1.5L
    - ✓ Continuous output>200-250ml/h X 2-4h
    - ✓ Clinical judgment
- R/O other areas of blood loss (Pelvis, extremities, externally)
  - ⇨ Stop bleeding

TRAUMA: PENETRATING CHEST

S: STABLE PATIENT

General
- ABCs
- IV, O_2, Monitor...

What is at risk of injury?
- External wounds → roll early
- Plain X-rays → missile localization and trajectory mapping

Check for specific areas of injury

PNEUMOTHORAX
(See Blunt Chest Trauma Algorithm)

Diagnosis
- Lung U/S as part of FAST
- R/O pneumothorax:
  - ⇨ Initial CXR
  - ⇨ If CXR negative → Repeat CXR @ 3 hours (J Trauma 2008;65:549-53)
  - ⇨ Previously would repeat CXR @ 6 hours → No additional benefit gained from CXR at 6 vs 3 hours

PENETRATING CARDIAC INJURY

Diagnosis
- Clinical exam, CXR, EKG, Pericardiocentesis → poor sensitivity and specificity
- Cardiac U/S
  - ⇨ Annals of Surgery 1996;223(6):737-746 → Sens 100%, Spec 100%
  - ⇨ Annals of Surgery 1998;228(4):557-567 → Sens 100%, Spec 99.3%
  - ⇨ J Trauma. 2000 Dec;49(6):1159 → Sens 100%, Spec 97%
- Conclusion
  - ⇨ Ultrasound should be the initial diagnostic adjunct for precordial wounds
  - ⇨ US is highly sensitive for cardiac injury, and immediate surgical intervention when positive
- ECHO: If US equivocal, may need formal Cardiac ECHO

Treatment
- OR immediately for sternotomy
- ER thoracotomy if too unstable for OR
- Pericardiocentesis if unable to perform thoracotomy

TRANSMEDIASTINAL INJURY

Traditional approach
- Unstable → OR
- Stable → pan-endoscopy, contrast swallow, angiography, echo

CT as screening approach (J Trauma 2002;53:635–638)(Ann Thorac Surg. 2007;83:377-82):
- CT Negative → 100% NPV, no need for further testing
- CT positive → (Evaluate trajectory, trajectory proximity to structures, +injury) → 28% required OR

LEFT THORACOABDOMINAL REGION INJURY
(J Am Coll Surg. 1998;187:626-630) (Essentials 2011 "Diaphragmatic Injuries"-Mallon)

R/O Diaphragm injury
- Location:
  - ⇨ Superior: Nipple → scapula tip
  - ⇨ Inferior: Costal margin
- Delayed diagnosis
  - ⇨ If not diagnosed at time of trauma, diagnosis may be delayed many years
  - ⇨ Occult diaphragmatic injury in 26% of SW and 13% of GSW at laparoscopy
- CXR
  - ⇨ May show PTX, hemothorax, herniation of abdominal contents into chest or completely normal
  - ⇨ Usually non-diagnostic
- CT
  - ⇨ Accuracy 96% for diaphragm injury in one study (J Trauma 2007;63:538-43)
  - ⇨ Laparoscopy gold standard to exclude diaphragm injury
  - ⇨ LAC + USC Protocol:
    - ✓ 6-12 hour observation to r/o GI tract injury
    - ✓ Then laparoscopic eval +/- repair
    - ✓ R/O PTX as above

TRAUMA: BLUNT CHEST

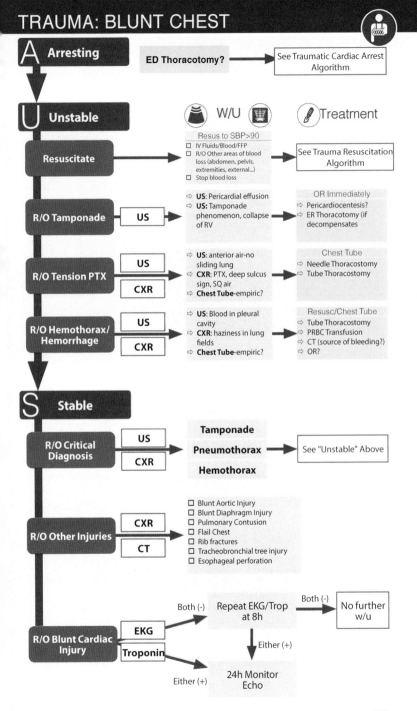

A **Arresting**

ED Thoracotomy? → See Traumatic Cardiac Arrest Algorithm

U **Unstable**

W/U   Treatment

Resuscitate

Resus to SBP>90
☐ IV Fluids/Blood/FFP
☐ R/O Other areas of blood loss (abdomen, pelvis, extremities, external...)
☐ Stop blood loss

→ See Trauma Resuscitation Algorithm

R/O Tamponade — US

⇨ **US**: Pericardial effusion
⇨ **US**: Tamponade phenomenon, collapse of RV

OR Immediately
⇨ Pericardiocentesis?
⇨ ER Thoracotomy (if decompensates

R/O Tension PTX — US / CXR

⇨ **US**: anterior air-no sliding lung
⇨ **CXR**: PTX, deep sulcus sign, SQ air
⇨ **Chest Tube**-empiric?

Chest Tube
⇨ Needle Thoracostomy
⇨ Tube Thoracostomy

R/O Hemothorax/ Hemorrhage — US / CXR

⇨ **US**: Blood in pleural cavity
⇨ **CXR**: haziness in lung fields
⇨ **Chest Tube**-empiric?

Resusc/Chest Tube
⇨ Tube Thoracostomy
⇨ PRBC Transfusion
⇨ CT (source of bleeding?)
⇨ OR?

S **Stable**

R/O Critical Diagnosis — US / CXR

Tamponade
Pneumothorax → See "Unstable" Above
Hemothorax

R/O Other Injuries — CXR / CT

☐ Blunt Aortic Injury
☐ Blunt Diaphragm Injury
☐ Pulmonary Contusion
☐ Flail Chest
☐ Rib fractures
☐ Tracheobronchial tree injury
☐ Esophageal perforation

R/O Blunt Cardiac Injury — EKG / Troponin

Both (-) → Repeat EKG/Trop at 8h → Both (-) → No further w/u

Either (+) → 24h Monitor Echo

Either (+) → 24h Monitor Echo

TRAUMA: BLUNT CHEST

A: CARDIAC ARREST

(Emerg M Clin N Am 2007;25:695 & 2012;28:377)(CMEDownload "Cedars Sinai 2012"-Braunstein)
(See Traumatic Cardiac Arrest Algorithm)

ED Thoracotomy indications:
- Trauma patient, CPR, no signs of life (SOL) +:
  - ⇨ Blunt trauma with CPR <10min
  - ⇨ Penetrating trauma with CPR <15min
  - ⇨ Penetrating trauma to neck/extremity < 5 min

Cardiac Arrest
- Resuscitative Thoracotomy (Open the left chest)
  - ⇨ Release tamponade and open resuscitation of heart
  - ⇨ Control bleeding
  - ⇨ Open Cardiac Resuscitation
  - ⇨ Cross-clamp aorta → Shunt blood up
- Right Chest Tube
  - ⇨ Blood? → Clamshell thoracotomy to control bleeding

Survival rates:
- Overall survival rate 7.4%, dictated by location & mechanism of injury (J Am Coll Surg 2000;190:288-98)
  - ⇨ **Thoracic injury 10.7% (Cardiac-19.4%)**, abdominal injury 4.5%
  - ⇨ Penetrating injury 8.8% (stab wounds 17%, GSW 4.3%) **blunt trauma 1.4%**

ED Thoracotomy Indications:
Trauma + CPR + no SOL +:
☐ Blunt trauma, CPR < 10min
☐ Penetrating trauma, CPR<15min
☐ Penetrating trauma to neck/ extremity < 5 min

No Signs of Life (SOL)
☐ No pulse
☐ No pupils
☐ No movement
☐ No breaths
☐ No PEA
☐ No cardiac motion (US)

U: UNSTABLE

CARDIAC TAMPONADE

Cause
- Blunt Cardiac Injury-Wall rupture, Coronary injury (See BCI section)

Clinical
- May be asymptomatic or non-specific
- Beck's Triad: Distended neck veins, hypotension/shock, muffled hear sounds

Beck's Triad
☐ Hypotension
☐ Distended neck veins
☐ Muffled heart sounds

Diagnosis
- Bedside US: Pericardial effusion
  - ⇨ Sensitivity 100% for detections of pericardial effusion in multiple studies
- ECHO

Treatment
- OR immediately for sternotomy
- ER thoracotomy if too unstable for OR
- Pericardiocentesis if unable to perform thoracotomy
- Closed chest CPR ineffective

PNEUMOTHORAX

Clinical
- Often asymptomatic
- Dyspnea, tachypnea, ↓breath sounds, poorly moving hemithorax, SQ emphysema

Chest Tube Stat!:
☐ Traumatic cardiac arrest
☐ No BP/Pulse during resuscitation
☐ Hypotension + ↑Ppeak or difficult to bag
☐ Hypotension or Hypoxia + decreased breath sounds or SQ emphysema

Diagnosis
- Upright CXR
  - ⇨ PTX, deep sulcus sign, SQ air
- Lung Ultrasound (Essentials 2013 #49)
  - ⇨ Diagnosis: Lung sliding, lung point
- True PTX? vs skin folds, blebs, peritoneal contents?

Treatment
- Chest tube: Unstable, hemothorax, multiple trauma
- Heimlich valve: stable, large PTX (>3cm)
- Observe & Oxygenate: stable, small-mod PTX (2-3cm; <20%)
- Occult PTX + Positive Pressure Ventilation (PPV) → if stable, can be observed

TRAUMA: BLUNT CHEST

Tension Pneumothorax
- Presentation:
  - ⇨ Classic presentation
    - ✓ Respiratory distress
    - ✓ Tachypnea
    - ✓ Deviated trachea
    - ✓ Hypotension/shock
    - ✓ Unilateral decreased breath sounds
  - ⇨ The reality (Emerg Med J 2005;22:8–16)
    - ✓ Tracheal deviation, hypoxia, and hypotension are inconsistent findings (<25% each)
  - ⇨ Course
    - ✓ Hypoxia with progressive respiratory compromise → hypotension → cardiac failure, respiratory arrest
  - ⇨ Ventilated pts
    - ✓ Sudden deterioration, hypoxia and hypotension (almost universal), increased Ppeak on vent, difficult to bag
- Treatment: Tension PTX
  - ⇨ Needle decompression (inconsistent and unreliable)?
  - ⇨ Immediate tube thoracostomy in mid-axillary line

SPONTANEOUS PNEUMOTHORAX (Chest 2001;119;590)
- Treatment
  - ⇨ ACCP recommends small bore (14F or smaller) catheter or 16-22 F chest tube connected to Heimlich valve or water seal
  - ⇨ If fails to re-expand → Chest tube
  - ⇨ May also do volume controlled re-expansion → Suction 200ml/hr from Heimlich and re-clamp
- **Re-expansion pulmonary edema** (mortality up to 20%)
  - ⇨ Risk factors: large size, long duration (>3days), rapid rate of re-expansion
  - ⇨ Clinical: 64% have symptoms within one hour, coughing, tachypnea, tachycardia and hypoxia
  - ⇨ Treatment: generally supportive, mechanical ventilation and hemodynamic support
- Dispo: may d/c with Heimlich valve if lung fully expanded (large ptx should be admitted, observe 24h)

HEMOTHORAX
(EM:RAP 11/12-Inaba)

Clinical
- Often asymptomatic
- Presentation: Dyspnea, tachypnea, hypovolemia, ↓breath sounds, poorly moving hemithorax, dull on percussion

Diagnosis
- Upright CXR: 150-200ml needed in pleural cavity to diagnose hemothorax
- Supine CXR: Sensitivity of 40-60% in ruling out hemothorax
- US: Can diagnose as little as 20ml of blood; Sensitivity of 96%

Treatment
- Small Hemothorax
  - ⇨ Observation option: (J Trauma Acute Care Surg 2012;72(1):11)
    - ✓ Consider as an option for small hemothorax (<300ml) but will likely need drainage
- Significant Hemothorax
  - ⇨ Chest tube: Drainage of hemothorax
  - ⇨ Tube size doesn't matter? (J Trauma Acute Care Surg 2012;72(2):422)
    - ✓ Size of tube is not a factor in causing complications (28-32F is equivalent to 36-40F)
  - ⇨ Auto-transfusion for large hemothorax
  - ⇨ Antibiotics prior to tube insertion (Cefazolin 2g IV)
- Unstable/Life threatening bleed
  - ⇨ Urgent thoracotomy: (J Trauma 2011;70(2):510)
    - ✓ More than 1,500 ml of blood immediately evacuated by tube thoracostomy
    - ✓ Persistent bleeding from the chest, defined as 150 ml/h to 200 ml/h for 2 hours to 4 hours
    - ✓ Persistent blood transfusion is required to maintain hemodynamic stability
    - ✓ Clinical stability of patient should determine whether or not patient needs OR (persistent shock etc...)

Complications
- Empyema- infection of retained hemothorax
- Retained fibrothorax-trapped lung
  - ⇨ Both may necessitate open thoracotomy and decortication

TRAUMA: BLUNT CHEST

S: STABLE

BLUNT AORTIC INJURY (BAI)

Epidemiology:
- Over 80% of patients die on scene

Mechanism:
- Rapid deceleration from high speed MVA, falls from height >3m, ejection from vehicle/motorcycle, crush between two objects

Evaluation
- All patients with significant mechanism of injury should have CT of mediastinum irrespective of CXR findings
- CXR: not sensitive to r/o aortic injury
- CT Chest: Normal CT essentially rules out aortic injury (J Trauma 1998;45(5):922)
- CT angiogram: sensitivity and NPV of approx 100%
- TEE: consider for patients too unstable for CT

BAI CXR:
☐ Widened mediastinum (>8cm)
☐ Apical capping
☐ Depressed L mainstem bronchus
☐ Widened L paratracheal stripe
☐ Loss of aortic knob contour
☐ Deviated NG tube

Treatment:
- Resuscitation
- Maintain low SBP <90 (β-blockers)
- Emergent surgical consultation

BLUNT CARDIAC INJURY (BCI)
(Essentials 2012 Cardiac Contusion: Does it Exist?)

Spectrum
- Structural
  - ⇨ Wall contusion (rarely clinically significant)
  - ⇨ Wall rupture (die at scene)
    - ✓ Incidence 0.045%, Mortality 89% (J Trauma. 2009;67(4):788)
  - ⇨ Septal rupture (die at scene)
  - ⇨ Valve disruption (die at scene)
  - ⇨ Coronary injury (die at scene)
  - ⇨ **Conclusion: Clinically significant structural injuries very rare in survivors**
- Electrical: Arrhythmias (Crit Care Clin 2004;20:57-70)
  - ⇨ Non-specific changes (50-70%):
    - ✓ Sinus tach/brady, PAC/PVC, conduction delays, ST-T wave changes
  - ⇨ Atrial arrhythmias (4-30%)
    - ✓ Atrial fibrillation most common arrhythmia to require treatment
  - ⇨ Ventricular arrhythmias (2-10%)

BCI Spectrum:
☐ Free wall rupture
☐ Septal rupture
☐ Coronary artery injury
☐ Cardiac failure
☐ Complex arrhythmias
☐ Minor EKG/cardiac enzyme abnormalities

Who is at risk?
- All patients with severe chest injury
- High risk mechanism: high speed, rapid deceleration, airbag, steering wheel damage, seatbelt restraint
- Associated chest trauma: fracture, contusion, hemothorax/PTX

Evaluation:
- Controversial: many approaches to rule out BCI
- Serial troponin/EKG (J Trauma 2003;54:45-51)
  - ⇨ Serial EKG/Trop at 0 and 8 hours → sensitivity 100%
  - ⇨ If either (+) → r/o ACS, 24h monitoring for arrhythmias, TTE
  - ⇨ If all normal, can d/c home

BLUNT DIAPHRAGMATIC RUPTURE
(Essentials 2011 "Diaphragmatic Injuries"-Mallon)

General:
- 50-80% on left side, right side rupture associated with liver injury (50%)
- Clinical symptoms are varied, subtle and non-specific
- Other injuries? Isolated diaphragm injuries from blunt trauma are rare

Mechanism
- Severe abdominal trauma → sudden, major increase of intra-abdominal pressure (MVC) → weak parts of diaphragm pull apart → +/- translocation of abdominal contents

TRAUMA: BLUNT CHEST

Diagnosis:
- CXR
  - ⇨ Classic: bowel in chest wall (<50% translocation), elevated hemidiaphragm, displaced NG tube, box-like R hemidiaphragm
  - ⇨ Usual: abnormal but non-specific
- CT → high specificity, sensitivity still low
  - ⇨ Collar sign on CT: Constriction of colon/stomach passing through tear
  - ⇨ If high clinical suspicion, may need surgical evaluation
- Delayed presentation:
  - ⇨ Most diaphragmatic ruptures missed on initial trauma eval → present later with bowel obstruction/incarceration

TRACHEOBRONCHIAL TREE INJURY

Upper Airway Injury
- Usually straightforward diagnosis
- Treatment: Relieve obstruction and secure definitive airway

Lower Airway Injury
- Clinical Presentation
  - ⇨ Rare and can be subtle (depending on size of defect, air leak, pleural communication)
  - ⇨ Small defect:
    - ✓ Mediastinal air on CT, SQ emphysema, hemoptysis
  - ⇨ Large defect:
    - ✓ Dyspnea, PTX, Persistent PTX after chest tube, air leak after chest tube
    - ✓ May need 2nd chest tube
- Diagnosis
  - ⇨ CT
    - ✓ Difficult to ID on CT → usually within 2cm of carina (right mainstem bronchus or trachea)
  - ⇨ Bronchoscopy
    - ✓ Locate injury to advance ETT beyond site of injury, possibly to unaffected mainstem bronchus
    - ✓ Diagnose location and size of injury → surgical repair
- Treatment
  - ⇨ High mortality from ventilation/oxygenation compromise
  - ⇨ Thoracic Surgery for repair

PULMONARY CONTUSION

Mechanism:
- High-energy mechanisms of trauma with rapid deceleration, compression, shear, or inertial forces
- MVC, falls from great heights, blast injuries

Pathophysiology
- Lung parenchyma damage → alveoli filled with mucus and fluid → decreased compliance, decreased oxygen diffusion, ventilation-perfusion mismatch, and shunting

Clinical
- May be asymptomatic
- SOB, hypoxia and increased work of breathing proportional to the degree of contused lung
- Symptoms progress over hours and usually peak at 72h

Diagnosis
- CXR
  - ⇨ Classical: infiltrates or consolidation
  - ⇨ Normal CXR in 50% pts on arrival → then progress to classic CXR at 24h
- CT scan
  - ⇨ More sensitive than CXR → may have parenchymal changes on CT with normal CXR

Treatment
- Mostly supportive
- Oxygen, pulmonary toilet, ICU monitoring
- Avoid over-hydration → may worsen lung edema
- NPPV may help avoid intubation in selected patients
- Intubation and PPV if other modalities fail
  - ⇨ Goal: optimize oxygenation while minimizing further lung trauma
  - ⇨ Low Vt (6ml/kg) and maintain low Ppl <30

TRAUMA: BLUNT CHEST

FLAIL CHEST

Cause
- Anterior or lateral double fractures of 3 or more adjacent ribs
- Flail segment moves in during inspiration

Diagnosis
- CXR
- Chest CT-in severe trauma to evaluate for pulmonary contusion or other associated injuries

Treatment
- Continuous pulse oximetry/ABG
- Analgesia
- Mechanical ventilation for severe trauma

RIB FRACTURES

Diagnosis
- CXR (costochondral junction fractures may not be seen)

Treatment
- Mild-moderate pain: oral analgesics
- Severe pain: IV pain medication or epidural
- Incentive spirometry

Associated injuries
- Pneumothorax/hemothorax
- 1st three ribs: subclavian vessels or major bronchi
- Pulm contusion/BCI/Aortic rupture/Diaphragm rupture

TRAUMA: PENETRATING ABDOMEN

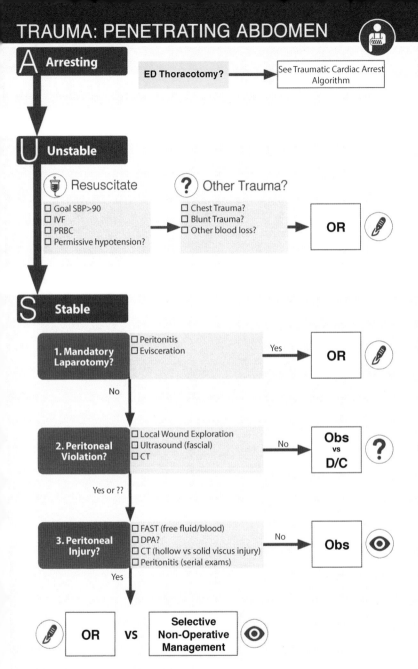

A Arresting

ED Thoracotomy? → See Traumatic Cardiac Arrest Algorithm

U Unstable

Resuscitate

- ☐ Goal SBP>90
- ☐ IVF
- ☐ PRBC
- ☐ Permissive hypotension?

Other Trauma?

- ☐ Chest Trauma?
- ☐ Blunt Trauma?
- ☐ Other blood loss?

→ **OR**

S Stable

1. Mandatory Laparotomy?
- ☐ Peritonitis
- ☐ Evisceration

Yes → **OR**

No

2. Peritoneal Violation?
- ☐ Local Wound Exploration
- ☐ Ultrasound (fascial)
- ☐ CT

No → **Obs vs D/C** ?

Yes or ??

3. Peritoneal Injury?
- ☐ FAST (free fluid/blood)
- ☐ DPA?
- ☐ CT (hollow vs solid viscus injury)
- ☐ Peritonitis (serial exams)

No → **Obs**

Yes

OR VS **Selective Non-Operative Management**

TRAUMA: PENETRATING ABDOMEN

A: ARRESTING

(Emerg Med Clin N Am 2007;25:713-733)

ED Thoracotomy indications:
- Trauma patient, CPR, no signs of life (SOL) +:
  - ⇨ Blunt trauma with CPR <10min
  - ⇨ Penetrating trauma with CPR <15min
  - ⇨ Penetrating trauma to neck/extremity < 5 min

Consider: Thoracotomy on left (Low utility in blunt trauma)
- Release pericardial tamponade
- Address hemorrhage inside chest
- Cross clamp aorta → diverts blood away from intra-abdominal hemorrhage
- Open cardiac resuscitation
- Chest tube on right, if + blood → clamshell

Survival rates:
- Overall survival rate 7.4%, dictated by location & mechanism of injury (J Am Coll Surg 2000;190:288-98)
  - ⇨ Thoracic injury 10.7% (Cardiac-19.4%), **abdominal injury 4.5%**
  - ⇨ **Penetrating injury 8.8% (stab wounds 17%, GSW 4.3%)** blunt trauma 1.4%

ED Thoracotomy Indications:
Trauma + CPR + no SOL +:
☐ Blunt trauma, CPR < 10min
☐ Penetrating trauma, CPR<15min
☐ Penetrating trauma to neck/ extremity < 5 min

No Signs of Life (SOL)
☐ No pulse
☐ No pupils
☐ No movement
☐ No breaths
☐ No PEA
☐ No cardiac motion (US)

U: UNSTABLE

Unstable = OR Immediately
- Mandatory laparotomy

Begin Resuscitation
- IVF, Crystalloids
- Consider permissive hypotension

R/O other causes for instability
- Chest trauma (PTX/HTX, cardiac tamponade)
- Neck trauma
- Other trauma/sources of blood loss

S: STABLE

1. Mandatory laparotomy?
- Hemodynamic instability (Unstable → see above)
- Peritonitis
- Evisceration
  - ⇨ Stab Wounds (J Trauma 2005;58:526-32)
    - ✓ Selective observation method? Small study showed 24/31 SW patients managed non-operatively discharged home without ex lap
  - ⇨ Gunshot wounds (Ann Emerg Med 2004;43:344)
    - ✓ Mandates laparotomy because of increase injury and contamination

2. Peritoneal violation?
- Work-up
  - ⇨ Local wound exploration
  - ⇨ Ultrasound (check fascial integrity)
  - ⇨ CT
- If (+)peritoneal violation
  - ⇨ Observation for development of peritoneal injury
  - ⇨ 30% of patients with peritoneal violation have no significant abdominal injury (Demetriades-"The Red Book")

3. Peritoneal injury?
- FAST (↑spec, ↓sens)
- DPA/DPL
- Serial examinations
- Laparoscopy
- CT

Selective Non-operative management

- Use if patient is clinically stable and no evidence of peritonitis/hemorrhage
- Not used in unconscious/spinal cord injury patients or receiving general anesthesia for other problem
    - ⇨ Mandates abdominal exploration
- Management
    - ⇨ Continue work-up of patient, r/o other injuries
    - ⇨ Monitor closely with serial examinations (vital signs, serial abdominal exams, serial H/H and WBC)
    - ⇨ Serial CT scans?
    - ⇨ IR for angiography/embolization? (depending on injury)
- Indications for laparotomy (OR):
    - ⇨ Patient develops signs of **peritonitis**
    - ⇨ Patient becomes **unstable/severe bleeding**

TRAUMA: BLUNT ABDOMEN

A Arresting

ED Thoracotomy? → See Traumatic Cardiac Arrest Algorithm

U Unstable

1. Abdomen Evaluation
- ☐ 1. Peritonitis
- ☐ 2. FAST (+)
- ☐ 3. DPA/DPL (+)

→ Yes → **OR**

↓ No

2. R/O Other Trauma

Other sources of Instability
- ☐ R/O Thoracic source: FAST, CXR
- ☐ R/O Pelvic source: PEX, Pelvic Xray
- ☐ R/O Extremity source: PEX, Xray
- ☐ R/O Neurogenic shock: PEX, CT Head
- ☐ R/O other causes (cardiac, drugs etc...)

3. Resuscitate

Resus to SBP>90
- ☐ IV Fluids/Blood/FFP
- ☐ Stop blood loss
- ☐ See Trauma Resuscitation algorithm

Stable? / Source? → **CT (when stable)**

S Stable

Non-Evaluable
- ☐ Clinical Exam
- ☐ **CT Abdomen Pelvis**
- ☐ Evaluate other injuries

→ **Obs vs OR** ?

Evaluable

→ **Peritonitis?**

→ Yes → **OR**

↓ No

- ☐ Physical Exam Concerning?
- ☐ FAST (+)?
- ☐ Bad Mechanism?

→ Yes → **CT**

↓ No

👁 **Observation**

179

TRAUMA: BLUNT ABDOMEN

A: ARRESTING

(Essentials 2010 -Inaba)

ED Thoracotomy indications:
- Trauma patient, CPR, no signs of life (SOL) +:
  - ⇨ Blunt trauma with CPR <10min
  - ⇨ Penetrating trauma with CPR <15min
  - ⇨ Penetrating trauma to neck/extremity < 5 min

ED Thoracotomy Indications:
Trauma + CPR + no SOL +:
☐ Blunt trauma, CPR < 10min
☐ Penetrating trauma, CPR<15min
☐ Penetrating trauma to neck/ extremity < 5 min

Consider: Thoracotomy on left (Low utility in blunt trauma)
- Release pericardial tamponade
- Address hemorrhage inside chest
- Cross clamp aorta → diverts blood away from intra-abdominal hemorrhage
- Open cardiac resuscitation
- Chest tube on right, if + blood → clamshell

No Signs of Life (SOL)
☐ No pulse
☐ No pupils
☐ No movement
☐ No breaths
☐ No PEA
☐ No cardiac motion (US)

Survival rates:
- Overall survival rate 7.4%, dictated by location & mechanism of injury (J Am Coll Surg 2000;190:288-98)
  - ⇨ Thoracic injury 10.7% (Cardiac-19.4%), **abdominal injury 4.5%**
  - ⇨ **Penetrating injury 8.8% (stab wounds 17%, GSW 4.3%)** blunt trauma 1.4%

U: UNSTABLE

Indications for OR
- Peritonitis
- FAST(+)
  - ⇨ Wide range of sensitivities for detecting intra-abdominal hemorrhage, depending on amount of fluid present
  - ⇨ ↑Specificity: Helpful if + free fluid → OR
  - ⇨ ↓Sensitivity: Unable to rule out free fluid/hemorrhage if negative
- DPA/DPL(+)
  - ⇨ Indication: Unstable patient and FAST (-) → r/o abdominal source as cause of instability
  - ⇨ Positive if 10ml of grossly bloody fluid is aspirated

R/O other sources of instability
- R/O Thoracic source → FAST, CXR
- R/O Pelvic source → PEX, Pelvic Xray
- R/O Extremity source → PEX, Xray
- R/O Neurogenic shock → PEX, CT Head
- R/O other causes (cardiac, drugs etc...)

Resuscitation (See Trauma Resuscitation algorithm)
- IVF, Crystalloids
- Hemostatic resuscitation-PRBC, FFP
- Goal: stabilize patient
  - ⇨ If stable and no evidence of intra-abdominal injury → CT AP

S: STABLE

Non-evaluable patient
- Definition:
  - ⇨ Intoxicated (alcohol/drugs), neurologic injury, multiple extra-abdominal injuries
  - ⇨ Non-alert patient that cannot be clinically evaluated for injury
- CT abdomen/pelvis
  - ⇨ Obtain CT regardless of clinical exam
  - ⇨ CT good for solid organ/vascular injuries, contrast extravasation, GU tract
  - ⇨ CT scan not good in identifying **hollow viscous injuries** & diaphragm injuries
- Clinical exam
  - ⇨ Even if CT negative, continue observation and clinical exams: labs, WBC, fever curves, tachycardia

DPA Indications:
☐ Hypotensive +
☐ Blunt trauma +
☐ Negative/equivocal fast

Evaluable patient
- Rely on PEX, FAST and mechanism (JAMA 2012 ;307:1517-27)
- Clinical exam (+):
  - ⇨ Severe abdominal pain, N/V
    - ✓ Absence of abdominal tenderness does not rule-out injury
  - ⇨ **Abdominal distention**
  - ⇨ **Hypotension**

High risk exam:
☐ Hypotensive
☐ Abdominal distention
☐ Peritonitis
☐ Seatbelt sign

⇨ **Peritonitis** (rebound,guarding)
  ✓ Immediate OR (47% with major vascular/solid organ injury)
⇨ **Seatbelt sign** (see below)
⇨ Gross hematuria (See pelvic trauma- GU algorithm)
  ✓ Microscopic hematuria is insignificant
  ✓ Concern for injury to urethra, bladder, kidney
  ✓ Post foley
    i. CT-r/o kidney injury
    ii. CT cystogram-r/o bladder injury
  ✓ Pre-foley
    i. Blood at meatus, perineal hematoma, abnormal prostate, inability to void/cath
    ii. Retrograde urethrogram (RUG)
- Work-up
  ⇨ Labs
    ✓ High risk: WBC, H/H, LFTs, UA, core temp
  ⇨ Serial US
    ✓ If FAST (+) → further work-up with CT AP indicated to r/o injury
    ✓ If FAST (-) → decreases likelihood but does not rule-out intra-abdominal injury
  ⇨ CT scan: (ACEP Policy Ann Emerg Med 2011;57:387)
    ✓ Indication: (+) PEX, (+) FAST, concerning mechanism
    ✓ CT reliably excludes liver and spleen injury
    ✓ CT **does not exclude** hollow viscus, diaphragmatic, or pancreatic injury
      i. Patient may still need observation even if CT AP negative
  ⇨ Observation option:
    ✓ Indication: Physical exam negative, FAST (-) and low risk mechanism
    ✓ Serial FAST US to increase sensitivity of US and serial abdominal exams
    ✓ Observation after negative CT → r/o hollow viscus injuries
  ⇨ OR indications:
    ✓ Patient becomes unstable, hypotensive from blood loss
    ✓ Pneumoperitoneum: indicative of hollow viscus injury
    ✓ Diaphragmatic rupture
    ✓ Persistent/significant GI bleeding
    ✓ Peritonitis: HD stable but with (+) peritonitis (Arch Surg 2005;140:767-72)
      i. Peritonitis is not always a hollow viscus injury
      ii. 47% with major vascular/solid organ injury
      iii. Stable patient with peritonitis → indication for OR

OR Indications:
☐ Hypotensive/unstable/ blood loss
☐ Pneumoperitoneum
☐ Diaphragm rupture
☐ Significant GI bleed
☐ Peritonitis

ABDOMINAL SEATBELT SIGN

(EM:RAP 11/08 - Shoenberger)(Essentials 2011-Trauma Course)

General
- Associated with increased rates of mesenteric, hollow viscous, pancreatic injuries and Chance fractures (Am Surg 1999;65(2):181)
  ⇨ Intra-abdominal injuries 23% (vs 3% without seatbelt sign) → 8x increase injuries
  ⇨ Children with seat belt sign are almost 3X as likely to suffer intra-abdominal injury (Acad Emerg Med 2005 12:808)

Work-up
- CT
  ⇨ Not adequate at detecting these injuries
  ⇨ CT indicated for patients with pain or tenderness
- FAST
  ⇨ Not adequate at detecting injuries (Cochrane Database Syst Rev 2005)
  ⇨ 78% of patients with injury had negative FAST (Arch Surg 2002;137:718)
- **Serial abdominal exams** needed to detect those with injuries
  ⇨ 90% of patients with an injury have abdominal pain or tenderness at presentation
  ⇨ Severity of pain more important than severity of mark
  ⇨ Most patients with injuries develop abdominal tenderness → OR

Associated injuries
- **BUCKET HANDLE MESENTERY INJURY**
  ⇨ Part of intestines separates from mesentery → peritonitis
- **CHANCE FRACTURE (Thoracolumbar fractures)**
  ⇨ Piking over seat belt → flexion-distraction forces posteriorly → thoracolumbar vertebral body fracture
  ⇨ Strong association between thoracolumbar fractures and intra-abdominal injuries

TRAUMA: BLUNT ABDOMEN

Neck Seatbelt Sign

General
- Shoulder belt rides up trapezius ridge → ecchymosis on neck

Work-up (See Blunt Neck Trauma algorithm)
- Blunt carotid injury (Mechanism of injury):
    - ⇨ Trauma → intimal tear can lead to:
        - ✓ Thrombosis → embolism → stroke
        - ✓ Dissection → vessel occlusion
        - ✓ Pseudoaneurysm → occlusion or rupture → hemorrhage or AV fistula
- Red flags
    - ⇨ LOC, GCS deficits
    - ⇨ Clavicle and 1st rib fractures
    - ⇨ Anterior neck triangle involvement
    - ⇨ Hoarseness, dysphagia, odynophagia
    - ⇨ Any neurologic findings or complaints-even transient
- Imaging the neck
    - ⇨ MR angio or CT angio
    - ⇨ Both superior to US duplex
    - ⇨ Look for intimal flap or pseudoaneurysm

Journal Club: Neck Seat Belt Sign

Mayberry et al (Arch Surg 2004;139:609)
- Rare diagnosis: 10 yrs & 35,000 blunt trauma patients → only 17 had BCI
- Most patients with BCI develop stroke symptoms within a few hours of presentation

DiPerna et al (Am Surg 2002;68:441)
- 2002 study at USC of 131 patients with neck belt sign
- Only 1 of 131 had abnormality (intimal flap with carotid artery stenosis → pt presented with lateralizing signs and GCS 8)

Rozycki et al (J Trauma 2002;52:618)
- Cervicothoracic seat belt sign PLUS abnormal physical exam provides effective screening
- Associations: GCS<14, ISS>16 and clavicle/1st rib fracture

TRAUMA: PELVIS

A — Arresting

ED Thoracotomy? → See Traumatic Cardiac Arrest Algorithm

U — Unstable

Resuscitate

Resus to SBP>90
☐ IV Fluids/Blood/FFP
☐ Stop blood loss
☐ See Trauma Resuscitation algorithm

→ See Trauma Resuscitation Algorithm

R/O Other Injuries → See Blunt Trauma Algorithm

Abdominal + Pelvic Injury

Abd Injury?
☐ Peritonitis
☐ FAST (+)
☐ DPA/DPL(+)

Pelvic Injury?
☐ AP Pelvis Xray
☐ Clinically unstable pelvis?

→ **Laparotomy + External Fixator + PPP (Preperitoneal packing)** → Persistent Unstable → **Angiography/ Embolization**

VS

Isolated Pelvic Injury → AP Pelvis Xray → **External Pelvic Stablilization** VS

IR → **Angiography/ Embolization**

OR → **PPP (Preperitoneal packing)**

Persistent Unstable?

S — Stable

CT Abd/Pelvis

Abdominal injury → **Laparotomy VS Observation**

Pelvic blush → **IR for Angiography/ Embolization**

No injury → ⇨ ICU for Observation ⇨ Continue Trauma evaluation

TRAUMA: PELVIS

A: ARRESTING

See Traumatic Cardiac Arrest Algorithm
Consider: Thoracotomy on left (Low utility in blunt trauma)
Survival rates:
- Overall survival rate 7.4%, dictated by location & mechanism of injury (J Am Coll Surg 2000;190:288-98)
  - ⇨ Thoracic injury 10.7% (Cardiac-19.4%), abdominal injury 4.5%
  - ⇨ Penetrating injury 8.8% (stab wounds 17%, GSW 4.3%) **blunt trauma 1.4%**

U: UNSTABLE
(EM:RAP 4/14)(westerntrauma.org)

Clinical Exam
- Unstable pelvis
  - ⇨ Do not rock pelvis: will open pelvis and cause further exsanguination
  - ⇨ Proper maneuver: grab iliac crests and push in evaluate for bony stability of pelvis
  - ⇨ **Earles sign**: palpation of fracture line on rectal/vaginal exam
- Pelvic bleeding
  - ⇨ **Destot's sign**: hematoma over inguinal ligament into scrotum (large pelvic bleed)
- GU injury?
  - ⇨ Blood at meatus, hematuria before foley, abnormal/boggy prostate, perineal bruising
  - ⇨ Inability to urinate or pass foley

Classification (Shock Trauma classification-Young and Burgess) (J Trauma 1989;29:981)
- Stability Types
  - ⇨ Hemodynamic stability-first concern in any pelvic fracture
  - ⇨ Skeletal stability- based on classification (AP vs LC vs Shear)
- **LC (lateral compression)**
  - ⇨ Mechanism: Most common mechanism of injury (e.g. t-boned by car)
  - ⇨ Pathophysiology: Pelvis shortens and implodes → usually not bleed
  - ⇨ Hemorrhage?
    - ✓ Not associated with hemorrhage (pelvic ligaments stay intact)
    - ✓ If hypotension → look elsewhere besides pelvis
  - ⇨ Associated with intra-abdominal bleeding, blunt aortic injury
- **AP (Anterior-posterior Compression)**
  - ⇨ Mechanism: Head-on impact (MVA), fall from horse
  - ⇨ Pathophysiology: Pelvis explodes (open book) → small or no bony component
  - ⇨ Hemorrhage?
    - ✓ Pure ligamentous rupture → Bleed!!!
    - ✓ Classic open book fracture
- **Vertical Shear (Malgaigne fracture)**
  - ⇨ Mechanism: Vertical force on lower extremity transmits force on hemipelvis (e.g. fall from height)
  - ⇨ Pathophys: Complete dislocation/fx of hemipelvis caused by at least 2 disruptions of pelvic ring which involve both the anterior (pubic symphysis/rami) and poterior pelvic ring (sacrum/SI joint/ileum)
  - ⇨ Hemorrhage: High risk for pelvic hemorrhage and abdominal injuries

Pelvic Xray:
☐ Look for disruption of posterior pelvis
☐ Concern for bleeding

Talk and Die Diagnosis:
☐ **Pelvic fracture**
☐ Epidural hematoma
☐ Sepsis
☐ MI → VF arrest
☐ Aortic dissection

Management
- Resuscitation (See Trauma Resuscitation Algorithm)
  - ⇨ Large volume crystalloid → not work well
  - ⇨ Blood, FFP early, T&C 6 units, prepare for massive transfusion
  - ⇨ Permissive hypotension?
  - ⇨ Hemostatic resuscitation
    - ✓ FFP and platelets early
    - ✓ PRBC:FFP in a ratio of 1:1?
    - ✓ Correct Coags (Coumadin, ASA)
  - ⇨ Tranexamic acid
    - ✓ Effective bridge in controlling hemorrhage
    - ✓ Dose: 100mcg/kg for severe bleeding
  - ⇨ Intubation
    - ✓ Pelvic binder prior to intubation because of possible drop in BP from sedation/paralytics
- Evaluate Pelvic injury
  - ⇨ Pelvic Xray → obtain in all unstable blunt trauma patients
- R/O Other Injury
  - ⇨ R/O Thoracic source → FAST, CXR
  - ⇨ R/O Extremity source → PEX, Xray
  - ⇨ R/O Neurogenic shock → PEX, CT Head
  - ⇨ R/O other causes (cardiac, drugs etc...)

- R/O Abdominal Injury (See Abdominal Trauma Algorithm)
  - ⇨ Workup: FAST, DPA, CT
  - ⇨ Stabilize Pelvic injury with external fixator
  - ⇨ Blunt force injury severe enough to fracture the pelvic ring can cause concomitant intra-abdominal injuries. (J Trauma. 1980;20:919-923)
  - ⇨ The frequency of abdominal injury, in association with pelvic fracture can range from 16% to 55%

Treatment, Pelvic Injury

- **External Pelvic Stabilization**
  - ⇨ Indication (Unstable pt)
    - ✓ Pelvis is clinically unstable to manual compression
    - ✓ Widening of the posterior pelvic ring
    - ✓ Pubic symphysis diastasis
  - ⇨ External Compression to reduce fracture fragments (up to 10%)
  - ⇨ MOA
    - ✓ Theory: Reduces volume → stops bleeding → stabilizes clot?
    - ✓ No evidence of decreased bleeding/transfusion requirements with pelvic binder
  - ⇨ Types
    - ✓ Pelvic binder: T-POD (Trauma Pelvic Orthotic Device)
    - ✓ Bedsheet crisscrossed across patient
    - ✓ MAST (Military Anti-Shock Trousers)
- **Preperitoneal Pelvic Packing (PPP)** (J Am Coll Surg 2011;212:628) (Injury 2009;40:54-60)
  - ⇨ General
    - ✓ OR/Pelvic packing of pelvis is as effective as pelvic angiography for stabilizing hemodynamically unstable pelvic fractures
    - ✓ PPP decreases need for pelvic embolization and post-procedure blood transfusions

Pelvic binder:
☐ Unstable patient +
☐ Unstable pelvis

    - ✓ PPP may reduce early mortality due to exsanguination from pelvic hemorrhage
  - ⇨ Indication:
    - ✓ **Hemodynamic instability** and **refractory hemorrhagic shock** and:
      - i. In a patient with concomitant abdominal and pelvic injury → can do laparotomy (for abdominal injury) and PPP (for pelvic injury stabilization)
      - ii. Isolated pelvic injury (depending on surgical team and availability of IR for angiography)
      - iii. Persistently unstable after angiography → immediate OR for PPP
- **Angiography/Embolization**
  - ⇨ Indication:
    - ✓ Patient remains unstable after PPP (preperitoneal pelvic packing)
    - ✓ Primary treatment for isolated pelvic injury

S: STABLE

Work-up

- Xray (J Trauma 1992;33:413)
  - ⇨ Questionable utility for screening asymptomatic stable blunt trauma patients if obtaining CT AP
  - ⇨ If patient awake and alert, no pelvic pain or tenderness → very unlikely to have pelvic fracture
- CT Abdomen/Pelvis
  - ⇨ Indication: Stable patient or stabilizes after minimal resuscitation
  - ⇨ Contrast extravasation?
    - ✓ Contrast extravasation or blush on CT → accuracy of 98% for identifying patients **requiring embolization** (Surgery 2000;128:678-685)
    - ✓ Site of extravasation corresponds to the site of bleeding at angiography → guide IR to the area of highest yield first
    - ✓ Treatment: IR for angiography/embolization
  - ⇨ No Injury on CT
    - ✓ Rule-out other injuries
    - ✓ ICU for completion of trauma evaluation and resuscitation

Stable Fractures (Minor Injuries)

- Pelvic Avulsion Fractures (Stable)
  - ⇨ Large muscle group causes avulsion
  - ⇨ Injuries: Greater trochanter (Gluteal muscles), Lesser trochanter (Iliopsoas), ASIS (Sartorius), AIIS (Rectus femoris), Pubic symphysis (Adductor group), Ischial tuberosity (Hamstrings)
  - ⇨ Iliac wing, single ramus fracture

TRAUMA: PELVIS

GU TRAUMA
(Essentials 2009 -Inaba)(Emerg Med Clin N Am 2011;29:501)

URETHRAL INJURY

- Anatomy
  - ⇨ **Anterior** (Bulbar and Penile urethra)
    - ✓ Straddle injury and Penetrating trauma
    - ✓ Associated with: Fractured penis, hematuria
    - ✓ Complications: fistula, stricture
  - ⇨ **Posterior** (Prostatic and Membranous urethra)
    - ✓ Blunt trauma, pelvic fractures
    - ✓ Associated with distended bladder, lower abdominal pain, dysuria, meatal blood, scrotal hematoma
    - ✓ Complications: Impotence, incontinence
- Clinical Signs (Injury 2009;40:984-6)
  - ⇨ Classic
    - ✓ Not sensitive or specific
    - ✓ Blood at meatus (20%), hematuria before foley (17%), abnormal/boggy prostate (2%), perineal bruising
    - ✓ No clinical signs (61%)
  - ⇨ Non-classical signs
    - ✓ Inability to pass foley
    - ✓ Inability to urinate
- Management
  - ⇨ Foley
    - ✓ If suspect urethral injury → no foley until urethral injury is ruled out
  - ⇨ Retrograde Urethrogram (RUG)
    - ✓ Use: to eval for urethral injury prior to foley
    - ✓ RUG(-):
      - i. OK to insert foley,
      - ii. R/O renal/bladder injuries
    - ✓ RUG(+):
      - i. **No Foley → Urology consult**
      - ii. Traditional tx vs IER (Immediate Endoscopic Realignment)
      - iii. R/O renal/bladder injuries
  - ⇨ Traditional management
    - ✓ Supra-pubic catheter (SP)
    - ✓ Delayed OR repair 3-6 mos, increased complications
  - ⇨ IER (Immediate Endoscopic Realignment) (J Trauma 2008;64:1443-50)
    - ✓ Once stable → Flexible cystoscopy, wire guided foley
    - ✓ Foley x3-4 weeks then RUG → if negative, remove
    - ✓ 78% success rate, improve time to void (35 vs 229 days), improve stricture rate (14% vs 100%), ↓surgical urethroplasty (0% vs 100%)

BLADDER RUPTURE

- Extra-peritoneal rupture
  - ⇨ Usually associated with pelvic fractures
  - ⇨ Adult: Pre-peritoneal rupture → FAST (-) → RUG + Cystoscopy
- Intra-peritoneal rupture
  - ⇨ From penetrating or burst injury at the dome because of sudden elevated pressures in a full bladder resulting from a direct blow
  - ⇨ Pediatrics: Intra-peritoneal rupture → FAST (+) → Immediate Ex-Lap
- Clinical Signs
  - ⇨ Gross hematuria: most reliable sign, present in almost 100% of cases
- Work-up
  - ⇨ **Retrograde cystography** (plain films) nearly 100% accurate for bladder injury
  - ⇨ **CT cystography** as accurate as plain film cystography, gives more detail
  - ⇨ Procedure: Bladder filled and distended with water soluble contrast + Xray or CT
- Treatment
  - ⇨ Blunt extraperitoneal rupture → immediate repair to avoid complications (fistula, abscess, prolonged leak)
  - ⇨ Intraperitoneal injury → immediate repair because injury is usually larger than what appears on imaging

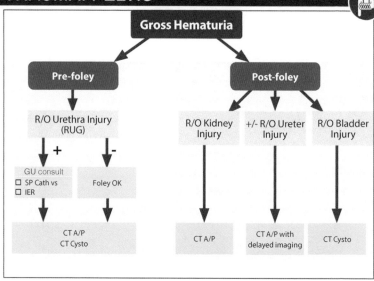

URETER INJURY

- Extemely rare injury, usually associated with other injuries (renal, bladder)
- Work-up
  - ⇨ **Delayed CT imaging**
    - ✓ Delayed images (5-20 minutes) after IV contrast
    - ✓ Dx: extravasation of contrast, peri-urethral urinoma or non-opacification of ureter
  - ⇨ Intravenous pyelography (IVP)- not very accurate, second line for diagnosis
  - ⇨ Retrograde ureterogam

KIDNEY INJURY

- Mechanism-sudden deceleration → damages renal vessels → renal pedicle avulsion, renal artery thrombosis, renal vein disruption
- Work-up
  - ⇨ UA: Hematuria not always present
  - ⇨ Imaging indications
    - ✓ Blunt trauma + gross hematuria
    - ✓ Microscopic hematuria + shock
  - ⇨ CT with contrast
    - ✓ High sensitivity/specificity → preferred imaging
  - ⇨ IVP-single shot-use intraoperative if patient going to OR for other injuries

---

WORK-UP: HEMATURIA + BLUNT TRAUMA

1. **R/O Urethral injury**
   - ⇨ No Foley
   - ⇨ RUG
     - ✓ RUG(-) → OK to insert foley
     - ✓ RUG(+) → No foley; Urology consult: traditional tx vs IER
2. **R/O bladder injury**
   - ⇨ CT cystography
3. **R/O renal injury**
   - ⇨ CT AP with IV contrast
4. **Consider r/o ureter injury**
   - ⇨ Delayed CT imaging

LOW BACK PAIN

1 General Red Flags

Red Flags **Action**

- □ **Age** (<20, >50)
- □ **Duration** (>6 wks)
- □ **Atypical pain** features (wake from sleep, intractable pain)

Consider further w/u:
⇨ Xray
⇨ MRI

2 R/O Emergent Dx

Vascular

AAA
- □ Acute epigastric/back pain
- □ **Wide pulsatile abd mass**
- □ Risk factors (age, male, smoking, CAD)

Ao Dissection
- □ Sudden onset, severe, tearing pain
- □ Risks: h/o Marfan, HTN, cocaine
- □ **Pulse deficit/Neuro deficit**

⇨ Screening test: Bedside U/S
⇨ CT – if stable
⇨ Vascular surgery C/S
⇨ β-blockade

Epidural Compression

- □ **H/O Cancer**
- □ **Focal neuro deficit** (B/L LE weak, sciatica change, gait disturbance)
- □ **Bowel/bladder incontinence**
- □ **Anal sphincter tone** diminished
- □ Sensory loss: **saddle anesthesia**, sensory level

⇨ Screening test: **PVR**
⇨ MRI
⇨ High Dose Steroids
⇨ Neurosurgery C/S

Epidural Abscess

- □ Classic triad (13%): **Fever**, Spine pain, Neuro deficit
- □ Risk Factors screen: **IVDA**, immunocomp, EtOH, spine procedure, distant infection, DM, CRF, CA, indwelling cath, spine fx

⇨ Screening Test: **ESR**
⇨ MRI

Vertebral Fracture

- □ **Trauma**
- □ Point Vertebral Tenderness
- □ **Steroid use**

⇨ Xrays
⇨ CT Spine

3 R/O Visceral Causes

Pyelonephritis

- □ Hematuria/Dysuria
- □ CVA- Tenderness
- □ Abdominal or flank pain/tender

⇨ Pregnancy
⇨ UA/U dip
⇨ Labs?

Nephrolithiasis

- □ Hematuria/Dysuria
- □ CVA- Tenderness
- □ Abdominal or flank pain/tender
- □ Colic type pain

⇨ UA/urine pregnancy test
⇨ Labs
⇨ CT vs US?

GI Pelvic

- □ Abdominal pain/tender
- □ BRBPR/melena
- □ Vaginal/urethal bleeding or discharge

Consider further w/u:
⇨ Labs
⇨ CT vs US?

4 Mechanical LBP

Herniated Disc

- □ Sciatica (radicular pain)
- □ SLR positive

⇨ Xrays L/S spine
⇨ MRI?
⇨ Surgery vs conservative tx

Lumbar Strain (70%)

- □ Diagnosis of exclusion
- □ No further w/u needed

⇨ Activity as tolerated
⇨ Analgesics/Muscle relaxants

LOW BACK PAIN

1. GENERAL RED FLAGS

(Emerg Med Clin N Am 2010;28:811) (EM:RAP 11/13)

General Approach
- Begin work-up by ruling out emergent/urgent conditions and evaluating/charting the absence of **red flags** that can signal the presence of an emergent condition
- Then consider other visceral causes of low back pain
- If no red flags are present and patient does not need further work-up, then the likely default diagnosis is benign mechanical (lumbar strain) LBP

Age
- **<20 years old**
  - ⇨ Increased incidence of congenital, developmental, bony abnormalities, and malignancy
- **>50 years old**
  - ⇨ Increased incidence of serious causes (AAA, vertebral fx, pancreatitis…)

Duration of sx
- **Acute** (0-6wks); **Subacute** (6-12wks); **Chronic** (>12wks), and recurrent
- **Non acute (>6wks)**
  - ⇨ Red flag because 80-90% sx should **resolve by 4-6wks** (Emerg Med Clin North Am 1999;17:877-93)

Atypical pain features
- **Awaken from sleep**
- **Intractable pain**
  - ⇨ Consider: infection, tumor, fracture, nerve impingement, or non-musculoskeletal causes

2. R/O EMERGENT CONDITIONS

AAA/AORTIC DISSECTION

(see Abdominal Pain-General/Chest Pain Algorithms for more details)

AAA (See Abdominal Pain-General Algorithm)
- Presentation
  - ⇨ Usually asymptomatic until rupture
  - ⇨ Acute epigastric & back pain
  - ⇨ Wide pulsatile abdominal mass
  - ⇨ Renal colic mimic (back pain, hematuria)
- AAA Risk factors (age, male, smoking, CAD/PVD, Fam Hx)

Aortic Dissection (See Chest Pain Algorithm)
- Presentation
  - ⇨ Sudden-onset, severe, "tearing" pain
  - ⇨ Pulse/neuro deficit
  - ⇨ New AI murmur
  - ⇨ Limb ischemia
- Risk factors: HTN, Marfan's, vasculitis, pregnancy, coarctation, bicuspid aortic valve, trauma, cocaine/meth

EPIDURAL COMPRESSION

(Essentials 2011 Cauda Equina vs. Peripheral Radiculopathy)

Causes
- Spinal cord compression, Conus medullaris syndrome, Cauda Equina syndrome

Clinical Presentation
- H/O cancer?
- Multiple myotomes/dermatomes may be involved
- **Focal Neurologic deficit:**
  - ⇨ Bilateral LE weak, sciatica change, gait disturbance
  - ⇨ Bowel/bladder **incontinence** caused by urinary retention (PVR >100-200ml)
  - ⇨ Decreased **rectal tone**
  - ⇨ **Motor** > Sensory loss
  - ⇨ **Sensory loss**: saddle anesthesia, sensory level
- **Age** (JAMA 1992;268;760-5)
  - ⇨ Age > 50 or h/o CA or unexplained wt loss or failure of conservative tx→Sens 100% for detecting mets to spine

LOW BACK PAIN

Work-up
- **Overflow incontinence**
  - ⇨ Cause (J Bone Joint Surg Am 1986;68:386)
    - ✓ Urinary retention (sensitivity 90%, specificity 95% for epidural compression)
  - ⇨ Abnormal PVR
    - ✓ Absence of **large PVR** (>100ml) has NPV 99.99%
    - ✓ In absence of significant neuro deficit → **normal PVR rules out compression**
  - ⇨ Post-void US: Volume = Length x Width x Height x (0.52)
  - ⇨ Anal **sphincter tone** diminished in 60-80%
  - ⇨ Saddle anesthesia has sensitivity 75%
- MRI
  - ⇨ Diagnose site of compression

Special Case: Patient with h/o Cancer (Emerg Med Clin N Am 2010;28:811)
- Group I: New/progressive neurologic sx
  - ⇨ Steroids (Dexamethasone 10mg IV)
  - ⇨ Xrays, emergent MRI
- Group II: **Stable neurologic sx**
  - ⇨ Steroids
  - ⇨ Xrays, urgent MRI (24h)
- Group III: **No neurologic signs/sx**
  - ⇨ Conservative tx
  - ⇨ Xrays, outpatient MRI

Treatment
- Emergent Neurosurgical Consult
- Steroids/Radiation if due to mets?

SPINAL EPIDURAL ABSCESS (SEA)

Other infectious causes
- Epidural abscess, Osteomyelitis, Diskitis, Transverse Myelitis

Clinical Presentation
- Classic **Triad** (Fever, Spine pain, neuro deficit)
  - ⇨ Triad present in only **13% patients with SEA and is usually a late finding**
  - ⇨ Must consider risk factor screening for r/o of epidural abscess. (J Emerg Med 2004;26:285-91)
- Progression of symptoms:
  - ⇨ Back pain → Radiculopathy → Sensory changes/motor weakness → Bowel-bladder dysfunction → Paralysis
- Risk Factors:
  - ⇨ IVDA, immunocomp, EtOH, spine procedure, distant infection, DM, CRF, CA, indwelling cath, spine fx
  - ⇨ Risk factor screening sensitivity 98%, for one or more risk factors

SEA Triad
☐ Fever
☐ Spine pain
☐ Neurologic deficit

SEA Risk factors
☐ **IVDA**
☐ Immunocompromised
☐ EtOH abuse
☐ Spinal procedure
☐ Distant infection
☐ DM
☐ Chronic renal failure
☐ Cancer
☐ Indwelling catheter
☐ Spine fracture

Work-up
- ESR (J Neurosurg Spine 2011;14:765-770)
  - ⇨ Used as screening test for value of >20mm/h (sens 100%)
  - ⇨ Useful as screening tool for ED patients with **spine pain**, **risk factor for SEA** and **no neuro deficits**
- Emergent MRI

Treatment
- Broad spectrum antibiotics (Staph/Strep/gm neg)
- Emergent Neurosurgical consultation

VERTEBRAL FRACTURE

Clinical Presentation
- Usually elderly with osteoporosis
- Trauma
- Point Vertebral Tenderness
- Steroid use
  - ⇨ A person with LBP on long-term steroids is considered to have a compression fracture until proven otherwise (Spec 99%)

Work-up
- Xrays/ CT Spine

LOW BACK PAIN

3. R/O Visceral Causes

UTI/Pyelonephritis
(Emerg Med Clin N Am 2011;29:539-552)

Definitions
- **Uncomplicated UTI**: young, healthy, non-pregnant women with structurally and functionally normal urinary tracts
- **Complicated UTI**: UTI associated with an underlying condition that increases the risk of failing therapy
- **Complicated pyelonephritis**: progression of upper UTI to emphysematous pyelonephritis, renal corticomedullary abscess, perinephric abscess, or papillary necrosis

Complicated UTI
☐ **Pregnancy**
☐ **Diabetes**
☐ **Male gender**
☐ **Immunosuppression** (AIDS, chemo...)
☐ **Functional** GU abnormality (catheter, neurogenic bladder...)
☐ **Structural** GU abnormality (stones, fistula, PCKD, transpant...)

Clinical Presentation
- Cystitis
  - ⇨ Urinary frequency and urgency, dysuria, and hematuria
  - ⇨ Suprapubic pain, low back pain
  - ⇨ New or increased incontinence in older patients or AMS/delirium
- Pyelonephritis
  - ⇨ Flank or abdominal pain, CVA tenderness on exam
  - ⇨ Fever/chills, N/V
  - ⇨ Complicated Pyelo (Sepsis, Renal failure)

Diagnosis
- Urine Dipstick/UA
  - ⇨ Either nitrite OR leukocyte esterase (LE) positive: 75% sensitive, 82% specific
  - ⇨ Nitrite AND leukocyte esterase positive: 35-84% sensitive, 98-100% specific
  - ⇨ Nitrite alone (95-98%) more specific than leuk esterase alone (59-96%) but S. saprophyticus, pseudomonas, and enterococci do not reduce nitrate
  - ⇨ False positive LE with vaginitis or cervicitis
  - ⇨ Pyuria and bacteruria may be absent if obstruction of the collecting system or ureters is present
- Urine Microscopy
  - ⇨ White blood cell casts are diagnostic of upper urinary tract infection
- Urine culture
  - ⇨ Helpful in guiding antibiotic therapy in pyelo or failed antibiotic treatment
  - ⇨ Positive: single organism isolated with ≥ 100,000 CFU
- Imaging
  - ⇨ Not routinely necessary
  - ⇨ CT abd/pelvis +/- IV contrast consider if:
    - ✓ R/O infected/obstructed ureteral stone
    - ✓ R/O pyelo complication (abscess...):
      - i. Consider if failure of response to therapy in 48-72 hours
    - ✓ Recurrence of symptoms within a few weeks of therapy
    - ✓ Suspicion for obstruction, gas, hemorrhage, masses
  - ⇨ US:
    - ✓ R/O hydronephrosis/obstruction/stone

Treatment
- Antibiotics
  - ⇨ Base antibiotic selection on previous culture data, local resistance patterns, patients history and medical problems
- Adjunctive pain control option: Phenazopyridine PO TID (urinary analgesic).
- See Current Guidelines (Clinical Infectious Diseases 2011;52(5):e103)

Complications
- Pyonephrosis
  - ⇨ Infection + obstruction (pus under pressure)
  - ⇨ Pyelonephritis with an obstructing stone, mass, or other obstruction
  - ⇨ Tx: emergent urology/interventional radiology consult for percutaneous nephrostomy tube or stenting
- Renal abscess
  - ⇨ Dx: CT with IV contrast; can be visualized on US
  - ⇨ Tx: Resuscitation, antibiotics, percutaneous drainage (depending on size and response to antibiotics)

LOW BACK PAIN

- Emphysematous UTI
  - ⇨ Define: necrotizing infection with gas formation in bladder (cystitis), renal pelvis (pyelitis) or kidney parenchyma (pyelonephritis)
  - ⇨ High mortality (20% to 40%) even with treatment
  - ⇨ 95% of cases occur in patients with **DM**
  - ⇨ Major risk factor is **infected obstructing stone**
- Papillary necrosis
  - ⇨ Define: coagulative necrosis of the renal medullary pyramids and papillae

Disposition
- Outpatient therapy appropriate if:
  - ⇨ Uncomplicated pyelonephritis
  - ⇨ Normal vitals, normal renal function, no urinary obstruction
  - ⇨ Pain control and hydration status adequate
  - ⇨ Able to tolerate POs

RENAL COLIC

Clinical Presentation
- Renal colic
  - ⇨ MOA: obstruction of urinary tract → ↑pressures → renal capsular distention (visceral pain/N/V) → ↑peristalsis of ureter (colicky pain)
  - ⇨ Unilateral flank pain → radiating to groin
  - ⇨ Migration of pain (depending on location of stone):
    - ✓ Back pain → flank pain → lower quadrant abdominal pain → penile/labial/testicular pain
  - ⇨ Colic pain: intermittent, waxes/wanes, patient writhing, unable to sit still
- Urinary sx: urgency, frequency, dysuria, gross hematuria
- Nausea/vomiting
- PEX: CVA- tenderness or lower abdominal tenderness

Diagnosis
- UA
  - ⇨ Microscopic hematuria only 85% sensitive for urolithiasis
  - ⇨ Use to rule-out infection/UTI and infected stone
  - ⇨ UA negative?: Patient may still have urine infection proximal to obstructing stone
- KUB
  - ⇨ 85-90% of stones are radioopaque (calcium, struvite, cystine) but KUB only 40-62% sensitive and 60-67% specific
  - ⇨ Little diagnostic utility; consider in patient with known hx radiopaque stones and typical presentation
- US
  - ⇨ Ureteral calculi
    - ✓ Sensitivity 45% and specificity 94%
    - ✓ More likely to see larger stones (>4mm), at the UVJ, or proximal near the renal pelvis.
  - ⇨ Hydronephrosis
    - ✓ Sensitivity 85-90% and specificity 90-100%
    - ✓ Not visualize stone itself but can demonstrate obstructive sequelae
    - ✓ Presence/absence of hydronephrosis is neither diagnostic nor prognostic
  - ⇨ Preferred initial test in pregnancy, children → no radiation
  - ⇨ Use to evaluate abdomen/pelvis for alternative diagnoses (gallstones, appy etc...)
- CT (Non-contrast):
  - ⇨ Study of choice to evaluate urolithiasis
  - ⇨ Indications:
    - ✓ 1st time diagnosis of urolithiasis
    - ✓ Atypical presentation
    - ✓ R/O infection
    - ✓ Not improving with conservative treatment
  - ⇨ Sensitivity 96-98% and specificity ~100%
  - ⇨ Useful in prognosis (size/location of stone, obstruction/hydronephrosis, perinephric stranding)
- No imaging?:
  - ⇨ Pt with known kidney stone, typical presentation, well appearing, no risks for complications and good follow/up
  - ⇨ May treat empirically (pain control, hydration)

LOW BACK PAIN

Treatment

- Conservative treatment
  - ⇨ Pain control, hydration, expectant stone passage.
- NSAIDs
  - ⇨ Inhibits prostaglandin-mediated process in urolithiasis
  - ⇨ As effective as opioids and fewer side effects of nausea and vomiting
  - ⇨ Ketorolac IV or Ketorolac + Opiate combination
- Opiates
  - ⇨ In addition to NSAID or if contraindications to NSAID
- Hydration & Diuresis
  - ⇨ No evidence that increased hydration or forced diuresis improves pain scores or rate of passage
  - ⇨ Use: replete volume in dehydrated patients or those with elevated creatinine only
- Medical Expulsion Therapy:
  - ⇨ CCBs (e.g nifedipine) or α-antagonists (e.g. tamsulosin)
  - ⇨ MOA: relax ureteral smooth muscle → allow passage of stone
  - ⇨ Conclusion: Trial of tamsulosin (0.4 mg qd x4 weeks) in stones <10mm is reasonable
- Emergent urology consult
  - ⇨ Urosepsis, obstruction with proximal infection, AKI, anuria, intractable pain/vomiting, stones >10mm
- Renal Stents
  - ⇨ Use:
    - ✓ Facilitate drainage of upper urinary tract and relieve obstruction
    - ✓ Temporizing while await stone passage or definitive urological procedure.
  - ⇨ Complications: pain, hematuria, urgency and frequency (more common), upward migration, infection, sepsis (rare)
- Infected kidney stone
  - ⇨ Treatment: decompression, emergently by urology or IR
  - ⇨ Admission, hydration, IV antibiotics
  - ⇨ UTI + non-obstructing stone: if well appearing, outpatient antibiotics, f/u urology

Size of stone	Rate of passage
1 mm	87%
2-4 mm	76%
5-7 mm	60%
7-9 mm	48%
>9 mm	25%

Disposition

- Admit
  - ⇨ Obstructing stone with a proximal infection, urosepsis, acute renal failure, anuria, or intractable pain, nausea, or vomiting
  - ⇨ Urology consult
- D/C Home
  - ⇨ Stable, tolerating po, pain controlled, nausea/vomiting controlled, outpatient urology follow-up
  - ⇨ Outpatient Urology follow-up:
    - ✓ Stone >10mm, failure to pass stone after conservative treatment, pain not controlled

Other: Consider GI and Pelvic Causes

Journal Club: Tamsulosin in ureteral stones (EM:RAP 9/11)

RCT (Arch Intern Med 2010;170:2021)
- Study: multicenter, placebo-controlled, randomized, double-blind study of tamsulosin vs placebo (good)
- **No difference in expulsion** delay within 42 days; (P = .30)
- **No difference in surgical procedure** or other secondary end points between groups
- Conclusion: "Tamsulosin **did not accelerate the expulsion** of distal ureteral stones in patients with ureteral colic"

Systematic review (Ann Emerg Med. 2007;50:552)
- Previous review suggested increase stone passage rate and decreased time to stone passage with tamsulosin
- Critique: Review had poor quality, unblinded studies, poor follow up

---

LOW BACK PAIN

4. MECHANICAL LBP

(EM:RAP (6/13) Notes from the Community: Back Pain)

SCIATICA

Define
- Peripheral radiculopathy caused by compression of nerve root, usually caused by disc herniation or spinal stenosis

Clinical Presentation
- Back pain + neuropathy (paresthesia, sensory loss) down one leg
- Unilateral symptoms that extend distal to knee
- Sensory > Motor
- Single myo/dermatome involved
- **SLR** (Straight leg raise)
  - ⇨ Pain when the straight leg is raised to an angle of between 30 and 70 degrees
  - ⇨ Pain must extend **below knee**
  - ⇨ Sensitivity 91%, Specificity 26% (Spine 25 (9): 1140–7)
- **Crossed SLR**: Raising the opposite leg causes pain on affected side (sensitivity 29%, specificity 88%)

Nerve Root	Muscle	Reflex
L4	Knee extension Ankle dorsiflexion	Patellar
L5	Great toe dorsiflexion Heel walking	-
S1	Foot plantar flexion	Achilles

Treatment
- 90% of acute sciatica responds to conservative treatment
- Conservative management: Tylenol/NSAIDS/continue daily activities
- Treat similar to lumbar strain except consider Xrays to r/o other causes of nerve compression (tumor, fx, spondylolisthesis, infection…)
- Emergent/Urgent Surgery
  - ⇨ Significant motor deficit (foot drop, unable to ambulate)
  - ⇨ Intractable pain
- Indications for outpatient surgery
  - ⇨ Definite herniation on imaging study +
  - ⇨ Corresponding pain syndrome +
  - ⇨ Corresponding neurologic deficit +
  - ⇨ No response to 4-6 wks conservative treatment

LUMBAR STRAIN

General
- Diagnosis of exclusion
- No further w/u needed

Treatment
- Activity as tolerated
- Analgesics/Muscle relaxants
- Continuing **normal daily activities** as tolerated leads to more rapid recovery than either bed rest or back immobilizing exercises (NEJM 1995;332(6):351-5)

OTHER CAUSES

- Inflammatory Arthritis, Spondylolisthesis, Paget's dz, Spinal Stenosis
- Treatment
  - ⇨ Conservative tx
  - ⇨ If no red flags, can be worked up as outpatient by PMD

JOINT PAIN

1 Periarticular?

- ☐ Tendonitis
- ☐ Bursitis
- ☐ Cellulitis

2 Fracture?

- ☐ Trauma
- ☐ Fall → Xray

3 Septic Joint?

	📋 H&P	🧪 Labs	💉 Action
Non-GC	☐ Acutely painful swollen joint ☐ Risk factors? ☐ Fever ☐ Minimal ROM	☐ ↑WBC ☐ ↑ESR, ↑CRP ☐ ↑Synovial fluid WBC, PMN ☐ Gm stain/Cx	⇨ Antibiotics ⇨ Ortho C/S ⇨ Culture results ⇨ Admit
Gonococcal	☐ Young, healthy sexually active F>M ☐ Migratory polyarthralgia ☐ Tenosynovitis ☐ Dermatitis ☐ Fever	☐ ↑WBC ☐ ↑ESR, ↑CRP ☐ ↑Synovial fluid WBC, PMN ☐ Gm stain/Cx	⇨ Pan-Cx every orifice ⇨ Antibiotics ⇨ Admit

4 Arthritis?

Mono-articular	→	☐ OA ☐ Gout ☐ Pseudogout ☐ TB/Fungal
Poly-articular	→	☐ RA ☐ Seronegative Spondyloarthropathies ☐ Lyme disease ☐ Viral

195

JOINT PAIN

GENERAL APPROACH

- The first step in evaluating a patient with joint pain is to ensure that the pain is in the joint and not the surrounding structures
- Then, rule out critical diagnoses such as fracture and septic arthritis
- We are then left with important, but non life/limb threatening causes of acute arthritis

1. R/O PERI-ARTICULAR CAUSE

CELLULITIS
- Superficial skin infection around area of joint (erythema, edema and warmth)
- Treat empirically for beta-hemolytic streptococci and methicillin-susceptible S. aureus (MSSA)
- Most patients with mild cellulitis and can be treated with oral antibiotics.
- Patients with signs of systemic toxicity or erythema that has progressed rapidly should be treated initially with IV antibiotics and possible admission

BURSITIS
- Inflammation of sac-like substances between soft tissue
- Caused by repetitive injury, trauma, crystal disease or infection
- May require aspiration of bursa for gram stain and CX to rule out infection
- Treatment: Rest, ice, heat, NSAIDS (if tolerated)

TENDONITIS
- Chronic pain from overuse

2. R/O FRACTURE

- History of trauma/fall?
- Rule out with X-ray if clinically indicated

3. R/O SEPTIC ARTHRITIS

SEPTIC ARTHRITIS: NON-GONOCOCCAL
(EM:RAP 3/13 "The Equivocal Arthrocentesis")

General: (Lancet 1998;351:197-202), (JAMA 2007;297:1478-1488)
- Must consider in any patient with an acutely swollen, painful joint
- Irreversible loss of joint function → 25-50% patients
- Case fatality rate 5-15%

Risk Factors: See Table (Arthritis Rheum 1995;38:1819-1825)

Clinical Exam:
- Classic exam is painful, swollen, red hot joint but:
  - ⇨ Joint pain → Sens 85%
  - ⇨ Joint swelling → Sens 78%
  - ⇨ Fever had Sens 57% → absence of fever does not rule-out infection

Laboratory evaluation (Am J Emerg Med 1997;15:626-629)
- Peripheral WBC, CRP, ESR have limited diagnostic utility because of low specificity
- Peripheral WBC >10,000 → Sens 90% (LR+ 1.4)
- ESR > 30 → Sens 95% (LR+1.3)

Risk Factor	LR+
Hip/knee prosthesis + skin infection	15
Recent joint surgery	6.9
Age >80	3.5
Hip/knee prosthesis	3.1
Skin infection	2.8
DM	2.7
RA	2.5
HIV	1.7

Synovial fluid analysis
- Because of history, physical and lab tests are unable to reliably change the pre-test probability (8-27%) that an acutely painful joint is septic arthritis → further work-up with arthrocentesis and synovial WBC/diff are often needed.
- Synovial WBC:
  - ⇨ Progressively higher WBC counts increase likelihood of septic arthritis
  - ⇨ Can still have septic arthritis with very low synovial WBC counts. (Acad Emerg Med 2004;11:276-280)
    - ✓ 10% of patients had synovial WBC counts < 10,000
    - ✓ Lowest value →168
  - ⇨ Gram stain positive in only 50%, Culture positive in over 90%

Synovial analysis	Specificity	LR+
WBC>100,000	99%	28
WBC>50,000	92%	7.7
WBC>25,000	73%	2.9
PMN≥90%	79%	3.4

- Synovial fluid lactate: (Acad Emerg Med 2011;18(8):781)
  - ⇨ Synovial fluid lactate > 10mmol/L has high LR+
  - ⇨ Virtually diagnostic of septic arthritis

JOINT PAIN

Decision rule? (Acad Emerg Med 2004;11:276-280)
- Retrospective study found that 100% of patients with septic arthritis had abnormality in at least one of the three tests
  - ⇨ Peripheral WBC
  - ⇨ ESR
  - ⇨ Synovial WBC
- If all 3 normal → very low likelihood of septic arthritis (Sensitivity 100%)

Treatment
- **Antibiotics**
  - ⇨ Empirically vs S. aureus & Strep or based on gram stain result
  - ⇨ Cephalosporin (3rd or 4th Gen) + Vancomycin
- Steroids (Pediatr Infect Dis J 2003;22(10):833)
  - ⇨ Significant reduction in duration and long term disability and joint dysfunction in this pediatric population
  - ⇨ Caution: Not been studied in adults
- Emergent **Orthopedics** Consultation
  - ⇨ Joint Drainage? Needle aspiration, arthroscopy, or open surgical drainage

SEPTIC ARTHRITIS: GONOCOCCAL

Clinical (Infect Dis Clin North Am 2005;19:853)
- Bacteremic Phase
  - ⇨ 2-3 days: malaise, fever, polyarthralgias with triad of symptoms
  - ⇨ **Tenosynovitis**: acute, asymmetric, on dorsum of wrists, hands and fingers
  - ⇨ **Arthritis**: asymmetric migratory polyarthralgia (most common presenting sx of disseminated GC)
  - ⇨ **Dermatitis:** pustular, macular, hemorrhagic on distal extremities; spares face, palms, soles
- Suppurative phase (3-6 days)
  - ⇨ ↑Articular findings, joint fluid purulent

GC Arthritis Triad
☐ Tenosynovitis
☐ Arthritis
☐ Dermatitis

Presentation
- Young, healthy sex active F>M
- Migratory polyarthralgia
- Tenosynovitis
- Dermatitis
- Fever

Diagnosis
- Synovial fluid Cx positive <50%, Blood cultures almost always negative→need to culture other sites
- Collect samples from endocervix (90% positive), urethra (50%), pharynx, skin lesions and rectum

Treatment:
- Antibiotics (Ceftriaxone 1gm) and admission to await Cx results

4. R/O OTHER ARTHRITIDES

GOUT

- Clinical
  - ⇨ Risk factors: Middle aged, metabolic syndrome, DM, HTN, Obese
  - ⇨ Recurrent abrupt onset monoarticular arthritis
  - ⇨ **Podagra**: 1st MTP involvement
  - ⇨ **Tophi**
  - ⇨ Labs: Hyperuricemia
- Diagnosis
  - ⇨ Joint aspiration
    - ✓ Definitive diagnosis and direct future urate lowering treatment
    - ✓ Exclude other causes of joint pain (e.g. septic arthritis)
  - ⇨ Crystals: **Negative birefringent crystals** vs pseudogout (positively birefringent crystals)
  - ⇨ Pearl: Crystals in synovial fluid does not rule out septic joint

Gout Pearl
Crystals in synovial fluid does not rule out septic arthritis

JOINT PAIN

- Treatment
  - ⇨ **NSAIDS**
    - ✓ Use for acute attack (Indomethacin 50mg PO q8H and taper)
  - ⇨ **Colchicine**
    - ✓ Use if unable to take NSAIDS or are contraindicated
    - ✓ Dosing: 1.2mg initial dose, then 0.6mg 1 hour later; then 0.6mg qd or bid for duration of attack
  - ⇨ **Glucocorticoids**
    - ✓ Use if contraindications to both NSAIDS and Colchicine (e.g. Prednisone)
  - ⇨ Urate lowering Tx (Allopurinol):
    - ✓ Should not be initiated during acute attack
    - ✓ If patient already taking → do not stop (reintroduction may predispose to another attack)
  - ⇨ **Opiate** analgesics for pain control

PSEUDOGOUT

- Joint aspiration: positively birefringent crystals
- Treatment similar to gout

OTHER ARTHRITIDES

LYME DZ (Med Clin North Am 2002;86:297-309)
- Clinical
  - ⇨ History of tick bite (weeks-years prior)
  - ⇨ Rash (ECM)
  - ⇨ Endemic area exposure
  - ⇨ Joint fluid (inflammatory with PMNs)
- Treatment
  - ⇨ If high suspicion → start empiric treatment (**Doxycycline** 100mg PO q12H) prior to results of serologic tests
  - ⇨ Early treatment shortens disease & prevents later disease

OA, RA
- Treat symptomatically with Tylenol, NSAIDS & appropriate referral (PMD, Rheum)

HYPOTHERMIA

1 Cardiac Arrest: HT IV

Futile?

Futility:
- ☐ Arrested before cooling?
- ☐ Asystole & Temp>32°C
- ☐ K+>12
- ☐ Irreversible injury?
  Trauma etc
- ☐ Chest not compressible

No or ???

ACLS (modified)
⇨ CPR, Intubation
⇨ Epinephrine (3 doses?)
⇨ Defibrillate x1 (VF) trial
⇨ **ECMO/CPB available?**

ECMO/CPB unavailable
⇨ Cont CPR/ACLS
⇨ Active external +
⇨ Alternative internal rewarming
⇨ Rewarm to temp>32°C (90°F)

Yes

Consider Termination of Efforts ☠

2 Resuscitation
(+pulse)

- ☐ Airway protection; Intubation?
- ☐ Warm humidified O₂
- ☐ IVF (warmed), antibiotics, labs, BCx
- ☐ Prevent myocardial irritation
- ☐ Treat cause: sepsis, trauma etc...

3 Re-Warming

Mild: HT I
(32-35°C)

Passive External Rewarming
⇨ Remove wet clothing
⇨ Warm sweet drinks
⇨ Warm room/blankets
⇨ Active movement (if possible)
⇨ Rewarm rate: 0.5-2°C/h

Moderate: HT II
(28-32°C)

Passive External Rewarming
+
Active external/Min Invasive
⇨ Avoid arrhythmias
⇨ Bair Hugger
⇨ Heat pads/blankets
⇨ Trunk only
⇨ Warm IV Fluids (38-42°C)
⇨ Rewarm rate:1-2.5°C/h

Severe: HT III
(24-28°C)

Passive External Rewarming
+
Active External/Min Invasive
+
ECMO/CPB?
⇨ Cardiac instability +
⇨ Refractory to medical management

4 Complications

Core-Temp After Drop
- ☐ Maintain horizontal
- ☐ Re-warm trunk (not extremities)

Re-warming Shock

Failure to rewarm (<1°C/hr)
- ☐ Adequate techniques?
- ☐ Underlying infection?

Bronchorrhea, Cold-induced
- ☐ Intubation?
- ☐ Airway protection → prevent aspiration

Arrhythmias
- ☐ Benign → Rewarm
- ☐ Malignant → ACLS as above, re-warm

Local Injuries
- ☐ Expose entire body (burns, trauma)

Coagulopathy
- ☐ Normal lab values
- ☐ Hypercoagulability (DIC)

Rhabdomyolysis
- ☐ Fluid resuscitation
- ☐ Renal function?

5 Cause?

- ☐ Exposure (Urban, Expedition)
- ☐ EtOH
- ☐ Hypoglycemia
- ☐ Hypothyroid
- ☐ Adrenal Insufficiency
- ☐ Sepsis (default diagnosis)
- ☐ All pts → Full sepsis w/u, antibiotics

HYPOTHERMIA

GENERAL

(N Engl J Med 2012;367:1930) (Am Fam Physician 2004;70:2325-32) (EM:RAP 1/14 & 2/09)

- Mild hypothermia → tachypnea, tachycardia, hyperventilation, ataxia, shivering, impaired judgment, "cold diuresis"
- Moderate → bradycardia, hypoventilation, CNS depression, loss of shivering, slow A-fib + other arrhythmias
- Severe → pulmonary edema, oliguria, coma, pupils fixed/dilated, ventricular arrhythmias, asystole

1. CARDIAC ARREST

Futile? Consider termination of efforts

- **Irreversible injury?**
  - ⇨ Decapitation, truncal transection, decomposition of the whole body, and a chest wall that is not compressible (the whole body is frozen solid)
- **K+>10-12**
  - ⇨ Serum K+>10 may be a valuable prognostic indicator for irreversible asphyxia and death. (Ann Emerg Med 1987;16:1042-55)
- Cardiac **arrest prior to cooling**
  - ⇨ Difficult to differentiate from a patient that **died and then became hypothermic** → resuscitation would obviously be futile
  - ⇨ Better outcome if patients were cooled before heart stopped
- Asystole and Temp > 32°C
  - ⇨ Hypothermia is then not the cause of arrest

Special Cases (trauma, drowning, avalanche)

- Trauma
  - ⇨ Hypothermia will decrease survival of blunt trauma
- Drowning
  - ⇨ Submersion
    - ✓ Patient under water immediately → drowns → hypoxic arrest → then cools down
    - ✓ Worse prognosis, case report of survival
  - ⇨ Immersion (rare)
    - ✓ Patient in water and continues breathing → cools → hypothermic arrest
- Avalanche (3 ways to die)
  - ⇨ Traumatic arrest
  - ⇨ Hypoxic arrest (airway filled with snow)
  - ⇨ Hypothermic arrest
    - ✓ Patient must be buried long enough to cool → then arrest
    - ✓ Rate of cooling 10°C/h so must be buried at least **35 minutes**

Continued CPR/Resuscitation

- Because of neuroprotective effects of hypothermia → complete recovery is possible even if prolonged resuscitation (hours)
  - ⇨ Survival and neurological recovery reported in temperatures as low as 13.7°C and cardiac arrest > 9 hours (Lancet 2000;355:375-6)
  - ⇨ Continue resuscitation until temperature is 32-35°C

Modified ACLS

- CPR, Intubation
- Rapid re-warming: ECMO/CPB
- Resuscitate until temp >32°C (90°F)
- Defibrillate x1 (VF) trial then rewarm
- Epinephrine x 1 trial then rewarm vs up to 3 doses
- ACLS recommendations
  - ⇨ European Resuscitation Council (Resuscitation 2010;81:1400)
    - ✓ **Defibrillations: up to 3**
    - ✓ Epinephrine: hold until core temp > 30°C then double interval between doses until temp > 35°C
  - ⇨ AHA Guidelines (Circulation 2010;122:Suppl 3: S829-S861)
    - ✓ Standard ALS protocol

ECMO/CPB

- Define: Extracorporeal Membrane Oxygenation(ECMO) / Cardiopulmonary Bypass (CPB)
- Indications:
  - ⇨ **Cardiac arrest (HT IV)**
    - ✓ Hypothermic patients who experience cardiac arrest have a survival rate of 50% when treated in an ECMO center but only 10% in a non-ECMO center
  - ⇨ **Cardiac instability refractory to medical management (HT III)**
    - ✓ SBP < 90, ventricular arrhythmias, temp < 28°C
- In patients with ROSC, multiorgan failure is expected → respiratory support with ECMO may be required.

Termination of CPR

- Consider termination if temp > 32°C and persistent cardiac arrest, not responsive to epinephrine and defibrillation

HYPOTHERMIA

2. RESUSCITATION

Intubation
- Risk of causing VF very low and outweighed by benefits of reliable ventilation, oxygenation, prevention of aspiration-especially if comatose or respiratory failure

Sepsis
- Treat all patients empirically for sepsis
- IVF(warmed), antibiotics, labs, blood cultures, lactate
- See Sepsis algorithm

3. RE-WARMING
(N Engl J Med 2012;367:1930) (EM:RAP 1/14 & 2/09)

General
- Degree of hypothermia and mortality will determine the aggressiveness of re-warming

Stage	Temp	Clinical
HT I	32-35°C	Conscious Shivering
HT II	28-32°C	Impaired consciousness, no shiver
HT III	24-28°C	Unconscious, no shiver, +VS
HT IV	<24°C	No VS

Stage HT I
- Clinical: conscious, shivering
- Treatment
  ⇨ **Passive External Rewarming** (0.5-2°C/h)
    ✓ Remove wet clothing
    ✓ Warm room/blankets

Stage HT II
- Clinical: Impaired consciousness, not shivering
- Treatment
  ⇨ Avoid arrhythmias
    ✓ Cardiac monitor
    ✓ Minimal/cautious movements
    ✓ Horizontal position and immobilization
  ⇨ **Active external/minimally invasive Re-warming** (1-2.5°C/h)
    ✓ Bair Hugger
    ✓ Heat pads/blankets
    ✓ Trunk only
    ✓ Warm IV Fluids (38-42°C)
    ✓ Indications (N Eng J Med 1994;331:1756-60):
      i. Cardiovascular instability, poikilothermia (T<32°C), failure to re-warm, comorbidities

Stage HT III
- Clinical: Impaired consciousness, not shivering, pt has vital signs
- Treatment
  ⇨ HT II treatments
  ⇨ Airway management as required
  ⇨ ECMO/CPB (cardiac instability refractory to medical management)

Stage HT IV
- Clinical: Cardiac arrest, no vital signs
- Treatment
  ⇨ HT II & III treatments
  ⇨ ACLS: CPR, Intubation, epinephrine, defibrillation
  ⇨ **ECMO/CPB if available** (N Engl J Med 1997;337:1500-5) (Resuscitation 2003;59:285-90)
    ✓ Rate of survival without neurologic impairment is 47 to 63% (vs 37% without ECMO/CPB)
    ✓ Cardiopulmonary bypass (CPB) for severe hypothermia and cardiac arrest showed survival rate of 47-63% with minimal to no cerebral impairment, even after prolonged cardiac arrest
  ⇨ Active external and alternative internal rewarming (ECMO/CPB not available)
    ✓ Thoracic lavage with chest tubes
    ✓ Bladder lavage?

HYPOTHERMIA

4. COMPLICATIONS

Rescue collapse
- Define: cardiac arrest that is related to the extrication and transport of a patient with deep hypothermia (stage HT III)
- Cause: circulatory collapse due to hypovolemia, cardiac arrhythmias triggered by interventions, and further cooling

Core temperature after drop
- Extremities and trunk are warmed simultaneously → cold, acidemic blood in periphery returns to core → drop in temperature and acidosis

Rewarming shock
- Peripheral vasodilation → hypotension, ↓coronary perfusion → fatal arrhythmias (VF)
- Prevention: maintain horizontal, re-warm trunk before extremities,

Arrhythmias
- Avoid jarring pt, no high central lines, gentle movement of pt → irritating myocardium may cause VF
- Most (A-fib, A-flutter) resolve spontaneously during re-warming
- Normal course: bradycardia → slow A-fib → VF → Asystole (refractory to conventional tx, must be re-warmed!)
- EKG changes with hypothermia
  - ⇨ Intervals prolonged: ↑PR, ↑QRS, ↑QT
  - ⇨ J point elevation (Osborne wave – characteristic but not pathognomonic: also seen in hypercalcemia and head injury)

Failure to re-warm
- Evaluate for adequate aggressiveness for severity of hypothermia
- Evaluate for reversible causes (hypoglycemia)
- Underlying infection?
  - ⇨ Rewarming rates <0.67°C/hr associated with underlying infection and increased mortality (Acad Emerg Med 2006;13:913–921)

Coagulopathy
- Cold directly inhibits enzymes of coagulation cascade and platelets → normal laboratory evaluation
- Hypercoagulability also present → can lead to thromboembolism; DIC

Cold induced bronchorrhea
- Intubation? Airway protection → prevent aspiration

Cold induced diuresis
- Usually diuresed 2-5L, replace with warmed IVF

Rhabdomyolysis
- Tissue ischemia and cellular destruction by freezing tissue

5. CAUSES

Environment
- Urban hypothermia
  - ⇨ Most common cause is environmental exposure with acute alcohol intoxication
- Expedition hypothermia

Sepsis/Infection
- Treat all patients empirically for sepsis
- Associated with slower re-warming rates (above)
- Begin empiric broad spectrum antibiotics and sepsis work-up

Adrenocortical insufficiency
- Consider empiric Hydrocortisone 100mg IV q8h or Dexamethasone

Hypothyroidism/Myxedema Coma (see Altered Mental Status algorithm)

BURNS

A Airway

Distress? →

Smoke Inhalation Injury
- ☐ Closed space fire
- ☐ Hoarseness/stridor
- ☐ Cough
- ☐ Dyspnea
- ☐ Facial burns
- ☐ Singed nasal hair
- ☐ Carbonaceous tongue/sputum

→ Consider Early Intubation
- ⇨ Early airway/prophylactic intubation
- ⇨ Fiberoptic/Machida scope
- ⇨ Large ETT
- ⇨ Succ or Rocuronium

B Breathing

Oxygenation →

Inhalation Injury?
- ☐ Thermal airway injury
- ☐ ARDS scenario

CO poisoning?
- ☐ Sat gap?
- ☐ COHb level

⇨ O₂ high flow
⇨ HBO therapy?
⇨ Pulmonary toilet
⇨ See Tox section

Ventilation →

Chest Wall burns?
- ☐ Full thickness burn → constrict chest

⇨ Chest escharotomy

C Circulation

Resuscitation →

- ☐ Large peripheral IV vs central IV
- ☐ Evaluate for hemolysis, SIRS, DIC

⇨ Aggressive fluid resuscitation (see formulas)

Pulseless Extremity →

- ☐ Circumferential extremity burn

⇨ Limb escharotomy

D Disability

Toxic Ingestion →

- ☐ CO → sat gap, COHb level
- ☐ CN → unexplained severe met acidosis, collapse on scene
- ☐ HS

⇨ See Tox algorithm
⇨ 100% O2
⇨ HBO (Hyperbaric oxygen) tx?
⇨ CN kit?

Trauma? →

Simultaneous Trauma Resuscitation

E Exposure

- ☐ Decontaminate/remove clothing
- ☐ Avoid hypothermia
- ☐ Evaluate burn severity
- ☐ Asses other injuries
- ☐ Evaluate for transfer to burn center

BURNS

1. Airway

(EM:RAP 9/06-Mallon; Essentials 2011-Menchine; 2009-Jeff Guy)

Respiratory distress
- Consider immediate intubation/airway control

Smoke inhalation injury
- Closed space fire
- Hoarseness/stridor
- Cough, dyspnea
- Facial burns, singed nasal hair/eyebrows
- Carbonaceous tongue/sputum

Treatment
- Timing
  - ⇨ Early airway management is key!
  - ⇨ When in doubt → intubate
  - ⇨ Patient may present well appearing, in no distress → then develop massive facial tongue edema minutes to hours → airway nightmare
- RSI Medication
  - ⇨ Ketamine
  - ⇨ Succinylcholine (2mg/kg) permissible for burns < 24hours
  - ⇨ Rocuronium (1mg/kg) always OK

Major Burn
☐ Partial thickness: >25% TBSA (adults); >20%TBSA (<10 or >50yo)
☐ Full thickness > 10 %
☐ Burns to face, eyes, ears, hands, genitals
☐ Inhalation injury, major trauma
☐ Chemical burn, electrical injury
☐ High risk patients

2. Breathing

Oxygenation
- Inhalation Injury
  - ⇨ Thermal airway injury
  - ⇨ ARDS?
- CO Poisoning (See Tox section)
  - ⇨ Check for saturation gap (SaO_2 significantly less on pulse oximetry than that calculated from the PaO_2 on the arterial blood gas), COHb level

Ventilation
- Chest wall burn
- Pathophysiology
  - ⇨ Chest wall constriction → ↓Compliance → ↑Increase PIP → Unable to ventilate
- Treatment
  - ⇨ Immediate problem: Must treat within a few minutes!
  - ⇨ Chest wall escharotomy

3. Circulation

Resuscitation
- Fluid resuscitation (Lactated Ringer's)
  - ⇨ Estimate burn surface area (rule of 9s, palms)
  - ⇨ Increase fluid requirements when inhalation or electrical injury present
- Place foley - should achieve a normal UOP (30-50ml/h in adults)

Pulseless extremity?
- Circumferential extremity burn
- Pathophysiology
  - ⇨ Burned skin contracts + SQ swelling → venous occlusion → arterial occlusion → Ischemia
- Treatment
  - ⇨ Limb escharotomy within a few hours

24h Fluid requirements-LR
☐ Parkland: 4cc/kg x %TBSA
☐ Consensus: 3cc/kg x %TBSA
☐ Modified Brooke: 2cc/kg x %TBSA
☐ Galveston (Peds): 5000ml/m^2 x %TBSA + 2000ml
☐ ALL formulas: ½ fluids in first 8 hours

4. Disability

Trauma
- Trauma present?
- Assess patient simultaneously for trauma (fall, blast Injury, MVA) and treat (C-spine, pneumothorax, internal bleeding!)
- Always attempt to obtain neurologic exam (including rectal/pupil exam) before RSI

Toxic inhalation
- CO: sat gap, COHb level
- CN: unexplained severe met acidosis, collapse on scene
- HS

BURNS

5. Exposure

Secondary survey:
- Remove clothing (operative for adherent clothing)
- Stop burning
- Provide first aid (avoid hypothermia with overuse of water to decontaminate wounds)
- Asses for other injuries, asses burn severity (below), consider transfer

General Assessment of Burn Severity (Emerg Med Clin N Am 2007;25:13-146)
- **Severity** of burn is multifactorial and depends on:
  - ⇨ Depth (use partial and full thickness to describe)
    - ✓ 1° epidermal injury, no blister, red, tender, painful (sunburn)
    - ✓ 2° **Partial thickness**
      - i. Superficial (no scar): involves superficial dermis→thin walled fluid blisters
      - ii. Deep (+scar): involves reticular dermis → red, blanched white, thick walled blisters
    - ✓ 3° **Full thickness**: epidermis, dermis → white, leathery, numb
    - ✓ 4° Skin, SQ, may involve fascia, muscle, bone
  - ⇨ **Extent** (only 2nd-4th degree)
    - ✓ Rule of 9s, palms for adults, palms + fingers for children (1%)
  - ⇨ **Location**: face, eyes, ears, hands, perineum
  - ⇨ **Age**: mortality = age + TBSA (if over 50yo)
  - ⇨ Etiologic agent (flame, contact, scald, flash, electrical, radiation, chemical)
  - ⇨ Presence of inhalation injury
  - ⇨ Coexisting injury or preexisting illness
- Classify burn according to severity (Major, Moderate, Minor) (AM Coll Surg Bull 1984;69:24)
  - ⇨ Major → need burn center
  - ⇨ Moderate → hospitalize for initial care, not necessarily burn center
  - ⇨ Minor → Outpatient management

Burn Center Transfer (ABA criteria)
☐ Partial thickness >10% TBSA
☐ Third degree burns any age group
☐ Burns to face, hands, feet, genitalia, perineum, major joints
☐ Electrical burns (including lightning)
☐ Chemical burns
☐ Inhalation injury
☐ Pre-existing medical condition that could complicate management
☐ Traumatic injury where burn poses greatest risk

MINOR BURNS

(BMJ 2004;328:1487-1489) (**Essentials** 2010 "Minor Burns; Again with Feeling")

Treatment
- Stop the burning process → Remove clothing (operative for adherent clothing)
- Cool the burn
  - ⇨ Effective within 20 minutes of burn
  - ⇨ Irrigate/immerse in tepid water (15°C) for up to 20 minutes (or soaked gauze)
  - ⇨ Do not use ice
- Analgesia: if severe, may require opioids, then NSAIDs; cover burn
- Cleansing/debridement (Br Med J 1987;295(6591):181)
  - ⇨ New burn is sterile
  - ⇨ Can clean with soap/water or mild antibacterial (chlorhexidine)
  - ⇨ Blisters
    - ✓ Controversial: can aspirate or de-roof **large blisters** and remove dead skin or leave alone
    - ✓ **Small blisters** should be left alone
- Topical antibiotics
  - ⇨ e.g. Silver sulfadiazene
  - ⇨ Cochrane review: (Cochrane Review 2010)
    - ✓ No effect on infection
    - ✓ Slows down healing in patients with partial-thickness burns
- Dressing Layers:
  - ⇨ Layer 1: Non-adherent dressing (xeroform, vaseline gauze, Adaptec)
  - ⇨ Layer 2: Consider antimicrobial layer (Silver sulfadiazene)
  - ⇨ Layer 3: Antishear layer (Kerlix and Ace wrap)
- Tetanus update; No empiric antibiotics
- Follow up: Recheck in 24h and dressing change

Minor Burn
☐ Partial thickness <15% TBSA adults; <10% (elderly, children)
☐ Full thickness: <2%TBSA
☐ No cosmetic/functional risk to eyes, ears, face, hands, perineum

Special types of burns
- **Sunburns** → if bad, may need IVF, H1/H2 blocker IV, NSAIDs, opiates
- **Oral commissure burns** (child bites electrical cord) → delayed facial artery bleed
- **HF (Hydrofluoric) acid** → need aggressive treatment with Ca (topical, IV, intra-arterial)
- **Flash burns** → may look bad but usually are not (rarely have inhalation injury)
- **Electrical burns** → may not look bad, but usually are (consider arrhythmias and rhabdo)
  - ⇨ Usually do not have delayed presentation of Vfib/arrhythmias
  - ⇨ Consider burn center transfer for electrical burns > 1000V
- **Tar burns** → like dissolves like (use butter, mayo, Bacitracin to remove after cooling)

DISEASE INDEX

DISEASE INDEX

DISEASE INDEX

Vital Signs

Systolic BP

<1 month	60 mmHg
1-12 months	70
1-10 years	70+(age x 2)
>10 years	90

Heart Rate (max)

<6 months	180-190
1-2 years	150
3-6 years	120-140
7-12 years	110

Respiratory Rate

<1 month	50
1 year	40
3 years	30
5 years	25
10 years	20

Weight (kg) = [age x 2 + 10]

<1 month	3 kg
1 year	10
5 years	20
10 years	30

Urine Output = 1-2 cc/kg/hr

Resus

ETT Size = [age/4 + 4]

<28 wks	2.5
28-32 wks	3.0
32-36 wks	3.5

Tip to Lip 3x ETT size

Laryngoscope

<2 years	Mac/Miller 1
2-10 years	Mac/Miller 2
>10 years	Mac/Miller 3

Intubation Drugs

Atropine 0.02 mg/kg min 0.1mg
Etomidate 0.3 mg/kg
Succinylcholine 2mg/kg

Vecuronium 0.1-0.2 mg/kg
Rocuronium 1 mg/kg

Ventilator Settings

Pressure support: TV 6-10cc/kg, Rate 20 (30 if <1 year)

NGT/Foley 2x ETT size
Chest tube 3-4x ETT size

Prep Drugs

Code Drugs

[Unstable bradycardia, V Fib/V Tach, PEA]
Epinephrine 1:10,000 = 0.01 mg/kg (0.1 cc/kg)
1:1000 ETT dose =0.1 mg/kg

[Bradycardia]
Atropine 0.02 mg/kg

[Torsades]

SVT

Adenosine 0.1 mg/kg max 1st dose 6mg, 2nd dose 12mg
Synchronized Cardioversion initial 0.5-1 J/kg, max 2 J/kg
Amiodarone 5 mg/kg over 20-60 mins
Procainamide 15 mg/kg over 30-60 mins

Shock

Dopamine 2-20 mcg/kg/min
Levophed 0.05-2 mcg/kg/min
Phenylephrine 0.1-0.5 mcg/kg/min
Dobutamine 2-20 mcg/kg/min

Seizure

Lorazepam (Ativan) 0.1mg/kg IV/IM q10min (Max: 4mg)
Diazepam (Valium) 0.3mg/kg IV (Max: 10mg); 0.5mg/kg PR
Midazolam (Versed) 0.1mg/kg IV, 0.3mg/kg IM
Phenytoin (Dilantin) 20mg/kg gtt at 50mg/min or 1mg/kg/min (pick slower)

Phenobarbital 20mg/kg (Max: 1g)
Depakote (valproate) 15-20mg/kg IV
Pyridoxine (INH tox) 1g IV/IM q30min, dose 1g per gram INH

Antibiotics

Amoxicillin (125 or 250mg/5cc) 80mg/kg/day div q8-12h
Augmentin (200 or 400mg/5cc) 40mg/kg/day div q12h
Bactrim (40mg/5cc) TMP 6-12mg/kg/day div q12h
Clindamycin (75mg/5cc) 10-30mg/kg/day div q6-8h
Keflex (125 or 250mg/5cc) 25-100mg/kg/day div q6h

Ampicillin 50mg/kg
Cefotaxime 50mg/kg
Ceftriaxone 50-100mg/kg

Gentamicin 4mg/kg q24h
Vancomycin 15mg/kg
Rifampin 20mg/kg

Pain/Symptom Relief

Tylenol 80mg/0.8cc or 160mg/5cc (15mg/kg) q6h
Motrin 100mg/5cc (10mg/kg) q6h
Benadryl 12.5mg/5cc (1mg/kg) q6h
Sudafed 15-30mg/5cc (1mg/kg) q6h

Interventions-Based Drug Regimens

Procedural Sedation

Ketamine (preferred)
1-2 mg/kg IV (10 min duration); 2-4 mg/kg IM

Propofol
0.5-2.0 mg/kg IV

Brevital
1 mg/kg IV

Etomidate
0.15 mg/kg IV

Code Adjuncts

Calcium Chloride
20 mg/kg IV/IO (0.2 cc/kg) Max: 1 g

Glucose

| 1 cc/kg D50 | 2 cc/kg D25 | 5 cc/kg D10 | 10 cc/kg D5 |

Narcan (opiate overdose)
0.1 mg/kg

Flumazenil (benzooverdose)
5-10 ug/kg (Max: 1 mg)

Mannitol
0.5-1 g/kg

Respiratory

[Croup]
Dexamethasone 0.3-0.6 mg /kg
Racemic Epi 0.25-0.5cc 2.25% nebulized in 3cc NS

[Anaphylaxis]
Epi 1/1000=0.01mg/kg IM/IV/IO q15min prn (Max: 0.5mg)
1/10,000=0.01mg/kg q3-5min (Max 1mg)
if hypotension - 0.1-1ug/kg/min IV
if refractory hypotension 0.1-1ug/kg/min IV

[Asthma]
Albuterol Neonate 0.15mg/kg/odse (Max: 5mg)
Atrovent <12yo = 250mcg, >12yo = 500mcg
Magnesium 50mg/kg (Max: 2g) over 20min
Terbutaline 10mcg/kg IV bolus then 0.1mcg/kg/min gtt
Epi 1/1000 0.1mg/kg IM q15min prn (Max: 0.5mg)
Steroids
Prednisone (15mg/5cc) 1mg/kg/day po
Methylprednisone 2mg/kg IV/IM (Max: 80mg) then
0.5mg/kg IV/IO q6h (Max: 120mg/day)

>10 years

Made in the USA
Lexington, KY
03 December 2016